Taking the Mystery Out of Medications

in Autism/Asperger Syndromes

A GUIDE FOR PARENTS AND NON-MEDICAL PROFESSIONALS

LUKE Y. TSAI, M.D.

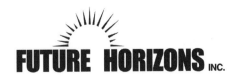

FUTURE HORIZONS INC.

All marketing and publishing rights guaranteed to and reserved by

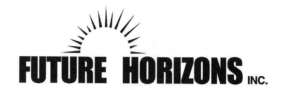

721 W. Abram Street
Arlington, Texas 76013

817-277-0727
800-489-0727
817-277-2270 (fax)
E-mail: info@FutureHorizons-autism.com
Homepage: www.FutureHorizons-autism.com

ISBN 1-885477-80-5

Dedication

I affectionately dedicate this book to:

My wife Merling,

My sons Stephen and Shane, and

The hundreds of families of children and adults with autism spectrum disorder who have taught me about Medication Therapy.

Table of Contents

Appendix A, "Basic Pharmacology," and Appendix B, "Basic Neuropharmacology," describe in detail how medications interact with body systems. These appendices provide scientific information on the biochemical and electrochemical processes that take place in the brain and other organs. You will see how and why medications are administered in different ways and how these medications interact with the body's systems. Appendix A and Appendix B are for those people who are more interested with the scientific and technical aspects of medicine and human biology.

THE UNIVERSITY OF NORTH CAROLINA
AT
CHAPEL HILL

Division TEACCH Administration and Research
Department of Psychiatry

(919) 966-2174
FAX: (919) 966-4127

CB# 7180, 310 Medical School Wing E
The University of North Carolina at Chapel Hill
Chapel Hill, North Carolina 27599-7180

Foreword

This wonderful book is long overdue, and I feel privileged being asked to write the foreword. Autism is a multidisciplinary field of study, and parents and professionals working with this population must know a variety of psychological, behavioral, educational, and medical approaches, among others, if they are to be effective. Until now it has been especially difficult for non-medical personnel to understand the medical aspects of the disability because of the complexity of the medical issues.

With this book the situation has now dramatically changed. Luke Tsai, a parent and professional who has been involved in research, teaching, and treating people with Autism Spectrum Disorders for almost three decades, is offering the fruits of his considerable experiences in a format that both medical and non-medical professionals will be able to understand and benefit from. The book will meet many important needs in the field.

This book is a gem for several reasons. Probably its greatest asset is that it reflects the man who wrote it being pragmatic, gentle, articulate, and comprehensive. Luke Tsai's pragmatism is evident throughout because the book not only deals with basic scientific information, it also describes in detail how this information should be applied in clinical and education settings. The applications are as thorough as the scientific information explains in detail how to manage some of the clinical realities that frequently arise and can interfere with effective medical management. The book reflects the splendid clinical skills that many of us have come to know and admire in Luke.

Not only does this book reflect great clinical skills but it also reflects the caring attitude Luke has always brought to his work. One feels throughout the book the deep concern and respect that this caring physician has for his clients. The human side of medicine is part of every problem and solution, and parents and professionals in the field will especially appreciate this emphasis.

The book is also extremely articulate and comprehensive, reflecting the intelligence, scholarship, and hard work that the author has always put into his professional activities. Many medical and scientific theories and practices will become much clearer as the reader progresses through this logically developed and clearly presented information. The amount of knowledge and detail that is contained in every page is indeed impressive.

All of us who have respected Luke for so many years will be delighted to have this wonderful addition to our professional libraries. For those who will be meeting Luke for the first time through this book, you are in for a real treat. I know you will appreciate this careful, comprehensive, and humane presentation of some of the critical issues in this important field. I am sure this book will also make you want to meet the man himself, and I hope that many of you will have that opportunity to experience his intelligence, versatility, and deep concern and respect for the work he does and the people he so capably serves. If you don't ever have the opportunity that I feel so lucky and privileged to have had knowing Luke over the past 30 years, this book, at least, will give you a glimpse into the scholarship and humanity of a great leader in our field.

Gary B. Mesibov, Ph.D.
Director, TEACCH Program

Preface

This book is the result of more than twenty years of clinical experience in working with, and learning from, more than one thousand individuals with autism spectrum disorder and their caregivers. I entered the field of child psychiatry in 1977. My mentor, the late Mark A. Stewart, M.D., was one of the few experts in the field of psychopharmacotherapy, which is medication therapy for neuropsychiatric disorders. Although Dr. Stewart was fully aware of the advantages and disadvantages of using medications in children with these disorders, he strongly emphasized non-medical treatments or interventions. I learned from Dr. Stewart about when and how to appropriately use medications to treat children with neuropsychiatric disorders, including those who have autism spectrum disorder (ASD). It is, however, those hundreds of individuals with ASD and their caregivers who have taught me how to practice state-of-the-art medication therapy. I have learned from them that medications can significantly improve the quality of life in those with ASD and related disorders. They have also taught me that medications can cause serious physical and psychological harm when used inappropriately. It is my concern with this latter aspect that is the major reason for writing this book.

Over the years, I have seen physicians unnecessarily prescribe medications for many individuals with ASD and related neuropsychiatric disorders. The patients not only did not benefit from any of the medications; many of them also suffered from serious adverse effects. I have observed physicians treat patients with inadequate dosages of multiple medications for many months without any therapeutic benefits when an adequate dosage of one of the medications could have helped the patients in a much shorter period of time.

One particular pattern of practicing medicine by some physicians gives me the most agony. These doctors would admit to the parents of the patient that they did not have any, or very little, training in treating individuals with ASD and related disorders. Yet they would still treat the children with psychotherapeutic medications that they had not previously prescribed for anyone. A few of the physicians would issue prescriptions after just a brief telephone consultation with someone who had some experience with ASD and related disorders. Most of them did so because some parents requested it. Nonetheless, most of these physicians very rarely would make a further consultation to ensure the appropriate and effective use of the medications that he/she prescribed. Even worse, many physicians prescribed psychotherapeutic medications without consulting anyone. Such a practice of medicine not only delayed some individuals' needed treatment, it also caused serious side effects. In fact, in my special clinic, I spent an enormous amount of time helping individuals with ASD and their families clean up the "drug mess" caused by some physicians.

I appreciate that it is often difficult for parents to find a physician who has adequate training and experience in ASD and related disorders. I wonder, however, how many parents would want a physician without adequate training and experience in cancer treatment to treat their child's leukemia or any other form of cancer. I also wonder how many family physicians or general pediatricians without special training in cancer treatment would prescribe cancer medications for children with the disease. Although ASD and related disorders are not cancers, they are quite grave disorders.

I am fairly sure that most ethical and responsible physicians will not treat patients that have medical conditions that are unfamiliar to them. But there are some physicians who may consider ASD and other "mental disorders" as "disorders of second-class citizens" or disorders without much hope for improvement or recovery. Therefore, they could feel that quality care of these patients is not essential.

How can we improve the quality of care for our children with ASD and related disorders? I have learned from the business world that "empowerment of the consumers" is the most effective way to make the manufacturers produce high-quality products. When consumers know the "standard of quality" for a product, manufacturers will maintain and improve quality control.

I have written this book to empower you with the knowledge of the standard of medication treatment of ASD and related disorders. It may sound arrogant to say that this book will provide the "standard" of medication treatment of ASD and related neuropsychiatric disorders. The truth is that the guidelines in this book are far from the ultimate "standard of care." Nonetheless, I hope this book will at least help raise the standard of using psychotherapeutic medications in children with ASD and related disorders.

Physicians have a bad habit of taking it for granted that everyone else understands their rather specialized terms. Unless I am careful, I tend to fall into the same trap. I have included a medical glossary that should help you understand medical terms that are not specifically explained in the chapters.

Some may find Appendices A and B especially difficult to understand. However, these appendices contain important information about how our bodies interact with medications. You may want more in-depth knowledge of the interactions in order to ensure effective medication treatment for your child. You may need stamina, patience, and determination to read through these appendices.

Finally, I want to give special thanks to Nancy Aseltine, Joanna Armour, and Veronica Palmer for their helpful suggestions and editing, and to Polly McGlew, who edited the final version of this book.

Luke Tsai, M.D.

Chapter 1

The Autism Spectrum

In 1943, Dr. Leo Kanner at Johns Hopkins Hospital in Baltimore, Maryland, described a group of eleven children as having the following characteristics: an inability to develop relationships with people, extreme aloofness, a delay in speech development, non-communicative use of speech, repeated simple patterns of play activities, and islets of unusual ability. Dr. Kanner, however, believed that only two features were of diagnostic significance: autistic aloneness and obsessive insistence on sameness. He used the term *infantile autism* to describe this previously unrecognized disorder.

Research in the past five decades has changed the original concept of a single disorder (i.e., infantile autism) to the current concept of a spectrum disorder: pervasive developmental disorder (PDD), as defined by the American Psychiatric Association. PDD has several subtypes, including autistic disorder, Rett disorder, childhood disintegrative disorder, Asperger Syndrome, and pervasive developmental disorder not otherwise specified, including atypical autism (PDDNOS/atypical autism). This book focuses on the three commonly seen subtypes of PDD. These are the autistic disorder, Asperger Syndrome, and PDDNOS/atypical autism. Both Rett disorder and childhood disintegrative disorder are very rare neuropsychiatric disorders, and the majority of non-medical professionals working with individuals with developmental disabilities will not encounter them. Because autistic disorder, PDDNOS/atypical autism, and Asperger Syndrome share many clinical features and interventions, including medication therapy, the term autism spectrum disorder (ASD) is used in this book to cover the three subtypes of PDD.

As this book is a comprehensive medication guide for parents and non-medical caregivers, the author assumes that the readers are familiar with the clinical features of ASD; therefore, the assessment and diagnosis of ASD will not be covered.

Research on the use of psychoactive, psychotropic, or psychotherapeutic medications to change or improve troubling behaviors, disturbed emotions, or impaired cognitive function in persons with ASD has focused primarily on autistic disorder. Nonetheless, the information and guides described in this book are also applicable to persons with Asperger Syndrome and PDDNOS/atypical autism.

Co-Existing (Comorbid) Neuropsychiatric Disorders

The core clinical features of autistic disorder include impairment in social interaction; impairments in verbal and non-verbal communication; and restricted, repetitive, and stereotyped patterns of behavior, interests, and activities. In addition to the core symptoms, however, many investigators have reported other behavioral and/or psychiatric symptoms in persons with the disorder:

- Approximately 60% had poor attention and concentration

- 40% were hyperactive

- 43%-88% exhibited morbid or unusual preoccupation

- 37% had obsessive phenomena

- 16%-86% showed compulsions or rituals

- 50%-89% demonstrated stereotyped utterance

- 70% exhibited stereotyped mannerism

- 17%-74% had anxiety or fears

- 9%-44% showed depressive mood, irritability, agitation, and inappropriate affect

- 11% had sleep problems

- 24%-43% had a history of self-injury

- 8% experienced tics

In the past, the medical community considered these additional symptoms "associate features" of autistic disorder. Several reasons may explain such a concept. First, those who had less experience with this population tended to dismiss these additional abnormal behaviors or symptoms as stemming from the cognitive and communication deficiencies, ignoring the possibility of concurrent nervous system and psychiatric (neuropsychiatric) disorders. Second, difficulties in language, self-evaluation, and concept development in persons with ASD made it more difficult for clinicians to obtain an accurate history, identify precipitating or stressful events, and evaluate thought disorder. The individuals with ASD were less able to report subjective distress and mood disturbances, such as anxiety, depression, and other abnormal states. Third, it appears that some of the neurobehavioral syndromes and aberrant behaviors seen in ASD do not fit neatly into the current classifications of psychiatric disorder [e.g., American Psychiatric Association's Diagnostic and Statistic Manual of Mental Disorders, 4th edition (DSM IV)].

Today, however, there is an increasing number of investigators who argue for considering these behaviors and symptoms as features of co-existing neuropsychiatric disorders, such as attention deficit hyperactivity disorder (ADHD), affective disorders (AD), obsessive-compulsive disorder (OCD), and Tourette syndrome.

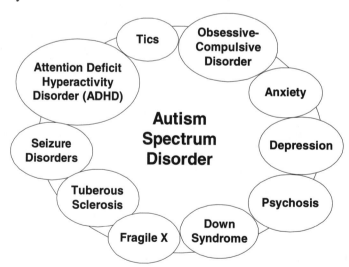

Figure 1-1 Co-Existing Neuropsychiatric Disorders of ASD

In 1991, a British study reported that thirty-five percent of a group of eighty-five adults with Asperger Syndrome also had psychiatric disorders. Of this group, four had mania only, four had mania and depression, two had depression psychosis only, three had schizophrenia, four had hallucinations, one had epileptic psychosis, five had depression only, four had anxiety only, two had depression and anxiety, and two had obsessive-compulsive disorder.

There is no currently available research on co-existing neuropsychiatric disorders among individuals with PDDNOS/atypical autism. Clinical experience indicates that individuals with PDDNOS/atypical autism also have the same types of co-existing neuropsychiatric disorders as those observed in autistic disorder and Asperger Syndrome. (See Figure 1-1).

Treatment Considerations

Behavioral and biological studies suggest complex neurobiological causes of ASD. The degree of abnormality varies among individuals and involves multiple brain regions. So far, researchers have not identified any specific biological cause of ASD. Hence, there are no physical treatments for ASD that are specifically based on cause. Nevertheless, comprehensive intervention, including parental counseling, behavior modification, special education in a highly structured environment, sensory integration training, speech therapy, social skills training, and medication therapy, has demonstrated significant treatment effects in many individuals with ASD.

Parents and non-medical caregivers of persons with ASD rarely have any grave concern over accepting the comprehensive, non-medical intervention approach. However, they often feel uneasy about medication therapy for their children. Such a feeling, no doubt, comes from past abuses of perception- or behavior-altering medications in individuals with developmental disabilities, as well as from the lack of clinical data supporting the efficacy of medication therapy. Many parents and non-medical caregivers view medication therapy as the treatment of last resort, to be used only when other types of intervention have failed to adequately improve the symptoms.

Can Medication Change Behavior and Emotion?

In the past, people believed that individuals were in complete control of their feelings and behaviors. Our understanding of the causes of troubling behaviors or emotions in humans continues to change. Neurobiological and neuropsychological studies in the last three decades have demonstrated that the causes of behaviors and feelings are extremely complex. It is quite clear that the body and the mind are not two separate systems; rather, there are complex interrelationships between the two. Many problem behaviors and disturbed emotions may be partially caused by neurobiological dys-function. For example, there is evidence that disturbed emotions or abnormal behavior involves subnormal neural communication resulting from the malfunctioning of neurotransmitters. Neuro-transmitters are chemical substances responsible for the transmission of signals between synapses. Researchers are identifying which neurotransmitters travel through specialized networks in the brain. See Appendix B.

Neuroscientists have identified several types of neurotransmitters, including epinephrine, norepi-nephrine, dopamine, serotonin, acetylcholine, gamma-aminobutyric acid (GABA), and certain other amino acids and neuropeptides. Emotional states like arousal, rage, fear, anxiety, pleasure, stress response, motivation, and exhilaration apparently involve epinephrine and norepinephrine. Neuro-transmitters also impact cardiovascular and respiratory function, eating and drinking, neuroendocrine regulation, activity level, selective attention, movement, memory, cognition, and learning.

Dopamine is crucial to every voluntary movement and is also involved in cognition, eating and drinking, neuroendocrine regulation, sexual behavior, selective attention, etc. Serotonin seems to play a crucial role in sleep and wakefulness, certain types of sexual activity, and perhaps in modulating and balancing a wide range of synaptic activities, such as body temperature, pain, sensory perception, immune response, motor function, neuroendocrine regulation, appetite, learning, memory, etc.

Every behavior or emotion can involve several neurotransmitters. At present, however, it is acceptable to emphasize a one-to-one relationship in terms of further understanding the neurobiological causes of various neuropsychiatric disorders, as well as developing effective medication therapy based on such a relationship. Neuroscientists have found that altered central dopaminergic function in the midbrain is the principal neurotransmitter system in the development of Tourette syndrome. Psychotherapeutic medications like Haldol® (haloperidol) and Orap® (pimozide) are dopaminergic blockers, which may restore the balance of dopamine in the particular neural circuit and decrease the tic symptoms.

In individuals with too much norepinephrine (adrenaline), everything gets pumped up (increased heart rate and blood pressure), and every stimulation demands a response. Beta-blockers, such as Inderal® (propranolol), block receptors for norepinephrine. With less norepinephrine igniting their brain circuits, patients can calm their anxiety. On the other hand, a shortage of norepinephrine seems to rob people of the ability to pay attention to what is important. The well-known stimulant Ritalin® (methylphenidate) can increase the availability of norepinephrine in children with ADHD, thus restoring their ability to pay attention to what is important.

Shortage of serotonin in the frontal lobes and in the brain's limbic system (where emotions come from) seems to relate to impulsivity. Individuals with inadequate serotonin are unable to connect dis-agreeable consequences with what provoked them. A serotonergic defect involving the three clusters of nerve cells at the base of the brain (basal ganglia) may cause obsessive-compulsive symptoms in some people. Prozac® (fluoxetine) is a serotonin reuptake inhibitor (SRI) that can increase the avail-ability of serotonin in the particular neural network relating to obsessive-compulsive disorder (OCD).

Developments in Drug Therapy

The use of psychotherapeutic medications to control or change human emotions and behaviors is not new. In the past, physicians used a range of sedating drugs like barbiturates, paraldehyde, and opiates to suppress problem behaviors or disturbed emotions. Since the mid-1980s, however, medication therapy in mental disorders has become increasingly popular, respected, and scientific. Neuroscientists have learned much more about the workings of the brain. This is partly due to the increasing sophistication in methods of studying it:

- Magnetic resonance imaging (MRI) or positron emission tomography (PET) scans to investigate brain structures and brain cell function

- Brain mapping to pinpoint areas of the brain that become active during particular thoughts or mental states

- Chemical analyses to study nerve cell receptor physiology

More than twenty years of studying psychotherapeutic medications has shifted emphasis from practical experience to neurotransmitter theory for neuropsychiatric symptoms or disorders. Neuro-scientists now have fairly good ideas of how medications work in some disorders and, therefore, what the underlying nervous system mechanisms might be. The pace of neuroscience research is accelerating, and neuroscientists are learning more about the relationships between neurotransmitters and receptor systems. Someday it will be possible to selectively target a specific area responsible for a certain behavior with medication. Such an approach will make psychopharmacotherapy, which is psychoactive medication therapy, more exact and effective.

Advances in psychopharmacology have also provided better information about dosing levels, concentration of the drug at the effector site (pharmacokinetics), and the end response (pharmacodynamics). The balancing of these variables will enable doctors to selectively use many drugs to treat psychiatric symptoms or behaviors not previously thought to respond to medications.

Medication Therapy in ASD

Certain psychotherapeutic medications are quite effective as a first-line treatment for some disorders (e.g., ADHD, AD, OCD, tic disorders, anxiety disorder, seizure disorders, and sleep disorders) that may develop during the course of ASD in some individuals. The psychopharmacological field has also compiled extensive knowledge of the side effects that these medications may cause.

The study of neuropsychiatric disorders in the last twenty years has certainly helped the field of ASD. Many of the "behavioral problems" or "disturbed emotions" may be clinical manifestations of co-existing neuropsychiatric disorders, as described above, or side effects induced by the drugs taken by individuals with ASD (See Chapters 6 and 8). Early detection and effective treatment of these co-existing neuropsychiatric disorders and side effects are critical. Improving the symptoms will also improve the patient's response to other forms of intervention. Rational use of psychotherapeutic medications will enhance the individual's ability to participate in educational, social, vocational, and family settings.

Not a "Cure"

Like most drugs used in the practice of medicine, psychotherapeutic medications correct, or compensate for, some malfunction in the body. They do not cure ASD or alter the core social and linguistic features of it, but they often can reduce the frequency and intensity of associated affective and behavioral disturbances, including:

- Agitation

- Anxiety

- Mood instability

- Hyperactivity

- Impulsiveness

- Aggression

- Self-injury

- Repetitive, stereotypic, and compulsive behaviors

Life for some individuals with ASD and their caregivers can be enhanced through the knowledgeable, humane, and careful use of psychotherapeutic medications.

Who Should Prescribe the Medications?

The decision to use psychotherapeutic medications in persons with ASD should not be taken lightly—these medications can cause serious side effects. Some of the behavioral problems or disturbing symptoms in ASD may be learned or maladaptive behaviors (e.g., self-injury to get attention or avoid tasks) that usually do not respond to psychotherapeutic medications. A complete functional behavioral analysis must be completed before starting medication therapy (See Chapter 3). The physician must consider the functional behavior information to determine *whether* to prescribe medications and must also decide *which* drugs to prescribe.

Because behavioral problems or symptoms are often multiple, the doctor must specify the medication treatment for each targeted behavior or symptom. For example, when an individual has hyperactivity and inattentive behavior, as well as maladaptive self-injury, the medication treatment plan should make clear to everyone involved in the care of the patient that a particular medication is only for symptoms of hyperactivity and poor attention, and that it is unlikely that the self-injurious behavior would respond to the same medication. Such an approach provides a more realistic expectation of the results of prescribed medications.

Psychoactive drug therapy in ASD is just part of a comprehensive treatment plan. There should be a multidisciplinary treatment approach. The responsible physician must take into account the input of the patient, parents, and other caregivers, including psychologists, special education teachers, speech and language pathologists, occupational therapists, and physical therapists.

The inclusion of non-medical professionals in the treatment team recognizes the large psychosocial component of intervention in ASD. The prescription and management of medications, however, must be managed by a physician specialized in developmental, behavioral, and psychiatric disorders (i.e., a developmental neurologist, developmental/behavioral pediatrician, or psychiatrist). The physician must work closely with the individuals with ASD and their parents and other caregivers. This is the only way to ensure that the most effective use of psychotherapeutic drugs is achieved with a minimum risk of side effects.

Qualifications of Physicians

Many parents and caregivers are not sure about what type of physician they need. General psychiatrists and child-adolescent psychiatrists spend several years in residency training in mental disorders. Behavior and developmental pediatricians spend a significant amount of their residency training in childhood behavior and developmental disorders in addition to the training in childhood physical diseases. Internists, family practice physicians, general neurologists, and pediatric neurologists may receive some training in mental disorders during their residency training. If the medical centers or hospitals where these physicians were residents do not have a special program for ASD, the physicians may have very few, if any, opportunities to learn how to provide medication care to persons with ASD.

Unfortunately, learning about the medical and mental health care of persons with ASD occupies a very low status in the training priorities of pediatricians, neurologists, and psychiatrists. Furthermore, credentials alone do not make a good physician. A good physician should be compassionate, committed, open-minded, and willing to learn from anyone, including parents and non-medical professionals. You should ask about the physician's prior experience in using psychotherapeutic medications in persons with ASD or other developmental disorders.

If you are unable to find resources that exactly meet your needs in your geographic area, you may want to consider locating nearby physicians who have experience in helping individuals with developmental disabilities.

Avoid Overmedication

More people with ASD receive medication now than in the past. In 1995, the Autism Society of North Carolina did a survey of medication patterns. The study found that one-third of people with autistic disorder took some psychotherapeutic medications or vitamins for autism or associated behavioral or psychiatric problems. The study found that the following factors increased the likelihood of the individual receiving some form of psychotherapeutic medications: age, living in sheltered housing, and severe mental retardation. The care providers' satisfaction ratings on the psychotherapeutic medications showed significant variation. The data appeared to indicate that not all the medications were effective. Some individuals may have received the wrong or ineffective medications or were taking the wrong dosages. This supports the growing concern of some professionals that increased reliance on medications may be an attempt to find a quick cure of the emotional and behavioral problems as a substitute for comprehensive intervention.

The study also found that the younger these individuals were, the less frequently doctors prescribed psychotherapeutic medications. Such a finding seemed to indicate that doctors were reluctant to prescribe medications for younger patients with ASD. The finding also indicates the possibility that certain symptoms warranting medication in young children with ASD were misdiagnosed and left untreated.

To effectively advocate for persons with ASD, you need to learn why, when, and how the psychotherapeutic medications should be prescribed, and you must also learn when to resist pressures from others for getting medications for your children. You should keep in mind that unnecessary medication therapy not only does not help, it can also promote chronic illness. Your child may come to believe that his problems only respond to medication, and the more medications are taken, the stronger the misconception becomes.

It is important that you be well-informed about psychotherapeutic medications for ASD. Despite the immense medical and mental health needs of persons with ASD, there is a great shortage of experienced and sensitive physicians. Highly skilled, non-medical professionals specializing in direct assessment, education, and behavioral management of persons with ASD have assumed primary diagnostic and therapeutic responsibilities. When physicians are available, many of them serve as part-time consultants whose responsibilities are largely confined to the prescription of psychotherapeutic medications, often with little or no direct observation of the patient. This pattern of practice has contributed to the widespread overuse of psychotherapeutic medicines in patients with ASD. The careful integration of medication into a comprehensive intervention program, with good communication between the physician and parents/caregivers, is the rare exception and not the rule. This is a national phenomenon.

From this book, you will gain more knowledge of *why* medications can be a part of the comprehensive treatment of ASD. You will understand *when*, *what*, and *how* psychotherapeutic medications can help your child, and you will learn proper ways to evaluate whether the medications are helpful and safe.

Chapter 2

Your Right to Make Informed Decisions about Medication Therapy

Are Psychotherapeutic Medications Safe?

The use of psychotherapeutic medication in persons with ASD continues to be controversial. On one hand, there are those who argue that any form of psychotherapeutic medication for people unable to give informed consent is totally unethical and unjustifiable. On the other hand, some maintain that any medicine provided by a physician must be beneficial—otherwise, the physician would not have prescribed it. As usual, the truth lies somewhere in between. With thousands of children and adolescents with ASD taking new psychotherapeutic medications that were designed for adults, there is the concern about the effectiveness and safety of these drugs when given to children younger than sixteen years.

The U.S. Food and Drug Administration (FDA) evaluates the drug companies' tests of the effectiveness and safety of new medications. The companies conduct the trials primarily on adults. They rarely test children. More than eighty percent of all psychotherapeutic medications are not specifically approved for use in children. However, once the FDA approves a drug for adults, physicians may freely use it on anyone, even if the drug company has done no special testing. One major problem with this is that physicians do not have good data on the correct doses for children or on the serious side effects. Nonetheless, once adults have taken the medication for some years, the odds are that the drug will be safe for use in children and adolescents. Until we conduct more clinical research of these medications in children, the best working model for understanding the effects in children is the adult model.

There are significant gaps in what we know about the effects of the medications on children and adults with ASD. Although there are clinical reports supporting the efficacy and safety of these medications, physicians need to be cautious about prescribing the medications for children and adolescents. Until more research is done, you must carefully consider the relative risk-to-benefit ratio when considering psychotherapeutic medications for your child. The majority of persons with ASD are vulnerable because they cannot make informed decisions for themselves. You must know how to get adequate information so that you can decide what is best for your child. One way is through informed consent.

What Is Informed Consent?

In medical and mental health practice, the patient or his parent/legal guardian should have the following information:

- The purpose of the treatment and the potential benefits
- A description of the treatment process, including the procedure or name of the medication, duration, and costs
- An explanation of the risks of the treatment, or the unknown risks in a new treatment
- The alternatives to the proposed treatment, including no treatment

- The right to refuse the recommended treatment

People usually receive this information verbally, although some hospitals, and even some state laws, require written consent. One exception is in the case of an emergency. The physician can proceed with needed treatment without consent, but he should contact the family as soon as possible. A second exception is "therapeutic privilege;" a physician may withhold information he thinks is detrimental (physically or psychologically) to the patient. For example, if both the child and his parent/legal guardian are in extremely unstable mental conditions and are unable to make a sound decision, the physician can give medications without providing the information.

A primary purpose of informed consent is to provide a basic minimum of opportunity for control to the patient or his parents/legal guardians. They should have ample opportunities to ask questions or to discuss issues of concern. The physician or his representative should not pressure or coerce them for permission.

What Does a Written Informed Consent Form Contain?

Most written informed consent forms contain the following information:

During a meeting with (name of parent/guardian) of the (child's name), it was explained that in the medical opinion of Dr._____ this child should be started on the following medication:

1. Drug Name:_____ Dosage:_____ Frequency: _____

2. It was further explained that the purpose of the medication is to treat, alleviate, or control the following symptoms: _____

3. It was also explained that the medication has side effects, and the person should be observed closely in case they should occur:

   a. Serious side effects that do require medical attention:
   _____

   b. Side effects that usually do not require medical attention:
   _____

4. The potential benefits of administering the medication were discussed. Those benefits are:
   _____

5. The potential risks of administering the medications were discussed. Those risks are:
   _____

6. The following alternative treatments were discussed: _____

7. The potential benefits and risks of no medication were discussed. The benefits and risks of no medications are: _____

8. Explanation was given regarding the fact that each individual reacts uniquely to a medication and a dosage level, and that the policy of Dr._____ is to begin each individual at the minimum dosage level, which might be increased as the clinical course requires. It was further explained that use of this medication is consistent with accepted medical practice and is not considered to be experimental in any sense. Moreover, it was explained that consent for this treatment may be withdrawn by the individual of concern, his parents, or legal guardian at any time.

9. A paper entitled Patient Information Leaflet, which explains proper use of the medication, precautions, and side effects, was given during the meeting.

The last page of the consent form is a treatment contract, which a parent or a legal guardian signs after reading and ag reeing to the following statements:

Dr._____ has informed me of the nature of the medication treatment and has explained the risks of the possible side effects, including _____. I understand that although Dr. _____has explained to me the most common side effects of this treatment, there may be other side effects, and I should promptly inform Dr._____ or any member of his/her staff if there   are   unexpected   changes   in   the   above-named person's condition.

I understand that I may not be compelled to consent to the administration of this medication to the above-named person, and I may request it be stopped at any time.

I also understand that although Dr. _____ believes that this medication will help, there is no guarantee as to the results that may be expected. On this basis, I authorize Dr. _____, or anyone authorized by him or her to administer this medication at such intervals as the physician deems advisable. The following signatures indicate consent for this medication administration discussed regarding areas on the first __ pages of this form. Signatures also indicate that an information leaflet was received or that there was an opportunity to asking questions regarding the medication.

_____

[Signatures of parents or guardians and physician and date]

A written consent form is a reassuring reminder of all the areas that need to be covered. A written form can enhance the patient or his parent's or/legal guardians' understanding of the process. If they are later uncertain about any aspects of medication therapy, they can quickly go back to the informed consent form for clarification.

Informed Consent in Individuals with ASD

To a large extent, obtaining informed consent from a majority of individuals with ASD, regardless of age, is very similar to obtaining informed consent from children. Therefore, the following is easily applicable to the ASD population.

Assent of the Child

Since a child generally is unable to give legally valid informed consent, parents or legal guardians become responsible for making the judgment. However, we now recognize the cognitive and judgmental capacities of children and their legal right to substantially contribute to the consent process. This includes the right to make certain decisions for themselves regarding surgery, medical treatment, abortion, and organ donation. The principle of "assent," therefore, helps parents or legal guardians and physicians to understand the fears, doubts, magical beliefs, and excessive hopes of children. Obtaining assent ensures that a child will receive attention, accurate information, and a chance to express feelings about the medication therapy. Sensitive and compassionate physicians or heath care providers usually ask assent from the child before obtaining the informed consent from his parents or legal guardians.

A child's assent for participation in medical research is advisable at the age of seven. This recommendation comes partly from common law, which traditionally views age seven as the "age of discretion." Modern cognitive psychology also supports this age. The physician, however, should periodically re-evaluate the children on long-term medication treatment. As a child develops, his capacity for understanding may alter earlier impressions and judgments. A child may regret a previous decision, or he may again agree to treatment with a deeper understanding and autonomy. It is critical to provide periodic opportunities for children to update their information and readjust their emotional involvement.

On the other hand, there is no consensus regarding at what age children can competently provide independent, informed consent. The courts have made decisions based on the medical or mental situation, life circumstances, family factors, and developmental capacities. There are differences in state laws and in regional practices. The U.S. Supreme Court has not supported a fixed age of competence below the age of majority. Courts, as well as clinicians, appear inclined to let individual circumstances determine the age of medical consent.

Parental Consent for a Child's Treatment

Before consenting to or refusing the recommended medication therapy for the child, parents or legal guardians should pay attention to the following:

- Clinical problems may arise when the child and parents disagree about the need for a treatment. The child may feel forced, or actually be forced, to take the medication. The parents and physician must deal with the child's anger.

- When the child agrees to the medication therapy, both parents have to agree to the treatment so that the child has the necessary support. The doctor cannot expect a child to comfortably take a medication when even one parent does not back the treatment.

- When a parent is psychologically symptomatic (anxious, depressed, psychotic, etc.), questions may arise about the legitimacy of his or her consent for the child's treatment. In some cases, it may be necessary to have a legally appointed guardian give consent to treatment.

Informed Consent in Individuals with ASD

Parents or legal guardians must make decisions for many lower-functioning individuals with ASD. Nonetheless, these individuals should be included as much as possible in the process of informed consent. Some high-functioning individuals with ASD are capable of fully participating in the process of consent. However, family involvement in this process can be quite valuable. If there is a doubt about the individual's ability to make an appropriate decision concerning medication, legal measures to determine competency may be required.

Assessing the Patient's Capacity to Consent

To determine whether a patient is capable or competent to make an appropriate decision, a professional who is not involved and will not be involved (directly or indirectly) in his care should consider the following:

- His ability to communicate, including asking questions

- His intact immediate and recent memory function showing his competence to take medications according to the instructions

- His intact orientation to time, place, and person

- His intellectual functioning for a response that shows evidence of abstract and logical processing

- His insight into his disability and need for treatment

- His perception of reality and actual understanding of the risks, benefits, and alternatives to treatment, including no treatment

- His ability to reach the reasonable, right, or responsible decision

Current Practice of Obtaining Informed Consent

A recent study in the *Journal of the American Medical Association* found that nine out of ten decisions made between primary care doctors and surgeons and their patients in routine office visits failed to include enough discussion to allow patients to make informed choices. This included decisions about lab tests and use of medications. The finding suggested that doctors did not routinely follow the ethical model of informed decision-making, and this was probably a widespread and persistent problem.

Among those physicians who do practice informed consent, many use a written consent form. Some physicians, however, do not use a written form because they are concerned that the routine use of such a form would turn an opportunity for free and spontaneous interaction between physician and the patient or his/her parents into a rigid procedure. Others do not use a consent form in order to avoid the implication that they have only given the information that is on the form to the patient or his parents/legal guardian. These physicians usually document the discussion in the patient's progress notes.

On the other hand, as the third-party provider organizations (HMOs, PPOs, etc.) apply greater pressure on physicians to use time "more efficiently" (i.e., to see as many patients as possible), physicians find it increasingly difficult to complete the informed consent discussion in the time available.

Legal Aspects of Informed Consent

Every state in the United States of America has passed laws concerning how physicians can obtain informed consent and how patients or their legal guardians can give or refuse consent. Before asking a patient or a parent/legal guardian to agree to any medical care or surgical procedure, *the physician is legally obligated to disclose the benefits and risks involved in the recommended care or procedure.*

If the physician does not obtain informed consent prior to a procedure or treatment, and some harm results because of the procedure, he or she may be liable for malpractice. From a legal point of view, the physician's disclosure is required, not the patient's or his parents/legal guardians' understanding. An informed consent may be sufficient for legal purposes, but not for ethical purposes.

Questions You Should Ask Before Consenting to Treatment

You need complete information when a doctor recommends psychotherapeutic medications as part of your child's treatment plan. As mentioned earlier, some physicians may not disclose all the information. By asking the following questions, you will better understand the recommended medications:

1. What is the name of the medication?

2. Is it known by other names?

3. How do body systems absorb and eliminate the medication?

4. What do researchers know about the medication's effectiveness in patients, especially in those with ASD?

5. How will the medication help my child?

6. How long does it take before we see improvement?

7. What side effects commonly occur?

8. What are possible serious side effects?

9. Is this medication addictive?

10. Can the child abuse this medication?

11. What is the recommended dosage?

12. How often will the medication be taken and at what time of day?

13. Are there laboratory tests, such as heart function or blood tests, that are needed before taking the medication?

14. Will any tests be required while using the medication?

15. Will a physician monitor my child's response to the medication, making dosage changes if necessary?

16. Who will assess my child's progress and how often?

17. How long will my child need the medication? What factors will lead to a decision to stop this medication?

18. Should my child avoid any other medications or foods while taking the medication?

19. Should my child stop participating in any particular activity while taking the medication?

20. What do we do if a problem develops; for example, my child becomes ill, he misses doses, or we see signs of side effects?

21. What is the cost of the medication (generic vs. brand name)?

22. Does health insurance cover it?

23. What type of financial assistance is available?

24. Do we need to tell the school staff (or supervisors at the job place) about this medication?

25. Can we obtain written information about the medication?

If, after the physician has responded to your questions, you still have other questions or doubts about the recommended treatment, you should seek another physician for a second opinion. Remember that the decision to place an individual with ASD on medication should not be made lightly or in a hurry. Physicians should give you as much time as you need for making this important decision. You have to carefully consider the information, even though you might have to "wrestle" emotionally with whether to accept medication therapy. If you do not take time to make the decision, you cannot make a sound decision. In some cases, you may want to delay treatment until you and your child have had a chance to grapple with questions generated by the treatment recommendation.

Chapter 3

Pre-Medication Treatment Assessment

Individuals with ASD exhibit a wide range of inappropriate and undesirable behaviors. People learn most of the challenging behaviors as they react to their environment and the people in it. Some of the behaviors, however, are symptoms of co-existing neuropsychiatric disorders. You must be able to distinguish between the learned challenging behaviors versus neuropsychiatric symptoms so that you can implement an effective intervention plan to improve these individuals' behaviors (see Table 3-1). The pre-treatment assessment is essential for establishing the baseline physical, psychological, behavioral, and cognitive status of the patient prior to medication treatment.

This chapter discusses the behavioral and medical assessment process before using medications to treat the behavioral and medical problems in individuals with ASD. You must be aware of the purposes and the process of such assessments because you will be, and should be, directly involved in the process. Your full understanding and cooperation will influence the choice of evaluation methods and the reliability of evaluation results.

Possible Causes	Behavioral Problem		
	Poor Attention	Self-Injury	Aggression
Attention Deficit Hyperactivity Disorder	Yes		
Attention Seeking		Yes	
Aversive Stimulation			Yes
Deprivation States			Yes
Excitement		Yes	
Fearful Situations			Yes
Frustration		Yes	Yes
Lack of Challenge	Yes		
Learning Disorder	Yes		
Medical Disorders		Yes	Yes
Neuropsychological Disorders		Yes	Yes
Obsessive-Compulsive Disorder	Yes		
Seizure Disorder	Yes		
Task Avoidance		Yes	
Tourette Syndrome	Yes		

Table 3-1 Possible Causes of Behavioral Problems

Purpose of Assessment

Behavioral and medical assessments have three primary functions:

1) Identify and classify a case on the basis of distinguishing characteristics

2) Determine the nature and causes of the problematic behaviors or symptoms

3) Provide guidelines for effective intervention

Both behavioral and medical assessments focus on the specifics of the behaviors or symptoms and take into account other factors, such as the characteristics of the individual, family, and environment that influence the behaviors or symptoms. The assessment should also pay attention to the strengths of the individual being evaluated. The combined behavior and medical interventions not only will decrease inappropriate and undesirable behaviors, they will also help increase appropriate and desirable behaviors.

Many unsuccessful attempts at changing an individual's behaviors or symptoms are due to an incomplete assessment, inaccurate assessment, or no assessment at all. Although a good assessment does not guarantee a successful outcome, it certainly can lead to a more effective intervention.

Clarify the Questions

If you and/or other caregivers of your child are concerned about the child's behavior and want to have a medical evaluation for further medication treatment, you must all agree on the issues *before* your child sees a physician. Your opinion of the child's behavior may be quite different from those of the other caregivers. Therefore, the first step in the assessment process is for the involved team members to meet to address the behaviors of concern. The team includes parents or legal guardians, teachers, a speech therapist, an occupational therapist or a job coach, a school administrator or the employer, and a psychologist or behavioral therapist. Since your child usually participates in various activities in different settings and is supervised by a variety of caregivers, you and all other caregivers should work together to pinpoint behaviors that are undesirable and need modification.

It is important that all caregivers agree on which behaviors to target. The target behaviors must be observable and measurable. The team should carry out a functional behavioral analysis to determine whether inappropriate behaviors or abnormal emotions are reactions to specific events, environments, or individuals, or whether these behaviors come from an internal source.

Conduct a Functional Behavioral Analysis

An experienced and qualified professional (usually a psychologist or a behavioral therapist) should conduct a complete functional analysis. A follow-up team meeting should review the results from this analysis. Referring your child for a medical assessment to obtain medication treatment is an appropriate process when the team members agree that the behaviors are related to a neurobiological disorder, or the behaviors have not responded to an intensive behavior intervention plan that was based on a previous functional behavioral analysis (see Figure 3-2).

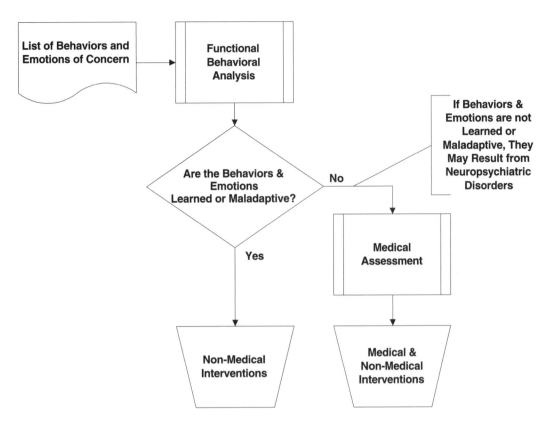

Figure 3-2 Making Intervention Decisions Based on a Functional Behavioral Analysis

What is Functional Behavioral Analysis?

Functional behavioral analysis is the process of gathering information that analyzes the purpose or function that specific behaviors serve for an individual. Functional analysis assumes that an individual's behavior is reasonable from his or her perspective. There is logic to a person's behavior, and functional behavioral analysis attempts to understand that logic. Nonverbal individuals will often use self-injury, property destruction, or aggression to obtain attention, food, drink, change of activity, change of staff, change of scene, or avoidance of a task or social interaction. Verbal individuals will often use undesirable verbal behaviors (e.g., cursing, arguing, etc.) as a way of avoiding social interaction, avoiding a task, obtaining negative attention, obtaining needed assistance, or changing an unwanted activity. Individuals with ASD might display a number of peculiar behaviors. However, even the most peculiar behaviors serve purposes for these individuals. Once we know the purpose of the behavior, we can design strategies that can provide the person with other ways of achieving his or her purposes.

A complete functional behavioral analysis will find what *antecedents (A)* precede the undesirable behavior, under what conditions the *behavior (B)* occurs, and what *consequences (C)* follow the occurrence of that behavior. This *ABC* analysis also determines what behavioral intervention plan is needed to manipulate specific situations and/or to apply new skills to change or perform target behaviors.

A complete functional behavioral analysis can also assess potential medical or physical conditions that may cause problematic behaviors in an individual. A wide variety of such conditions, including allergies; sinus, dental, or middle ear infections; premenstrual and menstrual cycle effects; urinary tract infections; chronic constipation; and sleep problems may exacerbate the occurrence of challenging behaviors. Many psychotherapeutic and seizure medications can cause side effects that may become challenging behaviors. To ensure an accurate determination of such variables, you need to contact a physician for further evaluation and intervention.

A good functional behavioral analysis guarantees neither a good intervention plan nor positive intervention results. Nonetheless, the analysis serves either as the foundation for a more effective behavior intervention plan or a more appropriate referral for further medication treatment.

How to Complete a Functional Analysis

Step 1: Interview All Caregivers

The responsible professional should interview those people who have direct contact with the individual and know him the best. These interviews are useful in defining and narrowing the range of variables that may affect the behaviors of concern. The information gathered in the interviews guides the assessing staff in focusing on the behaviors of concern. The interviewer should ask the following questions: *What* happens? *When, where, how*, and with *whom* does it happen? Do the behaviors occur:

- On particular days of the week?

- At a particular time of day?

- Before or after a specific activity or task?

- With certain people?

- At a certain place or setting?

- With certain materials?

- After a change in routine?

- With certain weather conditions?

Step 2: Direct Observation

Directly observe the individual in typical daily routines for an extended period of time. Collect data by observing him in the classroom, on the job, at home, in restaurants, in stores, or in any other setting in which the target behaviors tend to occur. The key elements of behavioral observation are:

- A data collection system is used

- Behaviors of concern are recorded in specified settings and periods

- Data is systematically checked for accuracy and reliability

- Baseline data are established for later comparison of behavior changes

Ideally, a qualified professional should carry out the observation and data analysis. If such a professional cannot spend an extended period of time observing the individual, then teachers or job coaches, parents, or group home support staff (already working with the person) should be trained to observe and collect data. Recognize the limits and priorities of these caregivers when designing the data collection procedures. The observation must be done in a manner that does not require extensive time or training.

Step 3: Systematic Manipulations

An intervention plan is complete after following these steps:

- The team identifies the "ABCs."

- After understanding the child's behavior pattern, the behavioral therapist predicts when the behaviors will and will not occur.

- The team members all agree that the behaviors of concern are severe.

If the functional behavioral analysis concludes that the behaviors require further medical assessment and treatment, the team should not develop the behavioral intervention plan.

The intervention plan generally outlines the strategies that will be used to change the challenging behaviors; that is, the therapist will manipulate the environment (the antecedent) to:

- Create situations (present difficult tasks, interrupt preferred activities, etc.) to test the accuracy of the cause-effect relationship as suggested by the functional behavioral analysis; or

- Increase more acceptable responses and decrease unacceptable behaviors to test the effectiveness of the behavioral intervention based on the functional analysis.

This approach is very expensive in terms of time and energy, but it ensures an adequate assessment of challenging behaviors.

Here is an example of behavioral analysis. A behavioral therapist conducted a functional behavioral analysis on Brian's challenging behavior—making noises and faces and pinching arms while he was working with his teacher assistants (TA), Ms. M and Ms. N, respectively. The staff used a structured diary method to collect several sets of data as shown in Table 3-3.

Date	Time incident began	Antecedents	Description of Behavior	Consequences
5/10	10:30 AM	Brian was asked to sit down to work on spelling with his TA (M)	Brian began to make noises and faces and pinched his forearm	Brian's TA told him to stop those behaviors. Brian continued those behaviors and was sent to the time-out room

Date	Time incident began	Antecedents	Description of Behavior	Consequences
5/15	10:30 AM	Brian was asked to sit down to work on spelling with his TA (N)	Brian began to make noises and faces and pinched his forearm	Brian's TA gently held Brian's pinching hand and helped him on the spelling. Brian's behaviors gradually subsided.

Table 3-3 Sample Data Collected for a Functional Behavioral Analysis

After the team had reviewed several sets of data and decided that Brian had a Tourette syndrome that tended to be exacerbated by stress and anxiety. M's intervention strategy apparently was ineffective because it caused more anxiety. On the other hand, N's intervention strategy seemed to be more effective. The team did in-service training to ensure all the staff helping Brian would use N's more effective strategy. Brian's "challenging behavior" responded to the intervention and subsided.

The behavioral assessment team must take into account the perspective of the concerned caregiver who may lack the information, or the ability, to assess the child's development. The caregiver may also have emotional problems or may be experiencing stress, all of which can distort his perception of the child's behaviors. For example, low tolerance of parents and other caregivers, high expectations for the child's behaviors, marital stress, and family problems can influence parents or other caregivers' perception of the child's behaviors.

The team should obtain cognitive and educational assessment records of the child, as well as screen the concerned caregiver's physical and mental health. The challenging behaviors might be caused by unreasonable expectation of academic or job abilities. Stress and frustration from an inappropriate curriculum or job placement could also cause challenging behavior. If this is the case, the focus of the intervention plan should be on revising the curriculum, changing the job, or helping the concerned caregiver gain a more accurate perception and expectation of the child.

Step 4: Assessing the Effectiveness of the Intervention

The behavioral assessment does not end when the intervention plan begins. Data collection and assessment on the antecedents and consequences continue throughout implementation of the intervention plan. This ongoing assessment provides data that can be used to evaluate the accuracy of the functional behavioral analysis and effectiveness of the intervention plan. The team can also use the data to evaluate the function of any new behavior that develops after the intervention.

Data Collection Methods for Functional Behavioral Analysis

Data collection methods must serve two purposes. First, the team must measure the occurrence or severity of the behavior. Second, the team must collect data for a functional analysis. Selection of methods will depend on the setting and staff resources. Ideally, a behavioral therapist should collect all the data needed for a complete functional behavioral analysis. If he or she is not available, and the primary caregiver is busy with instructional and behavioral programming, then data collection carried out by that caregiver must be kept to a minimum while still providing a basis for assessment.

Once the behaviors that need to be changed are pinpointed, methods for recording data can be chosen. The following are brief descriptions of strategies that have been helpful in assessing individuals with ASD.

Diary

Keeping a diary involves observing the individual in the target setting and continuously recording all onsets of events, interactions, and terminations of the behaviors. This is a labor-intensive assessment method usually used in low-frequency behaviors. A diary approach is cumbersome, but it can provide valuable information about the setting and the individual's interactions with that setting. The details available from the diary can often provide the basis for functional analysis.

Structured Diary

A structured diary is similar to a diary, but it is not as complete. It limits the type of information recorded, and it provides a format for collecting that information. The structured diary records the ABCs—the events that preceded the target behavior (antecedents), the behavior itself, and the events that followed (consequences). If the target behavior occurs in a typical classroom, home, group home, or job setting, the teachers or other caregivers can usually handle a structured diary if the behavior occurs less than five times a day. This method provides information on the frequency of the behavior and the functions of the behavior.

Frequency Counts

This method records the number of behaviors in a given category during a standard interval, such as a classroom period. Frequency counts are most suitable for behaviors that occur infrequently (e.g., tantrums, fighting, and property abuse). This method is economical because it does not require a behavioral therapist to spend an enormous amount of time collecting data on infrequent behaviors. Parents and/or caregivers can do the "frequency counts" that will provide information on the frequency of the behavior. They can learn how to complete the ABC forms.

Response Duration

This method measures the time during which the individual engages in a challenging behavior. It is most useful for long-lasting behaviors like tantrums, refusal of classroom tasks, etc.

Time Sampling

This procedure is appropriate when data cannot be collected continuously throughout the day due to limited resources. With time sampling, the team can collect data during designated periods of time on the assumption that the data will provide representative information. For example, collect data on Monday and Wednesday mornings between 9:00 a.m. and 11:00 a.m.

Tally Method

A tally counts the number of incidents of the target behaviors. A team uses this method when there are several challenging behaviors that occur too often (between five-to-ten times per day) for filling out ABC forms. The tally requires a timing device that signifies brief intervals (e.g., ten minutes) and an explicit coding scheme. The observer checks all categories of challenging behaviors that occurred in the previous interval. The frequency data might be used simply to provide information on how often the targeted behaviors occur. One example of the tally method is to use a counting device to record the frequencies of self-injurious behaviors like hitting head, biting hands, and slapping face during a time period.

Time Block

If a target behavior occurs at a high frequency (more than ten times per day) and is difficult to record accurately, then the caregiver may collect data during time blocks. In this procedure, the observer records whether or not the target behavior occurred in set periods of time—in twenty-minute blocks, for example. Using this method, the caregiver records whether or not the target behavior occurred in each twenty-minute block throughout the day and evening. For each twenty-minute interval, he or she simply records a " + " if the targeted behavior occurred and a " - " if it did not occur. The size of the interval should be large enough to allow the caregiver to record the target behavior and small enough to be able to assess progress. For example, if a behavior occurs almost continuously, a fifteen-minute time block might be necessary. However, if a behavior occurs only a few times each hour, a half-hour time block might be sufficient. Time blocks do not give as precise a measure as the tally method. However, this method saves time.

Combination Method

A time sample might be used for recording (on ABC forms) the first incident of the morning and the first incident of the afternoon, while only the most severe incidents in each hour are recorded. If the target behavior occurs between five and ten times per day, caregivers can take a tally, and structured diaries can be filled out on either a time sample basis or on a priority basis. If the behavior occurs more than ten times per day, a time block may be used to estimate frequency, and ABC forms can be completed on a time sample or priority basis.

Ratio of Responses to Opportunities

Some types of behaviors occur infrequently, being a direct response to environmental stimulus or opportunity (e.g., asking for help when a computer malfunctions). Assess such behaviors by examining the ratio of responses to opportunities. For example, if the target behavior is a "response to correction," the observer will record information on the type of response to each instance of correction. The total number of opportunities (instances of correction) then divides the total number of acceptable responses. This quotient is multiplied by 100% to result in a percentage of correct responses.

Productivity

Productivity measures are often the choice when concerned with off-task behavior that is due to self-stimulation, such as hand flapping, self-spinning, or rocking. Rather than concentrating on the off-task behaviors, focus on measuring productivity in terms of the work that the individual has produced (e.g., by counting the number of units produced).

Permanent Products

One might not directly observe aggressive, self-injurious, or destructive behavior, but the behavior can produce bruises, scratches, or cuts on the body; hospital bills; counts of destroyed property; bills for damaged property; frequency of neighbors' complaints, etc. Use these as measures of the behaviors.

Record Review

In some cases, the severity of the behavior requires immediate implementation of an intervention plan to control the damage. You can quickly review the records in order to estimate a baseline measure of the behavior. Sometimes, antecedent and consequence information is also in the records. Use the information to formulate a treatment plan to control the crisis.

What Data Should Be Recorded?

Antecedents

Assessment of antecedents involves listing all antecedents and events that might set off the challenging behaviors, no matter how innocent they appear. The following are examples of antecedents: being asked repeatedly to work on a task, giving or getting a toy with which to play, being asked a question that is difficult to answer, being teased or criticized, etc.

Setting Events

These are the events that most likely would cause challenging behaviors to occur given certain antecedents. Setting events can include the following:

- Hunger

- Lack of sleep

- Too much or too little caffeine

- Presence or absence of certain drugs, illnesses, allergies

- Presence or absence of a certain family member, caregiver, or peer

- Certain behaviors of parents, caregivers, or peers

- Staff and peer interactions

- Weather

- General environmental conditions such as the lack of space, lack of other activities, difficulty of tasks, and staff/client ratios

- Major events like a parent's illness, the parents' separation or divorce, a death in the family, or an impending move

Remember that inappropriate behaviors do not always stem directly from the child. The environment (setting event) often encourages a certain behavior. Knowing the setting events can answer the question of why the child usually responds well to the antecedent, but sometimes does not. List setting events that seem to relate to the concerned behaviors. Perhaps the setting events are more appropriate targets for intervention than the behavior itself. Often the individual's behavior improves with a change of setting.

Consequences

Information collected on consequences can reveal the individual's purpose for the behavior. Consequences that seem innocent may in fact make the behavior useful for the individual. When reviewing ABC forms, assume that any listed consequence might in fact explain the purpose of the behavior. Answer and record the following questions: Does the individual get what he wants? Does he get what he does not want? Does the individual get more caregivers responding to the behavior?

Duration

Use duration measurements when time is a critical factor. The observer must record the onset and ending of each incident of the target behavior (e.g., the length of severe, self-injurious behaviors).

Medical Assessment and Diagnosis

Medical assessment is a complex process that involves direct observation and recording of the individual's behaviors/symptoms and recording personal complaints or concerns. It also takes into account social, cultural, biological, and developmental influences on the individual. Therefore, assessing an individual's "behavioral problems" needs a multi-method, interdisciplinary approach. The team must work together to make a full assessment of an individual's weaknesses and disabilities, as well as his or her strengths and abilities.

The specific disciplines and types of in-depth assessments needed for each referred individual depend on at least three factors:

1. Areas of concern pinpointed during the screening process

2. Age and characteristics of the individual

3. Types of intervention needed following the assessment

The physician must understand a patient's complaints, use a diagnostic system to classify the behaviors or symptoms of concerns, find the cause or causes of medical disorders, and prescribe potentially effective treatment to eliminate symptoms or cure the underlying illness. The medical assessment and diagnosis in individuals with ASD involves the same basic techniques as in the non-autistic population, although greater reliance on gathering clinical information from family and caregivers may be necessary.

What Type of Physician Is Appropriate?

The course and the nature of the presenting problems always dictate the type of physician to which the individual should be referred for a medical assessment and treatment. For example, if a teenager with exemplary grades and excellent interpersonal skills has a sudden personality change accompanied by gross social disinhibition and headaches, a family physician, a pediatrician, or a neurologist should immediately examine him to rule out a medical/neurological disorder. On the other hand, an individual with chronic problems, such as long-standing anxiety, affective symptoms, or inappropriate behaviors, should see a behavioral or developmental pediatrician or a general or child/adolescent psychiatrist.

Specific to the medication assessment and treatment of individuals with ASD, the physician needs to know the following:

- Normal child and family development

- Assessment and diagnosis of ASD and comorbid neuropsychiatric disorders

- General theories and principles of behavioral, psychological, educational, occupational, sensory, and speech/language assessments and what assessment methods should be used

- How to communicate assessment results obtained by the non-medical colleagues to the child and his parents/caregivers

- How to provide intervention services to individuals with ASD and related disorders

How to Make a Referral for Medical Assessment and Diagnosis

Initial Contact

The initial contact is most often a telephone call requesting an assessment appointment. A staff member at the physician's office will screen the request, which is usually by a parent or a caregiver. The request must be specific concerning the type of evaluation desired and the reasons for making the request. The caller should also provide brief explanations of previous observations and information leading to needing a further medical assessment. If the referral is appropriate (i.e., the intervention team has completed a functional behavioral analysis and has agreed that a further medical assessment is necessary), a diagnostic interview session is the next step. The clinic will need the final report of the functional analysis and other available information before the first appointment (or the parent can bring the report to the first session). Such information can help avoid duplication of effort, define the nature of suspected problems, and determine which diagnostic procedures are most appropriate.

The staff will tell the referring person that the clinic will send questionnaires and rating scales to key caregivers to complete and return to the office before the initial visit. The physician's office should give you the option of not providing this information if you are uncomfortable in giving it. The questionnaires will provide information on the following:

- The family's socioeconomic status

- The developmental milestones of the individual

- Day care and school history

- Medical history

- The parents and/or caregiver's perception of the individual's problems and possible causes

- What has been done about the problems up to the point of making the referral (See Appendix D for examples of some commonly used questionnaires and rating scales)

If resources are available, the office staff will ask you to provide, either before or on the day of the first appointment, videotapes that record the incidences of the behaviors of concern. Information from the functional analysis reports, questionnaires, and videotapes sets the stage for the comprehensive assessment.

First Assessment Session

At the time of the first session, the physician should review the functional behavioral analysis report, returned questionnaires, videotape, and other available information. He or she then should make sure that you are all addressing the same problems. Assessment is useful only to the extent that there is agreement on the issues. Once the issues are clarified, the physician should then decide which assessment procedures will most appropriately address the issues.

The physician should explain the reasons for selecting the particular assessment procedure so that you understand what will occur and how you can assist in the assessment. The physician must obtain your permission before carrying out the assessment. Although the medical assessment employs various tests, a variety of information gathering and measurement devices are of value. The synthesis and analysis of all the assessment data lead to a diagnostic work-up that provides a fair, unbiased, and accurate evaluation of your child's strengths and weaknesses, abilities and disabilities.

The following sections describe the methods of gathering information for medical assessment and diagnosis in individuals with ASD.

Interviews and Observations of Behaviors.

Formal and informal interviews and behavior observation comprise one method for gathering in-depth information about the child, parents, caregivers, and the interaction among them. Child-rearing methods, discipline, and parental or caregiver's attitudes and perceptions of their child's behavior are important. Here are some common interview formats:

- Unstructured interview—This is the traditional way of using a free-floating interview that has some preconceptions and theoretical constructs as guides. Hence "unstructured" is a relative term.

- Structured interview—As the name suggests, this format usually consists of a series of questions, observations, or tests that must be carried out exactly as specified. Structured methods have advantages. They properly cover the diagnostic symptoms, minimize variations in how questions are asked, and leave little to individual interpretation. The disadvantages are that they are rigid, cumbersome, and user-unfriendly. These methods are particularly suited to research because they tend to yield good diagnostic reliability, but they are not likely to suit busy, experienced clinicians used to quickly homing in on the problem.

- Semi-structured interview—This is a compromise between unstructured and structured interviews. It allows for more flexibility and brevity, but it requires that the interviewer be trained and experienced enough to interpret the individual's response.

- Symptom checklists—These differ from the above in that while there is no structure to the interview, the clinician can go through a symptom checklist (similar to the systems inquiry in a physical examination) to ensure that he or she has covered the relevant areas.

- Computer-based interview—There is an increase in computer-based interview systems. Computer-based systems have the advantages of both diagnostic precision and the simultaneous compiling of standard, comprehensive, and legible patient files that can also be aggregated to provide statistics across patients. This interview, however, requires that the person being interviewed has sufficient computer skills to understand and respond to questions showing on the computer screen.

Interviewing Parents, Caregivers, and Child

Information gained from the completed questionnaires permits the physician to focus the beginning of the assessment on you and your child. Such an interview will allow your child to hear your concerns about his challenging behaviors. If your child's cognitive and communication skills are adequate, such an interview also gives him an opportunity to give his reasons for having the "challenging behaviors." However, due to being young or having limited cognitive and communicative skills, your child may not understand the reason for the assessment and may be unable to adequately express himself. Nonetheless, he should be respected as a participant and have the opportunity to listen to your concerns.

The interview also gives the physician the opportunity observe the interaction between you and your child. Most observations of such interactions include both structured and unstructured time. With younger children, for example, parents may have a variety of toys to play with the child as they would at home. After a few minutes, the doctor can instruct the parents to have the child put away all the toys. Older patients and their parents/caregivers can be play a board game, draw a picture together, or talk about a family vacation plan. The important dimensions of the interaction are:

- The extent to which the parent gives the child positive versus negative feedback, and whether that feedback is contingent on the child's behavior;

- The number of demands placed on the child;

- The number of questions asked; and

- The child's compliance or noncompliance to parental demands.

The interview room should be a spacious and comfortable setting with careful attention given to health and safety. The room should have ample toys, games, and books in good condition and appropriate for various ages. Some of these materials should be reachable so that the child can play with them without asking permission. Other materials should be visible but locked up. Observing the individual's behaviors in such a setting provides information on his developmental level in terms of cognition, social skills, and problem solving skills. With permission from you and your child, the staff can videotape the interaction session to use for later diagnostic feedback. It can also be used as the pre-treatment baseline that will be compared with the post-treatment changes.

Interviewing the Parents and Caregivers

Interviewing you and other caregivers out of your child's presence is of vital importance. It is a way to discuss more sensitive information. The physician must understand your/their perception of the problems and their influence on both the child and his environment (i.e., home and family life, classroom and learning, or job place and work performance). The parent and/or caregiver interview also follows up on information gathered from the previously completed checklists and questionnaires. The physician will review your child's developmental history:

- Past and present cognitive, physical, adaptive, and social functioning

- Past medical and psychiatric history (diagnosis and treatments)

- Family medical and psychiatric history

The physician usually will also review the basis for the diagnosis of ASD and may address how and when it was made. He may also ask you for further information about other areas that he may need to assess.

Past Medical History

A review of all previous medical illnesses of your child is important. For example, chronic ear infections may affect an individual's speech and language development. A history of rheumatic fever might relate to the development of obsessive-compulsive disorder. On the other hand, psychiatric disorders or challenging behaviors may be related to many medical or neurological disorders. The physician may want to know the following information to help determine whether the "challenging behaviors" are caused by medical or psychiatric disorders instead of the psychotherapeutic medications.

- Hospitalizations—The doctor needs to know the number and frequency of hospitalizations, nature and severity of conditions, and length of stay. This information may show a possible link between past illness and present behaviors of concern.

- Allergies—Are there any previous allergic reactions to medications, food, drinks, clothing, etc., with symptoms that resemble current challenging behaviors?

- Use of Substances—Use of alcohol or illicit drugs may relate to the development of the behaviors of concern.

- Current Medications—Medications for asthma, allergies, or seizures can cause side effects indistinguishable from psychiatric symptoms. For example, the use of phenobarbital for seizures can make children hyperactive, and the use of xanthines (such as theophylline) in the treatment of asthma can produce anxiety. Drug interactions may cause psychiatric symptoms or problem behaviors.

- Trauma—A history of head injury may relate to the behaviors of concern. Unexplained and/or multiple accidents or traumas could be the result of physical or sexual abuse that may be causally related to the psychiatric symptoms or challenging behaviors that the child has.

- Disorders of Central Nervous System—Symptoms of staring spells, fainting, dizziness, headaches, numbness, tingling, tremors, weakness, clumsiness, speech problems, pain, and motor or vocal tics may be related to seizure disorders or other brain disorders.

- Disorder of Eyes, Ears, Nose, and Throat—A history of chronic sniffing or blurting out obscene words might be a vocal tic that was misinterpreted as a challenging behavior. The medications could cause blurred vision and/or abnormal eye movements, thereby affecting the individual's mood and behavior.

- Dental Diseases—Cavities or gum infections might be related to an individual's headache, mood problem, and sleep disturbance.

- Disorder of Respiratory System—If an individual takes both anti-asthma medication and Inderal® (propranolol), the asthmatic symptoms may be exaggerated. A history of chronic coughing might be a symptom of Tourette syndrome.

- Cardiovascular Diseases—A history of having chest pain, fainting, or dizziness upon standing might be due to the individual's taking stimulants, antidepressants, or antipsychotic medications that have important effects on heart rate, blood pressure, and/or cardiac conduction and excitability.

- Gastrointestinal Disorders—Decreased appetite, poor eating habits, nausea, vomiting, diarrhea, constipation, stomachache, or jaundice might be related to affective illnesses (those influenced by or resulting from emotions), anxiety disorders, or side effects of psychotherapeutic medications.

- Urinary Tract—Individuals taking lithium may have to urinate more often, and the need to visit the bathroom may become a "challenging behavior." Some medications may cause a relapse of the involuntary discharge of urine (enuresis) or may exacerbate preexisting problems with enuresis. The problems of an individual in this situation may be misconstrued as being related to nervousness.

- Disorders of Genital and Reproductive Systems—The birth control pill can cause side effects with symptoms of affective illness. Similarly, antipsychotic medications can interfere with sexual functioning and cause some adolescents to experience complications such as menstrual disturbances and excessive flow of milk from the breast (galactorrhea) that in turn might cause mood disturbance.

- Musculoskeletal Disease—A history of multiple complaints of joint aches, muscle pains, or weakness might be related to musculoskeletal diseases. There are also important musculoskeletal side effects of certain psychotherapeutic medications (e.g., tics caused by stimulants and Parkinsonism caused by antipsychotics).

- Diseases of Skin—Psychotherapeutic medications can cause skin side effects. For example, photosensitivity caused by antipsychotics might be the reason to avoid outdoor activity.

- Endocrine System—The physician should consider the possibility of a thyroid disease if these symptoms are present: hot or cold intolerance, dry skin, rapid or slow heart rate, increased fluid intake, or growth abnormalities plus symptoms of affective (emotional) illnesses or attention-deficit hyperactivity disorder.

Family Neuropsychiatric History

Inherited neuropsychiatric disorders such as thyroid disease, Huntington's disease, obsessive-compulsive disorder, and Tourette syndrome may present with psychiatric symptoms. Side effects of drugs such as symptoms outside of the central nervous system (extrapyramidal) may be familial in some cases. The family neuropsychiatric history could help in the clinical diagnosis of the family.

Interviewing the Child

The individual diagnostic interview is often the most difficult obstacle for the physician who has little experience in evaluating individuals with ASD. The physician could have preconceived thoughts about people with ASD and could assume that the patient cannot provide useful or valid information about his challenging behaviors or symptoms. In fact, there are some individuals with ASD who are fairly capable of relating well verbally as long as the language is kept simple. Establishing rapport is vitally important. Knowing the cognitive-developmental characteristics of individuals at different ages and having appropriate interview skills are essential to conducting a successful interview.

The interview with a verbal individual provides valuable information on the individual's perception of himself, including his interests, fears, strengths, weaknesses, self-confidence, the environment (family, peers, school, job place, and co-workers), and the presenting problems. The physician can see how the child attempts to cope with and solve personal and interpersonal problems. The language used during the interview should be at, or just above, the child's cognitive/language level. The physician should provide the child with age-appropriate, unstructured materials (crayons, pencils, papers, books, Legos®, Play-Doh®, doll house, etc.). This will make the child more comfortable while talking to the physician.

When interviewing older children, the physician should introduce topics of interest that are developmentally appropriate (e.g., TV shows or cartoon characters, sports, popular songs, computer games, etc.). When the individual becomes more comfortable, the physician can slowly shift the focus of the interview to the concerns of the parents or caregivers.

A brief psychiatric review will help assess hallucinations, anxiety states, affective states, thinking problems, delusions, and compulsions. When suspected, the physician should address sexual activity and the possibility of pregnancy in teenagers and adults.

For those who are nonverbal, or have difficulty with the verbal interview, the physician should use nonverbal techniques for assessing the capacity for social interaction. In these cases, the physician can observe the individual's capacity to use alternate communication systems, such as gesturing, sign language, or communication pictures or symbol boards. If feasible, the physician should use these communication means to gather subjective information.

Observing the Child

Direct observation is the contemporaneous recording of spontaneously occurring, externally observable, behavioral events. It is highly objective and provides an accurate, relevant portrayal of the child. Direct observation can be repeated as frequently as required without practice effect (i.e., the performance score increase after each repeated testing), which tends to occur in using cognitive tests and rating scales to collect data.

Observing the child's selection of play materials and how he plays with them can be a valuable source of information about his intellectual and language development, special interests, leisure-time skills, social relationships and interaction skills, feelings, thoughts, worries, anxieties, etc. Such observation is particularly important and useful in gathering information from non-verbal, lower-functioning, or very disturbed and uncooperative individuals. However, there are certain disadvantages to direct observation.

- Direct observation requires extensive logistical and staff support, which is costly.

- The presence of an observer or video camera can distort the behavior of both the child and parents/caregivers.

- The sampling period may be too short or otherwise atypical.

The office staff can divide the interview room (playroom) floor into sections with tape or painted squares to measure grid crossings and toy changes. The child is typically observed in a free-play situation for part of the session. The child has to have the opportunity to interact with a variety of age-appropriate toys or games. After the free play (fifteen-to-twenty minutes), your child is told to stay in one sector of the room and play with only one toy or one game for about ten-to-fifteen minutes. The physician will then ask you to join in to play or interact with your child for another fifteen-to-twenty minutes.

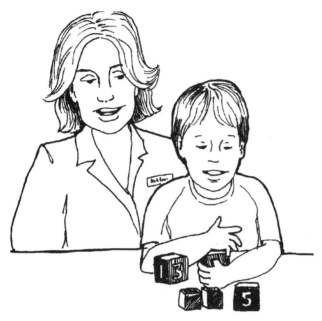

In the first part of observation, the observer assesses the grid crossings and toy changes and records the number of quadrants entered and the number of playing "forbidden toys" during restricted play. During this time, the child plays with toys like Legos®, a dollhouse, or simple rule-governed games. The observer can also determine the following variables: cognitive development, fine motor development, language development and skills, organizational skills, creativity, symbolic and pretend-play skills, attention span, distractibility, impulsiveness, compliance, persistence, use of help, frustration level, emotional expression, perceptions of family interaction, and problem solving skills. The information is useful for assessment of developmental disorders, ADHD, oppositional defiant disorder (ODD), and conduct disorder (CD).

Direct observation can also record behaviors such as crying or whimpering, inactivity, withdrawal, agitation, stuttering, tremors, and nervousness. These behaviors may relate to depressive and/or anxiety disorders. Observational data can identify the areas needing more formal testing.

Speech and Language Assessment

Given the potential of psychotherapeutic medications to alter speech and language skills, some baseline assessment is desirable. The physician can screen individuals for problems with speech and language by obtaining an accurate developmental history and informally interacting with the child. There is no single screening test for speech and language that serves all ages. When taking developmental history, the physician should look for particular items that could indicate dysfunction, such as problems with articulation or delayed clear speech development.

In addition to evaluating intelligibility of speech and articulation, the physician will look for items such as abnormal voice quality and pitch, limited syntax, failure to comprehend language, scarcity of speech, narration difficulties, inability to develop complex language structures, and perceptive language problems. If there are any doubts, a qualified speech language pathologist should conduct a full-scale evaluation of speech and language. At the very least, the mental status exam should include noting speech and language function.

Mental Status Assessment

The mental status examination focuses on the individual's appearance; mood or affect; orientation to time, place, and person; thought processes and verbalization; neuromuscular integration; awareness of problems; and cognitive function. The above interviews and observations would have collected much of this information.

Physical and Neurological Assessment

Because different behavior problems, symptoms, or side effects of medications may mimic other medical or psychiatric disorders, the physical and neurological assessment may reveal medical problems or disorders previously missed; new, unrelated medical problems or disorders; incorrect earlier diagnoses; or adverse effects associated with various treatments. An accurate differential diagnosis is essential in order to determine what medication and dosage is needed. The other major reason for a careful and complete physical and neurological assessment is to establish the baseline health status of the patient prior to medication therapy. This baseline is for monitoring and preventing the development of side effects.

Performing a complete physical and neurological assessment in some people with ASD can be a real challenge, and the physician needs special training and experience in working with them. This is particularly true in those patients with low cognitive and communicative functions. They may not be able to understand the examination procedure, so they will not cooperate during the assessment. Some individuals may resist any physical contact and even react violently to the usual examination procedure. The assistance of parents and/or caregivers who are familiar with the individual's behavior patterns and means of communication is most helpful. In some really difficult cases, the physician may have to concede the situation and focus on just obtaining the essential information. Or he may have to rely on a recent documentation of another physician's physical examination that occurred when the patient cooperated.

Laboratory Tests

Although laboratory tests can never replace clinical judgment in any medical specialty, they can play a significant role in explaining and quantifying biological factors associated with various medical and psychiatric disorders. Supplementary laboratory and diagnostic tests may be necessary when specific clues from the history, physical examination, or initial laboratory screens or tests suggest a medical or psychiatric condition that might have caused or exacerbated the behaviors or symptoms in the patient.

Avoid Unnecessary Laboratory Tests

Not all the laboratory measures and tests promoted by advocacy groups, non-medical professionals, or the media need to be done as routine screens or tests. Particularly, many are new tests that are not supported by scientific evidence showing that they meet minimum criteria of effectiveness. Inaccurate, false-positive results can cause profound anxiety and require additional testing that can be increasingly invasive and costly. The tests can also deplete society's limited medical resources. Physicians can (and should) refuse to order tests that would violate their medical and ethical judgment.

Some physicians who do not have much knowledge, training, and experience in working with individuals with ASD may order unnecessary tests. Ask about the reasons for the tests and how the results aid in the assessment and/or intervention of your child. Physicians have a responsibility to inform you of the limitations and risks of the tests. If you are not satisfied with the explanations the doctor gives you, and there is no life-threatening urgency, you should seek a second opinion before agreeing to the tests. It is the physical condition of your child and the physician's medical knowledge and experience that determine which laboratory tests should be done. Avoid wasteful laboratory tests that have limited clinical utility.

Current laboratory tests cannot confirm the majority of the diagnoses of mental or psychiatric disorders. Doctors should only order laboratory studies for specific diagnostic considerations (e.g., thyroid studies to evaluate depression), and baseline assessment where the proposed medications could alter organ systems (e.g., assessment of thyroid function before lithium is prescribed).

The following section focuses only on the usefulness of the more commonly considered laboratory measures in evaluating behavioral problems. The main function of these tests is to support or confirm the clinical diagnoses of certain medical and/or neurological disorders that also have behavioral symptoms. The other function of these tests is to confirm that the behaviors of concern are side effects of psychotherapeutic medication(s) taken by the individual with ASD.

- **Electrocardiogram (ECG)**—Cardiac monitoring via the ECG is an integral part of assessing anxiety disorder and drug-induced side effects, such as those that occur in children and adolescents treated with tricyclic antidepressants.

- **Electroencephalography (EEG)**—You should ask for a complete EEG and neurological consultation when there is a deteriorating course, clear history of seizure, or when the medical history and neurological examination indicates a tumor or infectious brain symptoms. The symptoms include staring or spacing spells, fainting spells, dizziness, headaches, numbness, tingling, tremors, weakness, clumsiness, speech problems, pain, and motor or vocal tics. Thus far, however, researchers have not identified specific EEG patterns that can accurately aid in the diagnosis of a particular psychiatric condition.

- **Catecholamine and Enzyme Assays**—Catecholamine is a class of molecules that serve as neurotransmitters and hormones. Catecholamines are assayed (analyzed) in a twenty-four-hour urine collection in individuals with anxiety. Accompanying abnormal levels of autonomic (involuntary) function should be screened for pheochromocytoma, a type of kidney tumor. In individuals taking antipsychotic medications and are being evaluated for the development of neuroleptic malignant syndrome (NMS), the physician needs specific tests. Fever, muscle rigidity, stupor, and autonomic dysfunction characterize NMS. The physician should check the blood levels of creatine phosphokinase, which is a muscle protein. The white blood cell count is also important.

- **Brain Imaging**—Imaging studies are not routinely necessary for people with behavioral disorders. Computerized tomography (CT) or magnetic resonance imaging (MRI), however, is clinically useful for ruling out brain tumors and for mapping signs of increased intra-cranial pressure, changing or degenerative neurological signs, craniofacial malformations, suspected syndromes, or inherited syndromes that include CNS structures. Positron emission tomography (PET) is helpful in the pre-surgical evaluation of individuals with intractable epilepsy.

- **Lumbar Punctures**—Clinical pictures of altered mental status consistent with cerebral spinal fluid (CSF) infection warrant examination of CSF with a lumbar puncture. This procedure removes spinal fluid from the spinal canal.

- **Electromyogram (EMG) and Nerve Conduction Studies**—These may help individuals when the doctor suspects muscle or muscle tissue diseases (myopathies). These studies can also ascertain whether there are problems with the nerves outside the brain and spinal cord— peripheral neuropathies—which may be misinterpreted as psychiatric symptoms.

- **Polysomnography (PSG)**—PSG refers to sleep recordings that monitor various physiological parameters. PSG is useful in the investigation and diagnosis of sleep disorders, especially sleep apnea and narcolepsy.

- **Metabolic Screening**—Many metabolic disorders may cause behavioral and emotional changes. For example, Wilson's disease, a recessively inherited disorder of copper metabolism, may cause incongruous behaviors, personality change, cognitive impairment, anxiety, and depression in adolescents. Its symptoms are a low serum ceruloplasmin level, low total serum copper level, and raised urinary copper excretion. Detection is critical because Wilson's disease is a treatable metabolic disorder.

- **Thyroid Function Tests**—If the physician suspects that thyroid disease is contributing to a disorder that has symptoms including anxiety, depression, mental retardation, dementia, restlessness, mental status change, and psychosis, he should conduct screening tests of thyroxine and triiodothyronine resin uptake. If results are abnormal or barely normal, the doctor should check thyroid-stimulating hormone levels. The doctor may want a thyrotropin-releasing hormone stimulation test if initial studies are ambiguous.

- **Liver and Kidney Function Tests**—When the physician questions whether particular medications are affecting the individual's liver and/or kidney functions that in turn might cause the behaviors of concern, he or she should evaluate the functions of these organs.

- **Serum Measures**—Children on newer drugs like Clozaril® (an antipsychotic medication) should always have regular, complete blood counts. Tests for serum amylase (an enzyme) and electrolyte values may be useful in the assessment and follow-up of bulimic patients.

- **Chromosomal Analysis**—A deficit in cognitive development may be influenced by abnormal numbers of X chromosomes. There have also been associations between increased numbers of Y chromosomes and increased risks of behavioral problems, most notably impulsiveness and immaturity. Genetic measures may be helpful. Testing for a fragile X chromosome may be helpful in individuals with mental retardation and abnormal physical characteristics.

- **Illicit Drug Screening**—For individuals with new-onset behavioral changes or psychotic symptoms, the doctor may want to test for drug abuse.

- **Toxicology Screening**—Lead ingestion, though rare, can be measured as a potential cause of behavioral difficulty.

Further Assessment

By this point in the assessment process, the doctor should have a fairly good idea about the nature of the problem and what other information is needed. Further assessment may include:

- **Home and School Observation**—Some individuals may not exhibit the challenging behaviors or symptoms at the physician's office or the behaviors shown in the videotape. If the physician has a well-trained staff member who specializes in behavior observation and assessment, she can ask the staff member to observe the child's behavior at home, in school, or on the job.

- **Problem- or Disorder-Specific Questionnaires/Rating Scales**—At this point in the assessment process, the physician may have some idea of a diagnosis. He may want additional "problem- or disorder-specific" questionnaires or rating scales completed by the individual's teachers or job supervisors. This is to facilitate the assessment process and enhance the diagnostic accuracy. Examples of the problem/disorder specific questionnaires or rating scales are in Appendix D.

- **Referral to Allied Health Professionals for Further Assessment**—If the nature of the problem is not yet completely understood at this point, the physician may need expertise from other disciplines. In this case, the physician can refer the individual to other appropriate allied professionals for further evaluation. These professionals include a pediatrician, pediatric or general neurologist, child or general psychiatrist, neuropsychologist, occupational therapist, physical therapist, speech/communication disorders specialist, and audiologist. In-depth testing and information gathering provide the basis for the final decision on the diagnosis and recommendation of a comprehensive treatment plan.

Diagnosis

Given these multiple sources of information, diagnostic evaluation requires more than a simple compilation of data. An analysis and synthesis that brings together the results of all the data analyses by each of the interdisciplinary team members results in an accurate picture of the individual's condition. Much of the information related to the behavior of concern has been assessed prior to the referral for a medical assessment and diagnosis. If the team believes the conclusion from a previous assessment is accurate and acceptable, it should focus on information gathered during the medical assessment process. However, the team should take into account that how the individual performs in a variety of settings or contexts may be quite different from the performance observed by professionals during structured testing sessions. The assessment information must be interpreted in terms of the individual's total functioning, including abilities or strengths, and disabilities or weaknesses.

Diagnostic Classification

At present, the most commonly used diagnostic system for mental disorders in the United States is the fourth edition of the Diagnostic and Statistical Manual of Mental Disorders (DSM IV), published in 1994 by the American Psychiatric Association. Health care providers worldwide use the tenth edition of the International Classification of Disorder (ICD-10), published in 1955 by the World Health Organization, to diagnose medical disorders, including neurological disorders. Both DSM IV and ICD-10 classification systems are relatively new and have not been thoroughly critiqued for their usefulness. Nonetheless, both represent a great improvement because they specify inclusion and exclusion criteria, duration of symptoms, and time of illness onset. These types of diagnostic systems should help facilitate communication between researchers and clinicians by clearly identifying those patients or diagnostic subgroups that responded to a particular intervention.

Initial Diagnostic Impression

Having obtained the necessary information from subjective and objective sources, the next step is to develop a preliminary diagnostic impression based on ICD-10 or DSM IV. This labels and refers to either the individual's complaints or the parents/caregivers' concerns. Although we have not yet attained the ideal of specific drugs for specific diagnostic categories, we do know which classes of existing drugs are likely to be effective in certain diagnostic groups and which of the existing drugs are contraindicated for certain medical and psychiatric disorders. See Chapter 10 for more details.

Developing an Intervention Plan

The interdisciplinary team of specialists then prescribes a comprehensive intervention plan that may include psychotherapy, behavior therapy, speech therapy, occupational therapy, activities therapy, and medication therapy for the individual. Often there is the need to consider and treat more than one challenging problem or symptom. The intervention plan should prioritize the identified challenging behaviors or symptoms and decide which behavior or symptom is the first priority.

Communicating Findings and Recommending Treatment

When the physician communicates and interprets the findings of the assessment to you and your child, he provides the critical link between the assessment and intervention processes. This can motivate you to obtain or provide the services required to effectively meet the needs of your child. The physician should communicate the information to you and your child through both feedback conferences and written materials (reports and letters).

Feedback Conference

The purpose of the feedback conference is not only to share information, but to also engage you and your child in problem solving. The physician should be empathic, objective, and truthful. His role is to facilitate expressions of feelings about the information presented and promote good coping responses on the part of you and your child. He should engage both of you in collaborative goal setting. He will ask you and your child (if he is capable) to specify and prioritize his and your goals for intervention. The physician then adds and prioritizes his goals. Thus, you, your child, and the physician work together to determine which goals will be addressed first.

Written Reports

The written reports should summarize the data gathered in the assessment, interpret the data in order to answer the referral question(s), make recommendations for intervention, and document the responses of you and your child at the feedback conference. Written reports provide a permanent record of the assessment process. They also serve as the baseline information that can be used to check the effectiveness of the intervention plan. You and your child have a legal right to any of this information. The physician and any other professionals who also participated in the assessment process should give you a copy of the written report. Such an approach helps prevent miscommunication and will promote follow-through on your part and that of your child's.

Chapter 4

General Principles of Medication Therapy

The first part of this chapter describes the scientific aspect of medication therapy (pharmacotherapy), such as choosing the initial medication and the different ways physicians can administer medications. The latter part of the chapter describes the general principles of practicing daily medication therapy, which should help you understand the general guidelines that physicians should follow. Knowing the general principles of medication therapy will empower you to work with your child's physician to ensure the highest quality of care.

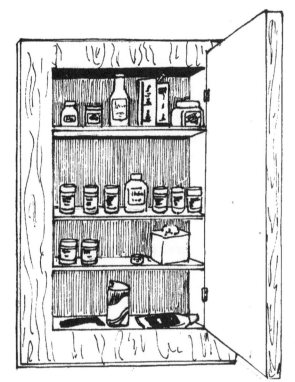

Pharmacotherapy as a Science

Clinical investigators have greatly advanced the concepts of pharmacotherapy. Over the past three decades, the techniques for evaluating pharmacotherapy have progressed to the point that medication therapies are now dominated by objective and scientific evaluations (see Chapters 3 and 5).

Physicians of every discipline have long recognized that individuals show wide variability in response to the same medications. The following sections discuss the strategies that deal with variability in clinical settings.

Individualized Medication Therapy

The safety or effectiveness of a medication in an individual is never assured. Because individuals differ in their responses to medications, each treatment must be considered an experiment with a hypothesis that can be tested. The scientific basis of the hypothesis comes from the database generated from controlled clinical trials during drug development and clinical experience obtained after drug approval (see Chapter 7). For example, a physician may assume his patient's problems with obsessive-compulsive disorder are due to impairment of serotonin regulation. To test his hypothesis, the physician will use a medication (e.g., Prozac) that usually increases the amount of serotonin going through the neuron synapses. If his patient's symptoms improve significantly with Prozac, the hypothesis is supported by the result.

When the physician thinks pharmacotherapy is a necessary intervention for modifying your child's behaviors or symptoms, he or she faces two important decisions: 1) the initial choice of a specific medication, and 2) the initial dosage. Optimal treatment results are achieved only when the physician knows the child's diagnosis, severity and stage of the problem/disorder, and presence of concurrent disorders or medication treatment, as well as his or her knowledge of variation in treatment response. Most of the considerations in the discussion of clinical trials of the medication must be applied to your child (see chapter 7). Of utmost importance is that prior to the therapy, the physician must establish well-defined goals of treatment and the means to assess the achievement of those goals. Otherwise, medication therapy is likely to be ineffective and continued longer than necessary.

Choosing an Effective Medication

In most clinical settings, the choice of medication is substantially influenced by the confidence the physician has in the accuracy of the diagnosis, estimates of the extent and severity of the disease, and previous experience with certain disorders and medications used to treat those disorders. Based on the best available information, the physician must decide on an initial medication from a group of reasonable alternatives. Many factors will influence selection of medications.

- A cost-benefit analysis of diagnostic tests of the effectiveness (e.g., test for blood level)

- Monitoring side effects (e.g., EKG monitoring for cardiac side-effects)

- Availability and specificity of alternative therapies (e.g., melatonin for certain types of sleep problems)

- Likelihood of a reduction in future use of expensive health care (e.g., use lithium to prevent the relapse of mania and readmission to an inpatient un it)

In choosing medications, the physician must consider the ways different medications move through the body and how the way the medication is administered (by mouth, by injection, etc.) affects the this. For some medications, the variability of these factors greatly affects the patient's response to the drug. Measuring the medication concentration in the blood can be helpful in individualizing medication therapy.

Individualizing Dosage

To design a rational dosage regimen, the physician must have some knowledge about rates of absorption and distribution, steady-state concentration, and half-life of the medication under consideration. Moreover, he or she must judge what variations in these parameters might be expected in a particular patient.

Determining Dosage Regimen

The initial dosage regimen is determined by estimating the pharmacokinetic properties of the medication in the particular individual. (See appendix A for more information on pharmacokinetics). The physician must base the estimate on an appreciation of the variables that are most likely to affect the action of the particular medication. Subsequent adjustments may be made based on medication concentrations in the bloodstream. Ultimately, the physician should base the dose on whether the medication positively changes the individual's behaviors or symptoms without inducing serious side effects. The usefulness of a medication is its ratio of benefits to risks.

Dosing Interval

In general, marked fluctuations in drug concentrations between doses are not beneficial. To maintain a steady drug concentration, the dosing interval is usually equal to the half-life of the medication. For example, the half-life of Ritalin is about two-to-four hours, and Ritalin is commonly taken every four hours.

If a medication is relatively nontoxic so that concentrations many times than necessary for therapy can be tolerated easily, the doctor can use a maximal dose strategy. In this case, the dosing interval can be much longer than the elimination half-life. For example, when Adderall® 10 mg is effective for about four hours, giving 15-20 mg may increase the effective interval to about six hours. For medications with a narrow therapeutic range, it is important to estimate the maximal and minimal concentrations that will occur for a particular dosing interval to avoid toxicity.

Titration

Most medication treatment begins by administering relatively low doses (most likely therapeutically ineffective). The doctor then increases the dose by increments every few days to a point at which the dose either reaches therapeutic effectiveness or starts to cause unwanted side effects. If therapeutic effects are not obtained at the highest recommended dose, or if severe side effects emerge and interfere with the desired changes, the next step is usually to use another drug from the same general class of medication.

Loading Dose

The "loading dose" is one or a series of doses that the physician may prescribe at the onset of therapy with the aim of rapidly achieving the target concentration. A physician may use a loading dose if the time required to achieve a steady state by dosing at a constant rate is long relative to the time sensitivity of the condition being treated. For example, in acute mania, 10 mg or more of Haldol may be given every one-to-two hours to stabilize the patient. After that, the doctor may prescribe 2 mg to 5 mg of Haldol for every four-to-six hours.

The use of a loading dose has significant disadvantages. First, a particularly sensitive individual may be abruptly exposed to a toxic concentration of a medication. If the drug has a long half-life, it will take a long time for the concentration to fall if the level was excessive. This increases the risk of adverse side effects.

Fixed-Dose Combinations

The use of two or more medications at the same time adds to the complexity of individualizing medication therapy. The physician must adjust dose of each medication to achieve optimal benefits. Combining medications is advantageous only if the ratio of the fixed doses corresponds to the needs of the patient. In the United States, a fixed-dose combination of medication is considered a "new drug," and must be approved by the FDA before it can be marketed. This is even though the individual medications are available for concurrent use. To be approved, the combined drugs must act to achieve a better therapeutic response than either medication alone; or one medication must act to reduce the incidence of adverse effects caused by the other.

<u>Dosage Adjustment</u>

When long-term therapy is needed, there may be questions such as how often to change the dosage and by how much. There is a simple rule of thumb: change dosage by no more than 50% and no sooner than every three-to-four half-lives at a time. For example, if an individual has been on 4 mg of Risperdal® (half-life of 24 hours) for a few months, the next dosage increase should not be more than 6 mg. The individual should be on that dosage for at least 96 hours before a further adjustment. On the other hand, some medications have very little dose-related toxicity, and maximum efficacy is usually desired. For these medications, doses well in excess of the average required will ensure both effectiveness and prolonged medication action.

Monitoring Dosage Regimen

Monitoring a patient's response to the medication by using predefined goals for acceptable effectiveness and toxicity requires close attention. Some adverse events are avoidable if therapy is individualized. However, other serious adverse reactions are related to an interaction of the medication with variables unique to each individual. When a medication is first marketed, it has been tested in only a limited number of well-characterized patients. Hence, the information on drug interactions is usually not available for newly marketed drugs.

<u>Monitoring Therapeutic Concentration of Medication</u>

Determining the therapeutic concentrations of medication in blood, serum, or plasma are particularly useful when:

- There is a demonstrated relationship between the concentration of the medication and the desired eventual effect and/or the toxic effect that must be avoided.

- There is substantial individual variability in disposition of the medication that makes the prediction of the drug concentration from dose alone almost impossible.

- Medications are used for preventing an intermittent, potentially dangerous event. E.g., measuring the concentration of medication in the blood may aid adjusting the dosage of anticonvulsants.

- There is an overlap in the concentration-response relationship for desirable and undesirable effects of the medication of an anticonvulsant dosage may be aided by.

- An individual causes therapeutic failures by not taking the correct dosage.

<u>Therapeutic Range</u>

In some medications, the desirable ranges of steady-state concentrations have been determined (i.e., therapeutic range). In general, the lower limit of the therapeutic range appears to be approximately equal to the drug concentration that produces about half of the greatest possible therapeutic effect. The upper limit of the therapeutic range is determined by toxicity, not by efficacy. Generally, the upper limit of the therapeutic range is such that no more than five-to-ten percent of patients on the particular medication will experience a toxic effect. For some medications, this may mean that the upper limit of the range is no more than twice the lower limit. These figures are highly variable, and some individuals may greatly benefit from drug concentrations that exceed the therapeutic range, while others may suffer significant toxicity at much lower values. Physicians usually target the center of the range.

For some medications with a narrow therapeutic range, the physician must carefully adjust the dose and choose a target level of steady-state concentration. Subsequently, he measures drug concentrations and adjusts the dose if necessary to approximate the target more closely.

In most clinical situations, the clinician administers medications in a series of repetitive doses or as a continuous infusion in order to maintain a steady-state concentration of medication in plasma within a given therapeutic range. Calculation of the appropriate maintenance dosage is a primary goal. To maintain the chosen target concentration, the rate of medication administration is adjusted such that the rate of input equals the rate of loss. If the clinician chooses the desired concentration of medication in plasma and knows the clearance and availability for that medication in a particular individual, he can calculate the appropriate dose and dosing interval.

Monitoring Therapeutic Effect by Using Placebos

A placebo is indispensable in a controlled clinical trial. In contrast, a placebo has only a limited role in the routine practice of medicine. Generally speaking, it is unethical to give a patient a placebo unless the patient agrees to take part in an experiment. A supportive physician-patient relationship generally is preferable to the use of a placebo for promoting therapeutic benefits. On the other hand, relief or lack of relief of symptoms upon administration of a placebo is not a reliable basis for determining whether the symptoms have a "psychogenic" or "somatic" origin. See Chapter 5 for other aspects of placebo effects.

Factors That Affect the Outcome of Medication Therapy

Many factors can influence the individual's response to a medication including:

- The patient's age

- Disease of the drug eliminating organs (e.g., kidney and liver)

- The concurrent use of other medications, foods, and chemicals, any of which can cause drug interactions

- Previous therapy with the same or similar medication (i.e., medication tolerance)

- A variety of genetic factors that can influence the rate of change (pharmacokinetics) and toxicity of medications

Drug-Drug Interactions

Drug-drug interaction is when one medication alters the intensity of the pharmacological effects of another. The net result may be enhanced or diminished due to one or both of the medications or the appearance of a new effect that is not seen with either medication alone. See Chapter 8 for details.

Drug Tolerance

Drug tolerance happens when there is a diminished response to the effects of a given amount of medication due to previous exposure to the same medication or other mechanisms. The patient needs increasingly larger doses of the medication to receive the same treatment effect.

Typical Tolerance

This occurs due to repeated exposure to the same medication.

Genetic or Dispositional Tolerance

One medication may not affect one individual as much as other individuals because of genetic or dispositional factors. In individuals with ASD, it is not unusual that some need less of a medication while others need more to achieve the treatment goals.

Tachyphylaxis

This is a noticeable decrease in the individual's sensitivity to the medication. It occurs over a very short period of time, on the order of a few hours. In this form of tolerance, the same amount of medication administered on two separate occasions, a couple of hours apart, may induce greater effects with the first dose than with the second dose.

Cross-Tolerance

This is developing tolerance to one type of medication that results in decreased sensitivity to the effects of another type of medication, particularly one acting at the same receptor site. For example, a heavy drinker who has developed tolerance to alcohol's sleep-inducing properties may not even get sleepy when given a dose of a barbiturate that normally induces sleep in other individuals. When cross-tolerance develops, maintaining a given therapeutic effect requires increasing medication dosage.

Mechanisms of Tolerance

Drug tolerance occurs through many mechanisms, but no single mechanism can account for all phenomena associated with tolerance. Several mechanisms may be:

- The ability of the liver to synthesize drug-metabolizing enzymes may increase when exposed to the medication for some length of time. The liver metabolizes the medication at a faster rate than it could previously, thereby decreasing its duration of action.

- A depletion of neurotransmitters, either because they are used faster than can be replenished, or because the actual synthesis of the neurotransmitter is decreased. With fewer neurotransmitters available, the patient requires a larger drug dose. If the cycle continues long enough, this form of tolerance can lead to the medication becoming completely ineffective, regardless of the dose.

- Many forms of drug tolerance occur because of learning processes and behavioral adaptations that may happen while the patient takes the drug. For example, a child may initially benefit from Ritalin and gain a better attention span during working on certain academic tasks. However, if the reward for the work loses its effect, the attention span decreases even though the Ritalin dosage is the same.

Rate of Tolerance Development

The rate at which tolerance develops depends on medication dosage and the time between doses. The larger the dose and the shorter the time between doses can cause tolerance to develop more rapidly. Furthermore, there is a threshold dose for each medication below which tolerance would probably not occur.

Potential Clinical Problems

Most psychotherapeutic medications are not especially harmful in and of themselves when taken in reasonable quantities with sufficient time between doses. However, once tolerance to a medication's effects develops, a physician may administer larger and more frequent doses, causing toxicity. With this type of tolerance, the therapeutic index for the medications gets smaller and smaller while the individual actually becomes more sensitive to the side effects. For example, the ability of amphetamine to induce euphoria decreases with regular use, but the ability for amphetamine to induce psychotic-like effects may actually increase with regular use of large doses. However, there are also examples of the development of tolerance to the undesired effects of a medication and results in an increase in its therapeutic index. An example is tolerance to sedation produced by phenobarbital when it is used as an anticonvulsant.

Pharmacotherapy and Adverse Events

Any medication has the potential to produce adverse reactions. Although FDA's mandate is to ensure that medications are safe and effective, both of these terms are relative. The anticipated benefit from any medication must be balanced by the potential risks. Since only a few thousand patients are exposed to experimental drugs in more or less controlled and well-defined circumstances, medication-induced adverse events that occur as frequently as one in one thousand patients may not be detected prior to FDA approval.

In general, "mechanism-based," adverse drug reactions (e.g., a decrease in blood pressure when using Catapres to treat ADHD) are relatively easier to predict based on pre-clinical and clinical pharmacology studies. However, the relatively rare idiosyncratic adverse reactions (e.g., severe adverse effects on the skin, liver, or blood), which result from an interaction of the medication with unique host factors that are unrelated to the principal action of the medication, are more difficult to predict. In addition, the risk of the rare individual (idiosyncratic) adverse reactions is not distributed evenly across the population. Some individuals, because of unique genetic or environmental factors, are at an extremely high risk, while the remainder of the population may be at little or no risk. Understanding the genetic and environmental bases of idiosyncratic adverse events will certainly improve the overall safety of pharmacotherapy. More information on adverse reactions of psychotherapeutic medications is in Chapter 6.

General Principles of Administering Psychotherapeutic Medications

Before going into detail about the various medications that could help your child, you should have some understanding of the general principles of administering psychotherapeutic medications (psychopharmacotherapy) as aids in carrying out a sound medication therapy. These principles are only rules of thumb. You and your child's physician must keep in mind the unique needs and circumstances of your child.

Principle One

Psychopharmacotherapy should begin with a functional behavioral analysis followed by a thorough medical diagnostic assessment.

Persons with ASD may develop the full range of neuropsychiatric disorders or suffer from side effects from psychotherapeutic medications. The first goal of your child's physician is to make an accurate diagnosis. However, due to limited resources available to most physicians at their clinics, your child's physician can only achieve this goal after a complete functional behavioral analysis by a qualified and experienced professional. The physician must know that the challenging behaviors or emotional disturbances of your child are not learned maladaptive behaviors. He then can focus on the goals of psychopharmacotherapy.

On the other hand, you and your child's physician should keep in mind that most challenging behaviors and emotional disturbances wax and wane on their own or are self-limiting. Rushing in with medication treatment may be unnecessary and costly.

Principle Two

The physician needs a careful history, thorough physical and neurological examination, and some laboratory data for evaluation and use as a baseline preceding the medication treatment.

Because symptoms or side effects may mimic other illnesses, the clinical history and physical exam are crucial in making a diagnosis that directly impacts on the nature and course of medication to be prescribed. For example, tics may develop while a child takes Ritalin for his ADHD. It is critical to document the presence or absence of tics before beginning medication treatment. The examination should include recordings of neuromuscular signs, blood pressure, pulse rate, height, and weight. The laboratory data include blood counts; EKG and echocardiogram in certain instances; liver, thyroid and kidney function tests when indicated; and function of any organ system that might be adversely affected by the medication. The physical and neurological examination and laboratory tests should be performed regularly while the patient is on psychotropic medications (see chapter 3).

Principle Three

The physician should never use medication treatment as the first and only intervention.

After a proper diagnosis, the physician can determine whether the problems are significantly interfering with the patient's adjustment or happiness. If medication treatment is likely to be both effective and safe, the physician should consider it. Medication therapy, however, should be just a part of a comprehensive intervention program that includes psychosocial interventions (including family counseling and individual and group therapies), cognitive therapy, behavior therapy, special education intervention, occupational therapy, speech and communication therapy, sensory integration treatment, and music therapy. Without these additional therapies, the therapeutic gain of medication treatment usually disappears after prolonged use or after stopping medications.

Principle Four

The physician should reserve medication treatment for individuals with severe behavior problems or emotional disturbances that fail to respond, or only partially respond, to non-medical interventions.

Except in certain disorders like ADHD, psychoses, and Tourette syndrome, medications have weak or limited effects, whereas psychosocial interventions can be very powerful. Non-medication treatments, such as counseling, psychotherapy, and behavior modification are preferred first treatments. Even when the behaviors or symptoms reflect one or more underlying organic brain syndromes or neuropsychiatric disorders (Tourette syndrome, ADHD, etc.), the physician should first prescribe the non-medication treatments because they may offer significant relief. Only after non-medication treatment fails to produce desired results should the physician consider medication treatment.

Principle Five

When there are multiple behavioral problems or emotional concerns, the treatment team should determine the treatment. If at all possible, treatment should begin with one medication for the most urgent problem.

If your child has multiple behavioral problems or emotional disturbances, you might have to focus on the one of the highest priority. This is possible if there is no acute crisis that requires the simultaneous use of several medications to control all problems or symptoms of concern. Choose the one problem or symptom that is of the greatest concern and is the most likely to respond quickly to medication.

Use the following criteria to prioritize the behavior or emotional concerns:

1. The first priority is any behavior that leads to a direct hazard to the health or safety of your child or other people.

2. The second most serious category includes disruptive or destructive behaviors such as running or screaming in the classroom, house, or job place; throwing tantrums; and kicking, throwing, or breaking objects.

3. The third category includes behaviors that pose a severe threat to the self-esteem of the individual, such as poor social skills and extreme shyness at group times.

4. The fourth category includes any other behavior like wasting paper, baby talk, and stereotyped movements (e.g., hand flapping or clapping).

If one medication can do the job, using it is simpler than juggling two or three. The physician should begin with the one medication he believes to be the most effective with the fewest side effects. Such monotherapy is still the best practice in terms of enhancing compliance, avoiding drug-drug interaction, minimizing side effects, and measuring the treatment effect and side effects.

If one medication at the maximum recommended dosage reduces the severity of the behavior or symptom, but does not control it sufficiently, the physician may try another medication in the same class or may add a second medication of a different class known to complement the first medication (co-pharmacy). For example, when 50 mg of Prozac, a serotonin reuptake inhibitor(SRI), moderately helps reduce the intensity of obsessive-compulsive behavior in an older adolescent, then Paxil (another SRI) may be tried. When Prozac helps reduce the intensity of obsessive-compulsive behavior, but the child still has significant tantrums due to not getting all the time to "carry out" the compulsive behavior, the physician can add Risperdal to control the tantrums. (Risperdal is an atypical neuroleptic, a different class of medication.)

When using more than one medication, it is important to make adjustments with a single agent at any given time. Generally, one medication should start or stop at a time so that its results can be evaluated. The concurrent use of two or more medications has the potential to cause interactions between the drugs.

A trend is to give several medications simultaneously (polypharmacy), some of which are to counteract the side effects of others. In turn, these counter-side-effect medications tend to induce other side effects. For example, when Catapres is used to counter the rebound effect of hyperactivity caused by the use of Ritalin, it causes sedative side effects. Another common form of polypharmacy is giving different medications of the same class (e.g., giving both Mellaril® and Haldol) in the hope that they may reduce the risk of side effects because lower dosages of each medication are used.

However, there is little evidence, if any, that such polypharmacy works. Polypharmacy is not only costly and unnecessary, it reduces patient compliance because of its complexity. It also increases the chances of drug-drug interactions. The interactions may reduce the effect of the main medication or increase the risk of toxicity.

Principle Six

Appropriate selection of psychotherapeutic medication is based on multiple factors, including medical, patient and family, physician, social, and economic.

Medical Factor

The ideal course is to consider the symptoms as the behavioral manifestations of underlying brain pathology and then formulate the treatment plans on this assumption. Currently, a specific diagnosis dictates most medication treatments. Hence the selection of medication depends on the known effectiveness of a certain class of medications for that diagnosis. For example, a physician will usually select one of the SRIs as the first-line medication for obsessive-compulsive disorder. He or she may have to try several different medications in the class before finding a suitable one—or ruling out the SRI class altogether.

Usually, there are a number of options, both of classes and subclasses of medications, so it is important to choose the medication that has the best risk-to-benefit ratio. For example, studies show that stimulants, antidepressants, and neuroleptics all can improve ADHD. However, the stimulants have the best result qualitatively and the fewest side effects. There is little reason to use the others except when stimulants fail or produce unacceptable side effects like weight loss, growth retardation, and severe tics.

Physicians usually avoid prescribing those psychotherapeutic medications that are known to have a high rate of drug-drug interactions or have adverse effects in certain populations. For example, physicians usually do not prescribe Ritalin for low-functioning individuals with ASD and seizure disorder because of the high risk of adverse reactions. A physician's call for therapeutic medications usually can be satisfied by a thorough knowledge of one or two medications in each therapeutic category. Your child will benefit if his physician avoids the temptation to choose from many different medications for your child's treatment. You should also not demand that the physician prescribe a particular medication that you have heard about from other parents or caregivers, especially if your child's physician uses it infrequently or has never used it. If the clinical setting calls for a medication that your child's physician uses infrequently or has never used, he must learn about its effects, use great caution in its administration, and apply appropriate procedures in monitoring its effects.

When certain medications require preliminary and follow-up laboratory tests, the physicians tend not to select them as first-line medications because individuals with ASD tend to poorly cooperate with laboratory procedures.

Some medications are clearly indicated during an acute phase of treatment but not for maintenance or prophylactic purposes. For example, Haldol is effective for controlling agitation during the acute phase of manic-depressive disorder, but it is ineffective in preventing a relapse. Conversely, certain medications may not be very useful for acute management but are exceptionally beneficial for maintenance. For example, lithium is not effective in controlling the agitation during the acute phase of manic-depressive disorder or episodic temper outbursts with physical aggression, but it is quite effective in preventing a relapse of manic-depressive disorder.

Patient and Family Factor

Selecting the right medication requires comprehensive information about the patient, including current functioning and diagnosis, past medical and psychiatric history, and family medical and psychiatric history. You must maintain an up-to-date medical record. For example, many medications may lower the threshold for seizures or can interact with anticonvulsants to either enhance or diminish their treatment effectiveness. Therefore, the physician has to know whether your child has a history of seizure disorder, previous use of and response to any medication, and current medications. Such information aids in making the final decision about medication.

Prior personal (and possibly family) history of a good or poor response to a specific medication usually is an important factor in making the first-line choice for a subsequent episode. Physicians usually avoid prescribing a medication that had previous side effects in a child or his family members.

Physician Factor

Studies show that most doctors grow comfortable with a set of basic strategies at the beginning of their careers and then use them again and again. Medical research may continuously validate new medications, tests, and operations, but practicing doctors tend to lag behind, favoring known options instead. There are also physicians who practice evidence-based medicine and search the medical literature for specific research studies. They then choose the medication that has shown the strongest treatment effect for a particular disorder or syndrome.

Unfortunately, a doctor sometimes selects a medication by his or her personal need to project an image of competence and authority. He or she may like to use new medications that have very limited safety and effectiveness data. This person likes to be the first and only physician in the community who knows something about the new drug. If you have any concern that a physician's motive for choosing a new medication is only partly influenced by objective medical knowledge, you should always ask for a second opinion.

Social Factor

Some parents may be under pressure from the school or work place to do something about their child's problem behaviors or emotional disturbances. If certain non-medical professionals involved in the care of your child strongly believe in psychopharmacotherapy, they may advocate for certain medications—sometimes based on media reports. This factor may impinge on both physician and parents in selecting medication.

Economic Factor

Pharmaceuticals are a big business, and drug companies have a limited patent period in which to recoup their very large investments in developing new products. Drug companies use every legitimate marketing technique to sell their products, with an increasing emphasis on projecting an image of being interested in aiding physicians. This factor may influence the physician's choice of medications. On the other hand, third-party payers (insurance companies, HMO's, etc.) tend to encourage their participating physicians to use generic brands or less expensive brand-name medications (see chapter 9).

Principle Seven

Some people may respond better to one medication than another. Some may need larger dosages than others. Children differ significantly from adults in their pharmacokinetic capacities.

Since there is no certain way of determining beforehand which medication will be effective, your child's doctor may have to prescribe first one and then another, until one is effective. The doctor usually continues treatment for a minimum of several months.

Before starting a medication, you, your child, and the doctor should discuss a plan for reaching the optimal dosage. All involved in the medication treatment should agree on how quickly the dose will be increased and what the maximum level will be. Like any other medication, psychotherapeutic medications do not produce the same effect in everyone. Age, sex, body size, body chemistry, habits, and diet are some of the factors that can influence a medication's effect. For some medications, however, the optimal dose is unrelated to weight, age, or illness severity. The optimal therapeutic dose for many psychotherapeutic medications is subject to wide inter-individual variation.

To determine the optimal dosage, many clinicians prefer to titrate (adjust) dosage as described earlier. This approach relies on closely monitoring the changes of behaviors or symptoms. In addition to your own behavioral observations and ratings, observe your child's subjective feelings and reactions to the medication. Many individuals with ASD can verbalize their feelings when asked to do so. They may report a sensation of being slowed down, being irritable, or feeling calmer or more attentive at school or the workplace once a therapeutic dosage has been attained. If your child is younger or less verbal, his physician has to rely heavily on your reports to determine the optimal dose of medications.

Some physicians may prefer to employ standardized doses based on the individual's body weight; however, physicians can measure certain medications in the blood to guide their use. Generally, the doctor should use the lowest possible maintenance dose that is within the therapeutic range once he has determined its therapeutic effect.

A physician commits a major error by prescribing ineffectively low doses that expose individuals with ASD to many risks without the benefits. On the other hand, there is an insidious tendency in medicine to operate on the principle that *more is likely to be better*. Some physicians give persons with ASD an excessively high maintenance dose of medications that can interfere with intellectual function and, in the case of antipsychotic medications, may hasten the development of tardive dyskinesia, a neurological problem caused by the long-term use of neuroleptic drugs (see chapter 6).

There is often a lag of two-to-six weeks before a psychotherapeutic medication begins to act. The apparent lack of effect in this phase may lead to unwarranted increases in dosage or discontinuation of the medication.

Due to the relatively large liver size in proportion to body weight in children, children need higher doses relative to body weight when compared to adults. On the other hand, children tend to have less adipose tissue and less protein binding when compared to adults, and they may have more medication available for bioactivity, and, potentially, more side effects. Children are vulnerable because their bodies are developing at a very rapid pace and may therefore be physically more susceptible to the actions of medications. You need to be vigilant about the risk-to-benefit ratio of psychoactive medication therapy if your child is younger than four.

Principle Eight

Whenever possible, the physician should prescribe medication that the patient will take in a single, daily dosage.

Adequate compliance with treatment is a major issue affecting the potential for a successful outcome. A vast majority of patients and their parents do not routinely follow instructions for the use of medications or other aspects of treatment. Studies that about fifty percent of the prescriptions filled each year are not taken correctly. Although physicians usually emphasize that taking the medications as prescribed is important, individuals with ASD and their parents may be ambivalent or forgetful about this. Drugs not taken at the correct intervals do not have the same effect.

Previous studies show that people tend to forget to take their medications when doctors prescribe a multiple, daily dose regimen. When physicians ask patients to take their medications more than once a day, the patients tend to miss more doses. Many psychotherapeutic medications can be given once a day, either administered in the evening or first thing in the morning. Whenever possible, you should ask the doctor about taking medications in a single, daily dose. Taking medication once daily will facilitate compliance and spares your child the embarrassment of taking medication in front of schoolmates or co-workers. You and the doctor need to make sure that your child fully understands the doctor's order. Ask the doctor for a printed treatment plan that includes instructions for taking the medication. Help your child learn how to follow the instructions.

Principle Nine

Whenever possible, ask the pharmacist to dispense tastier medications to make taking them easier. Whenever the medications are taken orally, always take them with water or another liquid.

If your child has difficulty taking medication by mouth due to the taste or size of the medication, ask the pharmacist to use flavorings to sweeten a bitter taste, mask strong medicine with a pleasant flavor, or create a liquid form of the medicine. Pharmacists can also dye medications with a favorite color. This will add just a miniscule cost, but it may make life easier for both you and your child, as well as reduce the risk of non-compliance.

Some medical experts are concerned about a lack of federal oversight. They worry that flavorings can dilute a medication or dangerously alter its chemical structure. Pharmacists, however, consider the droplets they put in a bottle harmless and can actually help because the individuals are more likely to take the full dose. The FDA has not received any reports that flavored drugs have injured anyone.

One particularly risky and potentially dangerous practice is that of taking tablets or capsules without water or other liquid. Liquids assist the pills' progress to the stomach where they will dissolve and yield their contents. If possible, always use liquid medicine rather than pills for very young children. If the medicines are tablets or capsules, provide at least 100 ml (½ cup) of liquid (water or a favorite soft drink), otherwise pills could lodge in the esophagus and cause physical damage to its lining.

Principle Ten

Involve the child in the treatment process as much as possible, despite his age and level of functioning.

Your child is the center of medication therapy. He should be involved in the entire process as much as possible. Make every effort to help him understand the reason for taking the medications. Even a very young child can have the medication explained to him in ways he can understand. Encourage him to ask questions and express his feelings. If necessary, appropriate and sensitive counseling can help overcome any fear or worry that he has about taking medication that may take away his self-control or stigmatize him by having to go to the school nurse or taking a break at his job. When the patient understands why he takes medicine and the long-term treatment goals, he feels better about himself and functions better at school or at work.

The educational process should continue throughout the entire treatment. If this is done properly, your child becomes a helpful ally throughout the treatment. This approach prevents the development of a negative attitude or a misperception toward the use of the medication. If you can provide close supervision, give your child the responsibility of taking his own medications so that he takes an important role in the treatment process.

Principle Eleven

You should always be involved in the entire process, from initial evaluation through monitoring the medication effects and final termination of medication treatment.

Many parents do not like to give their children medications because they worry that drugs will stigmatize their children. However, once the decision is made for medication therapy, your attitude toward its use and your ability to work with your child and his physician is extremely critical to the medicine's effectiveness. You have to inform the physician about your child's functioning and response to the prescribed medications. You need to know the reasons for medication therapy, the likely therapeutic benefits, and possible side effects. Your active participation in the entire treatment course is essential. Tell the prescribing physician about your child's past medical history, present medications, and after some experience with a medication, whether it is causing side effects.

In many instances of medication therapy in ASD, the situations or problems of concern may not be clear-cut. The prescribing physician may have an extremely difficult task in choosing appropriate medications for your child. He may need to experiment with a variety of medications and dosages before he can establish an appropriate and effective regimen.

Serve as an independent observer. Your reports of the medication responses are critical if the physician is to have any chance of helping. On the other hand, a physician might not want to take the time to explain that he does not know what a proper dose is for your child. You have to pay close attention to how your child responds. Watch for side effects. Make sure the symptoms of the original illness do not intensify. If the medication is not working, you should discuss this with your child's doctor and make a decision to discontinue the medication and seek another intervention.

Ask the prescribing physician the questions described in Chapter 2. You need to remember that giving a safe and effective level of medication for your child requires close supervision and a good relationship with the prescribing physician and other caregivers.

You should not have a war with your child about his taking medications. This will only discourage him from taking what he needs. Learn how to make taking medicine a pleasant experience for your child.

It is essential that you confer with the physician and other caregivers so everyone has a thorough understanding of the treatment plan when any new medication is prescribed. Always keep in mind not to be overly optimistic about the benefits of medication therapy so that you will not have an unrealistic expectation of the treatment effects.

Principle Twelve

Valid and clinically meaningful measures should be implemented regularly to assess therapeutic effects and side effects of psychotherapeutic medications.

You and your child's physician should obtain baseline measures before starting any medication. Document any symptoms or signs that resemble psychotherapeutic medication-induced side effects like hyperactivity and tics. You should regularly get follow-up measures of symptom frequency and severity of the behaviors or symptoms being treated over an entire course of treatment. This is to document the clinical effects of the medications. In addition to direct observational procedures, use behavioral checklists. Several instruments developed for the general population have been modified for use among those with developmental disorders, including ASD. See Chapter 5 and Appendix D.

When certain medications (e.g., tricyclic antidepressants, lithium, and anticonvulsants) are used, the physician should regularly monitor the blood level of these medications. Such laboratory drug monitoring can provide the necessary information on how rapidly an individual eliminates the drug. The physician can adjust the dose to maximize safety and effectiveness.

While psychotherapeutic medications have important benefits, there is no effective medication that does not have side effects. Everyone involved in caring for your child must watch for adverse effects throughout the entire course of treatment and must make every effort to minimize side effects.

The effects of psychotherapeutic medications on a child's brain are not fully understood, and they may produce long-lasting and irreversible effects. You should regularly and systematically question your child, if he is verbally capable, about the development of any possible side effects. In addition, direct-observation procedures, side-effects checklists, and blood-level monitoring of certain medications should be done to check for side effects. See Chapter 6 and Appendix G.

Principle Thirteen

How frequently the physician should see your child and how long the child should keep taking psychotherapeutic medications depend on the phase and nature of your child's disorder or problems of concern, as well as on the action of the medication.

The phase (acute, relapse, or recurrence) of a disorder or a problem of concern is very important in terms of the initial intervention and the duration of treatment. During the initial acute phase of medication therapy, the physician should see your child at least once a week. Once the acute episode has been adequately alleviated—usually after several weeks of treatment—an ongoing medication maintenance program can begin to prevent a relapse. The doctor can then see the patient less frequently, such as monthly or bimonthly, to review therapeutic response and development of side effects.

Certain symptoms or behavioral problems may respond before others. For example, in a depressive episode, vegetative symptoms such as sleep and appetite disturbances often respond early in the course of treatment, whereas mood may take several weeks to improve. You should take the lead in analyzing the data before asking for a medication change. Medication adjustment is usually a trial and error technique. With the possible exception of stimulants in ADHD, medication response in ASD tends to occur slowly. Avoid changing medications or dosages before the necessary time has lapsed for a response. In general, if an individual has not responded to a medication within four weeks while the dosage is in the therapeutic range, it is unlikely he will respond at a later date. The medication should be discontinued gradually (over about two weeks) while a second medication is instituted and its dosage slowly increased.

There are no firm guidelines about when to discontinue medication treatment. Nonetheless, the nature of a disorder or problem may determine how long someone must take a psychotherapeutic medication. Many depressed and anxious individuals with compulsive hair pulling may need medication for a single period, perhaps for several months, and then never have to take it again. For some conditions, such as schizophrenia, manic-depressive illness, or Tourette syndrome, medication may have to be taken indefinitely or perhaps of an anticonvulsant dosage may be aided by intermittently. In the latter conditions, however, every effort should still be made to take drug holidays (i.e., stop taking the medication) every four-to-six months for those patients who have a positive response.

In cases with positive therapeutic response, medication treatment should continue at optimal dosage for periods of four-to-six months. The medication should be gradually reduced and then discontinued for at least one-to-two months to see if there is a need for continued treatment as well as to assess the development of side effects, such as growth changes or neuromuscular abnormalities.

This reassessment should not be made at the beginning of the school year. This ensures that your child has adjusted to the new classroom. You do not want to make decisions on the basis of a "honeymoon" effect with a new teacher. A better time to do the reassessment is two-to-three weeks after the summer break starts. If there is no significant difference in your child's behavior when he is on or off medication, then treatment may be discontinued for a longer period.

Principle Fourteen

The patient, his parents or legal guardians, or the prescribing physician may terminate medication treatment. At this juncture, the potential for recurrence should be clearly discussed in the context of the risk-to-benefit ratio.

If a person with ASD has taken medication for several months or years, withdrawal must take place very slowly. Sudden withdrawal from a medication can cause severe reactions. Sometimes it takes several weeks to get a person off a medication that he or she has taken for many years. If a new medication is tried for just a few weeks, and it is not effective or has bad side effects, it can usually be withdrawn immediately.

Chapter 5

Monitoring Medication Therapy

When using psychotherapeutic medications to treat challenging behaviors or symptoms of neuropsychiatric disorders in individuals with ASD, the ideal strategy is to achieve the maximum therapeutic response with a minimum dose of medication and minimum side effects. To accomplish this, you play an important role in making sure that your child takes his medication as recommended. You and your child should work closely with the physician. Carefully monitor the treatment to ensure the desired effect of the medications, as well as to prevent or detect the early signs of side effects that may impact behavior or learning. This chapter emphasizes the measurement of medication-related behavior or symptom changes. Side effects of psychotherapeutic medications are covered in Chapters 6 and 8.

Compliance with Medication

Psychopharmacotherapy is the use of psychoactive drugs to treat patients with various disorders. Noncompliance can be a serious problem in the medication therapy of individuals with ASD. The failure to take medication as prescribed is probably the most likely explanation for the individual's lack of response, unexpectedly poor response, or increased variability in response to a given medication. Noncompliance can range from altering the prescribed number of doses or the length of treatment to completely failing to take the medication.

Obviously, a patient will not experience any benefit from a medication if he does not take it. There are four common reasons for an individual's not taking prescribed medications:

- Limited cognitive ability and lack of reliable assistance from the parents or caregivers

- Experience with very unpleasant or frightening side effects coupled with the inability to tell his parents or caregivers

- Misunderstanding instructions

- Carelessness.

Be especially careful not to overestimate your child's compliance. Work with the prescribing physician to counsel and educate your child about why and how to take the medications. Closely monitor your child's compliance and watch for side effects. In some cases, due to communication difficulty, direct and objective measures of compliance (laboratory tests of blood levels of the medications), as well as indirect measures (pill counts), may be necessary.

Measuring Therapeutic Effects

Dosage regulation of any medication depends on reliable measurement of changes in targeted behaviors at fixed points before and during the medication therapy. In most cases of ASD, patients receiving medications are unable to accurately report their response to the treatment. On the other hand, a positive treatment effect may be a decrease in the frequency or severity of long-standing, challenging behaviors or psychiatric symptoms, and the change may not be readily apparent in the physician's office. Therefore, measuring treatment response must rely on objective techniques (repeatable over time or across observers) that reflect what is actually being measured by caregivers. The measures must be sensitive to changes produced by the medication. Use an established, well-defined set of monitoring and assessing tools rather than trying to implement an elaborate and difficult system. The measures should be user-friendly, practical, economical, safe, and ethical.

What is most important in assessing medication effect is that a decision is made based on systematic data, preferably from several sources, instead of relying solely on the physician's clinical assessment. The prescribing physician should know which array of methods is most suitable for the particular patient.

Physicians can use various measurement techniques and instruments in the medication therapy. The techniques and instruments for measuring behaviors or symptoms are in a variety of categories, depending on what they measure, how they measure, and who is doing the measurement. These techniques and instruments include:

- Medical and psychiatric review

- Direct observation of behaviors

- Physical and neurological examinations

- Standardized tests

- Learning and performance measures

- Mechanical movement monitors

- Self-reports

- Behavioral rating scales

- Global impression.

Some of the assessment methods described in Chapter 3 can be used as both pre-treatment baseline measures and on-going measures of medication effect. These measures, along with other measures specifically for assessing medication treatment effect, should be continued throughout the course of the treatment to ensure the effectiveness of psychopharmacotherapy.

The following sections describe strategies, techniques, and instruments that physicians commonly use for assessing the effect of medication. This does not mean that other good strategies, techniques, and instruments are not available. Whenever the physician decides to use methods not described in this book, you should obtain information about the methods so that you can prepare yourself to assist the physician in assessing the mediation's effects.

How Frequently Should the Physician Review Your Child?

The physician must continuously evaluate and monitor the therapeutic effect of the prescribed medications. As discussed in Chapter 4, weekly-to-biweekly clinic visits may be necessary at the beginning of medication therapy. When your child's behaviors or symptoms improve or become more stable, a monthly phone consultation, paired with a clinic visit once every two-to three-months, may be adequate. If the behavior or symptom does not improve, more frequent visits or changes of medications may be necessary.

There is no clear-cut guideline for the frequency of carrying out various measures to enhance the medication treatment effects and monitor and minimize the development of side effects. Some measures described in the following sections should be carried out each time the physician sees your child. Other measures may be done less frequently. On a case-by-case basis, the physician will decide how frequently to carry out certain measures as indicated by the clinical status of your child.

When you return to the physician's office for your child's follow-up appointment, or when you call to obtain another prescription, use a checklist of your questions about the medication effect. It is also a good practice to use a measure such as the Side Effects Checklist (see Appendix G) to review any questions you may have about the side effects in your child. Chapter 6 describes other measures to monitor the medication-induced side effects.

Medical Review

Your child's doctor will conduct a medical review before implementing the medication treatment. This review will establish the baseline rates of the existing challenging behaviors or psychiatric symptoms and document the absence of commonly observed side effects of the prescribed medications. The medical review can be of critical importance in individuals who tend to be anxious and have a high baseline rate of physical complaints. A careful review avoids attributing to the medication problems the pre-existing physical complaints or symptoms.

The physician should conduct the medical review each time your child visits him so that the early emergence of any drug-induced side effects can be detected and treated effectively. The following medical review is not meant to be complete, but rather highlights certain critical questions.

- **Allergies**—Some individuals may be allergic to certain psychotherapeutic medications. A pre-medication assessment and documentation of the finding are essential. Ongoing monitoring of any sensitivity to the medication is critical to prevent a serious allergic reaction.

- **General Health**—Psychotherapeutic medications can cause fatigue and changes in eating habits, growth rates, and sleeping patterns. Obtaining baseline information on general health is important.

- **Disorders of Eyes, Ears, Nose, and Throat**—Psychotherapeutic medications can affect vision, produce nasal symptoms, cause problems in ears, and induce throat problems. The doctor should assess these systems before starting the medication.

- **Respiratory System Diseases**—Stimulants and antidepressants may exaggerate the effect of antiasthma drugs. Inderal, a beta-blocker, may block widening of the air passage (bronchodilation). A careful pre-medication assessment and documentation of the presence or absence of wheezing or bronchitis is critical.

- **Cardiovascular Diseases**—Stimulants, antidepressants, and antipsychotics all have important effects on heart rate, blood pressure, and cardiac conduction and excitability. Pre-medication assessment should document the presence or absence of heart murmur, chest pain, fainting, or dizziness upon standing.

- **Gastrointestinal (GI) Disorders**—Given the common occurrence of GI side effects from psychotherapeutic medications (e.g., constipation by tricyclic antidepressants and stomachache by stimulants), a complete pre-treatment review of any history of nausea, vomiting, diarrhea, constipation, stomachache, or jaundice is needed. The GI system is commonly involved in affective illnesses and anxiety disorders, thus drug choice may be governed by side-effect profiles of medications.

- **Urinary Tract Disorders**—Psychotherapeutic medications may exacerbate or ameliorate urinary tract symptoms. This is especially the case in lithium treatment. Furthermore, some medications may exacerbate preexisting problems with the involuntary discharge of urine (enuresis), whereas others, such as tricyclic antidepressants, have reduced or eliminated enuresis.

- **Disorders of Genital and Reproductive Systems**—Antipsychotic medications can interfere with sexual functioning and cause some mature adolescents to experience complications like menstrual disturbances and galactorrhea.

- **Disorders of Musculoskeletal System**—There are musculoskeletal side effects of certain psychotherapeutic drugs, notably stimulant-induced tics and neuroleptic-induced Parkinsonism. Pre-drug assessments and documentation of baseline state are essential.

- **Skin Diseases**—The skin is a common target for psychotherapeutic medication side effects. Photosensitivity with antipsychotic medications is sometimes seen, especially with chlorpromazine. Many psychotherapeutic medications can cause skin rashes.

- **Disorders of Endocrine System**—Some medications can affect thyroid function. It is important to establish a baseline of thyroid function before implementing the medication treatment. Documentation should include the presence or absence of hot or cold intolerance, dry skin, rapid or slow heart rate, increased fluid intake, and growth abnormalities.

- **Disorders of Central Nervous System**—Since most psychotherapeutic medications can cause neurological symptoms, it is important to establish a baseline. The physician should ask about any history of seizures, staring spells, fainting, dizziness, headaches, numbness, tingling, tremor, weakness, clumsiness, speech problems, pain, and motor or vocal tics. The doctor may want an EEG if the history suggests absence (petit mal) seizures.

Psychiatric Review

A thorough psychiatric review is important in establishing pre-medication baseline rates of challenging behaviors or psychiatric symptoms such as hallucinations, anxiety states, affective state, thinking problems, delusions, obsessions, and compulsions.

Direct Behavior Observation

In assessing the medication effects, direct behavior observation usually records only the frequencies of select behaviors over fixed periods of time. The observer records the behavior as it happens, with frequent reliability checks. Assessment results are often graphed to aid interpretation. This type of assessment can be done in either an artificial situation (e.g., an individual taking an intelligence test) or a natural situation (e.g., an individual's home or classroom).

Direct behavior observation is a highly reliable, objective tool for assessing medication effects. The ability to tailor the tool to specific clinical needs is a major strength. Direct observation can be repeated as frequently as needed without problems with practice effects such as those caused by repeated performance tests (e.g., IQ tests or academic tests). This could be a valuable feature in determining the time of onset and offset of medication action. However, the presence of an observer may change the very behavior (e.g., aggression) for which the doctor has prescribed the medication. The major limitations with this procedure are that it is expensive if a highly trained staff member must carry out observations, and it is time consuming.

Physical and Neurological Examination

Many psychotherapeutic medications alter blood pressure and pulse. The doctor should record these parameters (such as standing and supine measurements of blood pressure) before starting medication and during the course of treatment. Blood pressure and pulse rate should be checked weekly, particularly when the medication treatment begins or when the dosage changes. Psychotherapeutic medications can affect an individual's height and weight. Stimulants cause weight loss, and antipsychotic medications produce weight gain. Measuring height and weight at regular intervals, before and during medication therapy, reassures both physician and parents or caregivers that the medication is not affecting growth. Weight and height should be recorded on a monthly or quarterly basis.

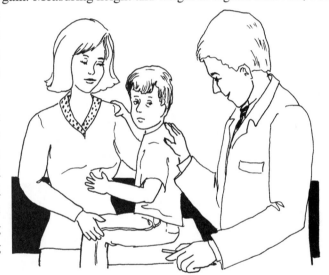

Psychotherapeutic medications can alter motor function. Everyone should pay particular attention to vocal and motor tics before the initiation of stimulants and during the course of treatment. Record symptoms of tardive dyskinesia, such as lip licking, tongue thrusting, and puffing or pouting of the lips when considering antipsychotic medications.

Cognitive Function and Speech/Language Assessments

Psychotherapeutic medications may affect an individual's cognitive function or performance (e.g., Pondimin® may retard discrimination learning). Medications, such as antipsychotics, stimulants, and tricyclic antidepressants, can alter speech production, rate, volume, and coherence. The initial symptom of mania caused by tricyclic antidepressants is often characterized by pressured or very rapid speech production. It is important to have a documented baseline of speech/language and cognitive functions during treatment and after treatment. A qualified, experienced speech pathologist and a psychologist should carry out these assessments.

Laboratory Tests

Laboratory tests play an important role in the medical work-up prior to medication treatment. The tests document the baseline and help the physician in answering specific questions about evaluation and medical management of individuals treated with medications. Judicious use of laboratory parameters during medication maintenance can enhance the medication effectiveness and minimize any toxicity or side effects.

The doctor should order laboratory studies for baseline and follow-up assessments For example, thyroid and kidney function tests before and during lithium treatment, serial EKG in medications with significant cardiovascular effects, and EEG in suspicion of a seizure disorder.

Some laboratory tests should be done on a regular basis during the entire duration of certain medication therapy. It is wise to repeat complete blood counts and differential blood counts, urinalysis, and basic chemistry screening at three months and every six months thereafter for each of the medications that may have a high risk of side effects of certain organs.

The doctor should not routinely order lab tests just because the patient is taking medication. Inquire about the procedures and rationales for ordering the laboratory tests if the doctor fails to provide this information.

Monitoring Blood Level of Drugs

In many branches of medicine, monitoring plasma levels rather than the dose of a drug is often the best way to reach the treatment goal. For many drugs, the plasma concentration is a reasonable index of the concentration at the site of action. Substantial data indicating large differences in plasma levels among patients treated with the same dose of a psychotherapeutic drug provide one reason for adjusting the dose to achieve the optimal clinical effect.

The plasma therapeutic range is the concentration range that has the highest probability of giving the desired response with a minimum amount of side effects. Researchers have defined the ranges for a number of psychotherapeutic medications, including anticonvulsants, antidepressants, and antimanic medications.

The therapeutic range is only a statistical concept and is not rigidly applicable to all patients. Some patients may have quite adequate clinical responses at drug concentrations below those considered therapeutic; likewise, some patients may require plasma concentrations that would be toxic for most. Remember that the ultimate goal is not achieving a plasma concentration within the therapeutic range— it is obtaining the desired therapeutic effect. Moreover, there is some disagreement among researchers as to whether there is a clear relationship between medication concentration in the blood and clinical response to that medication. Measurement of blood levels may be helpful in determining patient compliance with medication, providing a drug index that can be related to changes in specific behaviors, preventing serious side effects, and identifying non-responders. The best use of this technique remains for those circumstances in which the response is not adequate, or unexpected adverse events occur.

The physician should get blood samples in the elimination phase of drug dosing because these levels are more reproducible than those drawn during the absorption or distribution phases. For example, from one- to two-thirds of a dose of lithium is excreted during a six-to-twelve-hour initial phase of excretion. To determine the blood concentration of lithium, the blood sample is usually obtained at about ten hours after the last oral dose of the day. Determining the elimination phase requires knowing when the maximum concentration occurs, as well as the rapidity of fall-off due to redistribution. For most drugs, such monitoring should be after the patient has been on a stable dose for five-to-seven half-lives (steady-state blood concentration). After that, repeat monitoring is typically done only for causes such as:

- A change in drug efficacy or tolerability

- A change that might reasonably be expected to alter the clearance of the drug; for example, the addition of a second drug that could induce or inhibit the metabolism of the first drug, or the development of diseases that could adversely affect left ventricular, hepatic, or renal function

Using Performance Tests and Rating Scales to Monitor Treatment

Performance Tests

Psychotherapeutic medications may have an impact on learning, either by removing behavioral/emotional impediments (resulting in improvements) or by producing sedation, confusion, or other uncomfortable side effects (resulting in worsening of clinical conditions). For this reason, the physician may want to use performance tests to monitor a patient's progress while on longer-term medication treatment. A psychologist or speech pathologist will administer the performance tests before, during, and after medication therapy. See Appendix D for details of performance tests commonly used to monitor medication treatment.

Rating Scales

The most commonly employed method in modern psychopharmacology is the use of behaviors or symptoms rating scales. However, very few rating scales have been developed specifically for the assessment of medication effects in individuals with ASD. Physicians currently tend to use rating scales that have been developed for non-ASD populations.

Some experienced physicians may want to have caregivers complete a rating scale twice before instituting medication therapy. This is because caregiver-completed and patient self-rating scores tend to decrease in severity with repeated administration. This approach allows the physician to check the consistency of the particular caregiver, as well as to be able to obtain more accurate baseline measures. See Appendix D for details of rating scales commonly used in the assessment of medication treatment.

Customized Scales

One practical, all-purpose approach to assess medication treatment effects is to custom make instruments that reflect the principal target symptoms of the patient. For example, the physician asks the parents of a hyperactive child to list the four or five things about their child's behavior that they find most worrisome. These symptoms and their severity are then written down for subsequent rating by the parents each time they return for follow-up care. A similar approach might be to use DSM diagnostic criteria that are relevant for a given individual (i.e., identify those presenting behaviors or symptoms listed as diagnostic criteria) and ask parents and caregivers to assess the changes of those behaviors or symptoms after the implementation of medication treatment.

Another approach is to use the Maladaptive Behavior Scale (MABS), which requires the rater to estimate both the *frequency* of the behavior and its *intensity*. Frequency is rated on a six-point scale ranging from "Did not occur during preceding eight hours" to "More than twelve times during the preceding eight hours." Intensity is coded on a similar six-point scale that describes various degrees of severity. Each MABS form allows the rating of three target symptoms. The MABS was developed for use in residential-type settings, and the frequency and intensity scales may not be suited to outpatients, although variations could easily be made.

Powerful Placebo Effect

The word *placebo* originates in dual meanings from Latin roots. On the one hand, it means "I shall please" by satisfying the patient's needs, and on the other hand, it means "to placate" with deception or ignorance about both the disorder and the treatment prescribed. The placebo effect is often referred to as an "expectancy" effect because it stems primarily from the patient's and the physician's expectancy that the physician can help.

Today, we use the term *placebo* to describe beneficial effects that arise from the *act* of giving medication rather than the medication itself. It is usually demonstrated by giving a substance known to be inert or not known for its therapeutic effect in certain conditions but presented as if it were genuine. Placebo effects are commonly manifested as alterations of mood, other subjective effects, and objective effects that are under autonomic or voluntary control. The placebo effect varies significantly in different individuals and in any one patient at different times.

The non-medical public recognizes the placebo effect, but largely ignores it. This allows useless, mostly harmless, but occasionally potentially dangerous substances to stockpile the shelves of drugstores, health food shops, and supermarkets. This is because the placebo effect can be a powerful part of healing. Previous studies have demonstrated that for a wide range of ailments, roughly thirty-to-forty percent of patients experience relief after taking a placebo. Some studies suggest that only about twenty percent of modern medical remedies in common use have been scientifically proven to be effective. The rest have not been subjected to empirical trials of whether or not they work and, if so, how. It is not that these treatments do not offer benefits. Most of them do. But in some cases, the benefit may come from the placebo effect.

Today, parents and caregivers of individuals with ASD primarily seek psychotherapeutic medication treatment because: 1) other interventions have failed to improve or cure their children's autism and related problems, or 2) they believe in the healing power of some psychotherapeutic medications. Hence the decision to seek medical assistance restores some sense of control. The act of undergoing evaluation and treatment—seeing a medical expert, receiving a thorough medical evaluation, having a chance to discuss their children's conditions, getting a medical diagnosis and a plausible treatment plan, including taking a pill—helps the parents and caregivers feel better, less distressed, and more hopeful. These factors might significantly contribute to the parents' and caregivers' favorable ratings of the treatment effect of psychotherapeutic medications when, in fact, the medications might not have intrinsic value or have just an insignificant effect for the condition. Thus, it is critical to keep in mind the placebo effect when assessing the treatment response of psychotherapeutic medications.

Written Report

Although it is common practice to provide written feedback to parents and caregivers about the initial assessment and treatment plan, the physician must also give them a written summary after each clinic visit of the changes that have been made due to the prescribed medications. To this end, it is important to re-administer the pre-treatment assessment measures and, in a post-treatment session, to review the changes that have occurred. When possible, videotaped parent/caregiver-child interactions should be reviewed for pre- and post-treatment effect. This helps the parents to be more aware of changes that have occurred gradually throughout the treatment process.

Chapter 6

Monitoring Side Effects

Medication without side effects does not exist. All medications can have adverse effects if administered at a wrong dosage or under wrong conditions—even the age of the patient can cause some medications to have adverse effects. A medication may be therapeutic for one person but toxic for another. For instance, lithium carbonate has a calming effect on the mood of individuals with mania. However, when normal people take lithium, it produces a depressed mood. Like other medications, psychotherapeutic drugs may induce various side effects, although they do not produce the same side effects in everyone. Some people experience annoying side effects, while others do not. This chapter begins with a brief discussion of developmental neurotoxicity and then describes various measures to monitor medication-induced side effects.

Developmental Neurotoxicology

The growth of the human brain progresses until around the age of eighteen, although myelination continues through at least the third decade. The developing nervous system remains vulnerable as late as young adulthood.

There are a large number of medications, including psychotherapeutic medications, that may potentially influence brain development. While exposure during pregnancy is likely to produce structural changes in the body and brain, later exposure is likely to produce more subtle effects, including cognitive and behavioral alterations, (particularly inattention and hyperactivity). When young children take psychotherapeutic medications, behavioral toxicity often appears before any other side effects. The other side effects include extrapyramidal, autonomic, and endocrinologic side effects. The early emergence of behavioral side effects is a warning sign, and the doctor should consider whether to continue the medications. Continuing the medications may affect other body systems and may cause permanent harm. For example, long-term use of acutely sedating medications may have progressive and cumulative effects on arousal, behavior, and learning. Long-term use of stimulants into late adolescence may suppress physical growth and cause permanent stunting because growth of long bones stops between the ages of seventeen and twenty-one.

Medications used in adolescence for short terms may also cause long-term side effects (e.g., thyroid and skin effects from lithium and dental caries from anticholinergic medications).

You have to be vigilant when working with your child's physician in deciding when to start psychotherapeutic medications. Make a careful risk-benefit evaluation that includes calculating the risk of developmental neurotoxicity.

Recognizing Side Effects

The prevalence of side effects from psychotherapeutic drugs is difficult to calculate due to lack of universally accepted definitions of side effects. Clinicians find it difficult to determine where medical or psychiatric symptoms end and where the medication-induced side effects begin. Therefore, it is not possible to predict who is at risk for developing side effects from psychotherapeutic medications. Much information is available about the side effects of these medications. Understanding, preventing, assessing, diagnosing, and treating the side effects are essential in the clinical care of your child.

Recognizing side effects is crucial when using psychotherapeutic medications. One sees what one knows. Psychotherapeutic medication-induced side effects may range from a minor nuisance to a potentially fatal reaction. Unrecognized side effects can adversely affect both the medical and the psychiatric well-being of your child. If your child has limited cognitive and communicative abilities, he may not be able to comprehend or recognize the side effects. He may be unable to verbalize his feelings or alert you about the development of the side effects. Your child may become frightened or suspicious if a sudden change in his feeling about food (e.g., bitter taste of certain food), in his perception about his environment (e.g., visual hallucinations), or in dysfunction of certain body systems (e.g., hand tremors and muscle spasms) occur following the administration of psychotherapeutic medications. Such feelings may trigger tantrums or cause non-compliance with taking any medication. Psychotherapeutic medication-induced side effects are the reason for discontinuation in 25% to 33% of those who stop treatment. The importance of monitoring drug response cannot be overemphasized. To minimize adverse effects, you must be particularly vigilant in working with your child's doctor to prevent the development of side effects and to effectively manage any effects that do appear.

You need to know the full range of side effects of medications and how to manage some of them at home, school, the workplace, and in public. Learn when to take your child to a clinic or a hospital emergency room.

Nevertheless, the best approach to managing side effects is prevention. Follow the general principles in Chapter 4 and become familiar with measures your child's doctor may use to monitor and assess side effects.

Monitoring the Emergence of Side Effects

This section presents an overview of the techniques available to document baseline measurements and assess the side effects or adverse changes of psychotherapeutic medications. These tools are essential to more scientific and safer use of medications. Clinicians find them helpful in their daily practice, and you can use them to participate in the treatment of your child.

Physicians use checklists, rating scales, laboratory studies, physical and neurological examinations, and electrophysiological studies (EEG and ECG) in assessing side effects. Much of the current information on measuring and monitoring side effects is derived from adult data, and many of the instruments were developed for adults and are not necessarily appropriate for children. For young children, make a checklist of side effects that are commonly produced by the specific medication. You and other caregivers, including the prescribing physician, then use the "customized" rating scale to monitor the medication-induced side effects.

Use Rating Scales to Monitor the Side Effects

The use of subjective rating scales as a means of assessing side effects is important to the prescribing physician in terms of charting your child's progress on a specific medication, as well as in comparing medications. In daily practice, physicians tend not to use formal rating scales for the assessment of drug-induced side effects. Standardized and user-friendly rating scales for monitoring the various medication-induced side effects in ASD have not been developed. Nonetheless, there are a number of general and specialized rating scales that can be adapted and applied to the ASD population.

Rating scales are either global rating scales or multi-item scales. Although global rating scales usually have good validity and require little training, they may not always be reliable. The following are some general purpose rating scales:

- Adverse Drug Reaction Detection Scale (ADRDS)

- The Dosage Record and Treatment Emergent Symptom Scale (DOTES)

- Subjects Treatment Emergent Symptom Scale (STESS)

- NIMH Systematic Assessment for Treatment Emergent Events (SAFTEE-GI)

- Monitoring of Side Effects Scale (MOSES)

DOTES

Many central nervous system side effects, as well as some behavioral side effects, are contained in the DOTES, which was developed by the Psychopharmacology Research Branch of the NIMH for both children and adults. The DOTES is a systematic review of all body systems through both an inquiry and a simple physical exam. Judgments on intensity, relationship of symptoms to the medication, and action taken for each symptom occurrence are required. Daily medication dosages, ratings of symptom severity and subjective distress, and various adverse effects may also be recorded. One of the advantages of this scale is that dosage is readily related to side effects.

STESS

The STESS, developed by NIMH, also records drug-induced side effects. It is a thirty-two-item scale, rated on four points:

- Not at all (0)

- Just a little (1)

- Pretty much

- Very much

The scale is suitable for children up to age fifteen and elicits information about various complaints, including physical ones. The child, parent, or a caretaker can complete the STESS.

Other Scales

For the assessment of central nervous system side effects, checklists for untoward effects are available for specific medications, such as the Lithium Toxicity Checklist for lithium (LTCL), or specific neuromuscular side effects such as the Simpson Tardive Dyskinesia Rating Scale (STDRS) for tardive dyskinesia. Other neuromuscular side effect-specific scales:

- Abnormal Involuntary Movement Scale (AIMS)

- Barnes Akathisia Rating Scale (BARS)

- Dyskinesia Identification System Condensed User Scale (DISCUS)

The AIMS is a standardized rating instrument developed by NIMH for the assessment of tardive dyskinesia. It covers three groups of movements:

- Facial and oral movements (muscles of facial expression, lips and perioral area, jaw, and tongue)
- Extremity movements (upper and lower)
- Trunk movements (neck, shoulder, and hips).

   In addition, there are three items under the heading of global judgments:

- Severity of abnormal movements
- Incapacitation due to abnormal movements
- Individual's awareness of abnormal movements

   There are two under the heading of dental status:

- Current problems with teeth or dentures
- Whether the individual usually wears dentures.

   The items are measured on a five-point scale. "Tremor" is not part of this scale, perhaps because it is rare in individuals with marked tardive dyskinesia. The five points are:

- None (0)
- Minimal, may be extreme normal (1)
- Mild (2)
- Moderate (3)
- Severe (4)

   The best time to perform the AIMS is prior to long-term neuroleptic treatment, and then at regular intervals while the patient remains on drug therapy

   The Simpson Tardive Dyskinesia Rating Scales (STDRS) consists of 34 neuromuscular symptoms, plus 6 "other" symptoms. The symptoms are organized under movement of face, neck and trunk; upper and lower extremities; and those of the entire body. The scale includes the rabbit syndrome, which is actually a late-onset, extrapyramidal symptom. The symptoms are rated on a 6-point severity scale:

- Absent (1)
- Possibly present (2)
- Mild (3)
- Moderate (4)
- Moderately severe (5)
- Very severe (6)

All items are defined. The STDRS is a very comprehensive rating scale that has been widely used.

   The DISCUS is the only dyskinesia scale that has been systematically studied in the developmentally disabled population. The DISCUS includes fifteen separate ratings of 0–4 for involuntary movements (dyskinesia) covering seven body regions.

Use Videotaping to Monitor the Side Effects

In some instances, videotaping an individual in his usual activities, or during a rating evaluation, is quite helpful, especially if it is done before the medication treatment and then repeated at intervals.

Clinical Manifestation and Management of Side Effects

The following sections describe medication-induced side effects and management options. A single medication can cause multiple side effects, and the same side effect can be produced by many different medications. One general strategy for dealing with side effects is to change the medication. For example, when dealing with extrapyramidal symptoms (EPS), the physician can replace a high-potency neuroleptic medication (e.g., Haldol) with a lower-potency neuroleptic like Mellaril. Mellaril generally has a lower incidence of EPS. However, the lower-potency neuroleptics are more likely to be associated with a higher incidence and degree of anticholinergic side effects, such as dry mouth and constipation. The physicians need to weigh the benefit-to-risk ratio along with the potential risks associated with the disorder itself.

You can find expected physiological effects and specific side effects of commonly used psychotherapeutic medications, including anticonvulsants, in Appendices F and G.

Behavioral Effects

Psychotherapeutic drugs can adversely change almost any behavior. Behavioral side effects may develop insidiously over a long period of time (e.g., dependence) or may behave in an idiosyncratic and unpredictable fashion (e.g., a switch to mania). Manifestations of behavioral side effects can sometimes mimic the symptoms for which the medication was originally prescribed and are not an indication for a higher dosage.

Jitteriness Syndrome

This is an inner restlessness or a "wired" feeling, irritability, increased energy, and insomnia. Most individuals develop tolerance to this jitteriness once the initial dose is lowered or discontinued. Low doses of benzodiazepines may help to alleviate the initial jitteriness.

Sedative Effect

The sedative causes tiredness and initiates sleep. The patient should take the medication in divided doses during the day or switch to a less sedating medication.

Impaired Memory

Change to a medication with a lower risk.

Disinhibition, Hostility, and Aggression

Change to a medication with a lower risk.

Paradoxical Mood Effects

This is the direction opposite to the clinically desirable one. For example, a doctor may prescribe a benzodiazepine but it increases anxiety. Change to a medication with a lower risk.

Pendular Effects

This effect is in the desired direction but to a degree that the resulting mood state will be the opposite of the one for which the medication was initially prescribed (e.g., Thorazine depressing manic patients). The doctor should discontinue medication and replace it with a medication of a different class with a lower risk.

Switch Mania

Depressed individuals become manic. When depressed bipolar individuals are being treated with a tricyclic antidepressant (TCA) or a serotonin reuptake inhibitor (SRI), hypomania or mania may develop. The patient should simultaneously take a monoamine oxidase inhibitor (MAOI), which is another antidepressant, to reduce the risk of switching to mania.

Paranoid Psychosis

Initially, the psychosis manifests by paranoid ideas, auditory hallucinations, hyperactivity, and irritability. Prolonged use may cause a withdrawn, disorganized, dysphoric state. The psychotic state usually clears within one week of discontinuing the offending medication.

Work and School Phobia

The doctor should discontinue the drug and replace it with a medication of a different class that has a lower risk. If the problem continues, consider adding an anti-phobia medication if not contraindicated.

Sleep Disturbances

These include nightmares or disturbing dreams accompanied by temporary confusion and disorganization, somnambulism (appearing confused and walking about in a quick, detached, and clumsy manner), and quasi-hallucinatory, hypnagogic (drowsiness) episodes. The sleep disturbances may disappear spontaneously. If the disturbances persist, switch to daytime doses.

Initial and Middle Insomnia and Daytime Somnolence

Insomnia may respond to a short-acting hypnotic, antihistamine, or a sedating antidepressant like Desyrel.® Daytime somnolence (sleepiness) may require discontinuing the medication.

Withdrawal Reactions

Symptoms of withdrawal that may appear following discontinuation of psychotherapeutic medications include:

Nausea	Anorexia	Loss of appetite	Vomiting
Diarrhea	Abdominal cramps	Malaise	Cold sweats
Chills	Dizziness	Headache	Insomnia
Anxiety	Panic attacks	Tachycardia	Diaphoresis
Hypertension	Restlessness	Sleepiness	Fatigue
Hunger	Depression	Agitation	Irritability
Destructiveness	Aggression		

Table 6-1 Reactions to Withdrawal of Psychotherapeutic Medications

If the withdrawal symptoms are mild, they usually subside within two weeks. In more severe cases, the physician may prescribe a small dose of the discontinued medication and then taper it off over a period of one-to-two weeks. If necessary, symptomatic treatment with anti-anxiety medications (e.g., Ativan®) or adrenergic blockers (e.g., Inderal®) may help.

Dependence

Most psychotherapeutic medications do not cause dependence. Individuals taking drugs with a higher risk of dependence should be monitored closely and gradually tapered off the drugs.

Impaired Psychomotor and Cognitive Function

Discontinue the medication or replace it with a medication with a lower risk.

Neuromuscular Side Effects

Medication-induced side effects that affect neuromuscular systems include the following types.

Muscle Tension, Tremor, Twitching, Cramps, or Pains

These symptoms are usually mild. In severe cases with muscle cramps or pains, Benadryl® or Ativan® may help.

Myoclonus

This is the side effect of brief jerks of the lower extremities (usually in the evening during relaxation), repetitive jaw jerking causing stuttering, and sudden arm jerking, resulting in dropped objects. In most cases myoclonus is mild. In severe cases, Klonopin, ® Depakote, ® or Tegretol® may help.

Nocturnal Myoclonus

This is the nighttime, repetitive, violent, jerky contraction of the legs. It sometimes responds to dose reduction or to medications for myoclonus such as Tegretol, Klonopin, and Depakote. Individuals who fail to respond to the above measures need another medication.

Tremor of Upper Extremities

The tremor occasionally involves the tongue. If a dose reduction does not help, the doctor may try Inderal or similar medications.

Impaired Motor Functions

These include decline in speed, accuracy, attention and coordination (ataxia), falls, and impaired automobile driving. If a dose reduction does not help, change to a medication with a lower rate of such side effects.

Extrapyramidal Symptoms (EPS)

These symptoms come from disturbances in the brain structures that affect bodily movement, excluding motor neurons, the motor cortex, and the pyramidal tract. The symptoms of EPS consist primarily of the following:

Acute Dystonia or Acute Dystonic Reactions

Has sudden onset with intermittent or sustained muscular contraction or spasm that may produce an abnormal posture or involuntary movements (dystonia). The muscles of the head, neck, or trunk are rigid or cramping. Bizarre postures or gait may result from the involvement of extremities. Sustained contraction of the masticatory muscles can produce facial grimacing, opening of the jaw (trismus), and protrusion of the tongue. In oculogyric crisis, the individuals may have a fixed, blank stare, which is followed by an upward and lateral rotation of the eyes. Blepharospasm with sustained eye closure may occur. During these events, the head may be tilted backward (retrocollis) or side ways (torticollis) with the mouth opened, or the trunk may have a tetanic spasm (opisthotonus). Acute dystonic reactions occur in 2% to 5% of individuals treated with neuroleptic agents, although incidences of up to 10% have occurred.

The incidence of these reactions is highest among males under the are of 30 years. These reactions typically occur within 24-to-48 hours after the first dose, but they can also occur or recur when doses are increased. The slow-release, injectable neuroleptics, such as fluphenazine decanoate and haloperidol decanoate, usually produce reactions within 72 hours after an injection. These reactions may last from a few seconds to several hours. Acute dystonic reaction may be relieved quickly by anticholinergic drugs such as Cogentin® or Benadryl given orally (or intramuscularly for an acute crisis). Cogentin is then used for several weeks and discontinued gradually. In order to avoid acute dystonic reaction, antipsychotic medications, particularly the high-potency medications, need to start at a low, subclinical dose.

Acute Dyskinesia

This is among the earliest manifestations of extrapyramidal side effects seen with neuroleptics, as are the dystonias. The dyskinesias are clonic, involuntary spasms of muscle groups in the form of facial tics, blinking, chewing movements, lip smacking, tongue movements, shoulder shrugging, and pedaling of lower extremities. The management of this is similar to that for acute dystonia.

Neuroleptic-Induced Parkinsonism

This is characterized by bradykinesia (slowed movements) or akinesia (lack of movements), tremor, and rigidity. The finger/hand tremor is a coarse "pill-rolling" or "to-and-fro" rhythmical movement, which is greater at rest. Rigidity is most apparent in the limbs, where a cogwheeling resistance (slow, rigid movement of a body joint) or claspknife phenomenon (a body joint holding tightly) is noted during passive movement, and there is a lack of arm swinging when walking. A common sign of this syndrome may include mask-like face, soft and monotonous speeches, drooling, slow initiation of motor activity, shuffling gait, and flexed posture. The symptoms may show in varying degrees and combinations.

Neuroleptic-induced Parkinsonism occurs in approximately 20% to 40% of all individuals treated with neuroleptic medications. The age distribution closely parallels that of Parkinson's disease, with an increased incidence after age 40. However, drug-induced Parkinsonism is also individual-specific and dose-related so that young adults, and occasionally children and newborn babies, may be affected. Neuroleptic-induced Parkinsonism occurs at varying times after initiating neuroleptic therapy, but typically within the first two-to-three weeks up to 90 days. In some individuals, the symptoms persisted for some time, even after discontinuation of the medication.

Once the diagnosis is established, and the symptoms are not severe, the dosage can increase. The second option is to initiate or increase the dose of an antiparkinsonian medication. But atropinic side effects, such as behavioral disorganization, impairment of cognition, impaired attention and short-term memory, disorientation, anxiety, visual and auditory hallucinations, and other psychotic imagination may be induced by a high dose of antiparkinsonian drugs. Physostigmine given intramuscularly can reverse this central anticholinergic organic mental state. After four-to-six weeks, the physician can stop the antiparkinsonian medication with no recurrent symptoms. If anticholinergic effects are a problem, he may prescribe Symmetrel® instead of the antiparkinsonian medications. A third option is to stop the neuroleptic medication and change to a lower-potency neuroleptic drug.

Neuroleptic-Induced Catatonia

This is similar to catatonic stupor with rigidity, drooling, urinary incontinence, and cogwheeling. The physician will slowly withdraw the offending medication while using antiparkinsonian medications.

Acute Akathisia

The main symptoms are an inability to sit still, constant pacing, or an intense, subjective sense of restlessness and being driven. It may include feelings of fright, rage, terror, or sexual torment. Insomnia is often present. Akathisia is a common and distressing form of EPS. It usually occurs in the first five weeks of neuroleptic administration, but it may occur within a few hours after taking a high dosage of high-potency neuroleptic medication. Akathisia may persist even after neuroleptics are discontinued.

Akathisia occurs in approximately twenty percent of individuals receiving neuroleptics, although it may be less common in children and adolescents. The incidence ranges from five-to-fifty percent (or more) in individuals receiving moderate doses of high-potency agents. The incidence also increases with duration and increased doses.

If feasible, the physician should first try a reduction in dosage. Antiparkinsonian medications such as Artane or Cogentin may help. In resistant cases, Inderal, Valium, or Symmetrel may alleviate the symptoms.

Rabbit Syndrome

This has a late onset and is a rare subcategory of EPS. It is characterized by perioral muscular movements of muscles around the mouth that resemble the very rapid, chewing-like movements of a rabbit. Antiparkinsonian medications could reduce these abnormal movements.

Prevention (Prophylaxis) of EPS

Approximately ninety percent of acute neuroleptic-induced EPS occurs within the first two-to-three months of therapy. The use of antiparkinsonian drugs for prevention of neuroleptic-induced EPS is controversial. Because most of these reactions can be quickly controlled with anticholinergic medications or other anti-EPS agents, some clinicians prefer to treat EPS only after it occurs. If EPS recurs following discontinuation of the anti-EPS agent, it can be quickly controlled following re-initiation. Others, however, feel that anti-EPS agents should be used prophylactically for the first few months of psychotherapeutic medication therapy.

The best approach to the use of antiparkinsonian or other anti-EPS agents is to individualize therapy. If an individual becomes non-compliant due to EPS, prophylaxis may be beneficial. In patients with a history of EPS, prophylaxis should be considered.

The best prophylactic strategy is, however, to use the lowest effective dose of a high-potency agent, or use a low-potency agent where tolerable. Add anticholinergic agents when EPS occurs.

Treatment of Medication-Induced EPS

In some cases, EPS may be terminated or decreased by reducing the drug dosage. Switch from a high-potency to a low-potency medication that possesses more anticholinergic activity.

If the above strategies are inappropriate or ineffective, try the following agents: centrally acting anticholinergic agents like Cogentin, Artane, Benadryl, Akineton,® and Kemadrin;® dopaminergic agents like Symmetrel; benzodiazepines like Ativan, Valium, and Klonopin; and beta-adrenergic blockers like Inderal.

Tardive Dyskinesia

This is a frequent, repetitive, involuntary movement disorder that usually involves the lips, tongue, and face and extends to the neck, trunk, and extremities—even to the toes. Early manifestations include fine, worm-like movements of the tongue at rest, difficulty in sticking out the tongue, facial tics, increased blinking frequency, and jaw movements. Later manifestations can include lip smacking, chewing motions, mouth opening and closing, disturbed gag reflex, puffing of the cheeks, disrupted speech, and myoclonic (rapid, involuntary contraction) or choreoathetoid (jerking and writhing) movements of the extremities. Respiratory dyskinesia due to abnormal diaphragmatic activity, peculiar vocalizations, and grunts also occurs.

The abnormal involuntary movements may increase with emotional arousal or during activities requiring repetition of motor activities or attention to fine motor tasks. Attempts to consciously control the symptoms may increase the movements. The movements may decrease with relaxation. The movements can be voluntarily suppressed for short periods and are entirely absent during sleep. The abnormal movements have to be present for at least four weeks before a diagnosis can be made.

Although the prevalence of the syndrome appears to be the highest among the elderly, especially elderly women, it is impossible to rely upon prevalence estimates to predict which individual is likely to develop the syndrome, and if it develops, whether the individual will recover. Whether antipsychotic drug products differ in their potential to cause tardive dyskinesia is also unknown. However, the risk of developing tardive dyskinesia (and the likelihood that it will become irreversible) increases as the duration of treatment and the total cumulative dose of antipsychotic medications increases.

Tardive dyskinesia is usually seen months or years after starting neuroleptic administration. However, the syndrome can develop, although much less commonly, after relatively brief treatment periods at low doses. While tardive dyskinesias are most commonly associated with antipsychotic medications (neuroleptics), clinicians have also reported them with a variety of other psychotherapeutic medications, including antihistamines and antiseizure drugs. The syndrome affects ten-to-thirty percent of individuals who have undergone long-term neuroleptic therapy.

In individuals who require chronic treatment, the doctor should select the smallest dose and shortest duration of treatment producing a satisfactory clinical response. He or she should periodically reassess the need for continued treatment. If signs and symptoms of tardive dyskinesia appear in a patient on a neuroleptic drug, the doctor should consider discontinuing the drug.

Tardive dyskinesia may remit, partially or completely, if the patient no longer takes antipsychotic medications. Currently, there is no effective treatment for tardive dyskinesia. Several medications (Clozapine, Catapres, Inderal, benzodiazepines, Depakote, and vitamin E) have shown some treatment effect, but further studies are needed to establish their effectiveness in the treatment of tardive dyskinesia. As there are no proven safe and effective treatments available for tardive dyskinesia, prevention and early diagnosis of these potentially socially disruptive symptoms are essential. Physicians should examine patients regularly (every three-to-six months) for early signs of tardive dyskinesia.

Tardive Dystonia

This is an extrapyramidal side effect that is characterized by slow movements around the long axis of the body, ending in a spasm. It is usually seen together with tardive dyskinesia. The spasm of facial muscle, neck, limb, and trunk may last twenty-to-thirty seconds. It is usually quite disabling. Treatment is similar to the management of tardive dyskinesia.

Neuroleptic Malignant Syndrome (NMS)

This symptom complex includes the following:

- Severe muscle rigidity or catatonia

- Instability of the autonomic nervous system, including irregular pulse, hypertension or labile blood pressure, tachycardia or bradycardia, cardiac arrhythmias, dilated pupils, pulmonary congestion, prominent diaphoresis, and incontinence of feces or urine

- Hyperthermia (hyperpyrexia) in the range of 101 degrees to 104 degrees Fahrenheit

- Altered mental status ranging from agitation to stupor, or even coma.

There may be associated choreiform movements (jerking of multiple body parts), dyskinetic movements, a hastening gait, and flexor extensor posturing. Additional signs include elevated creatine phosphokinase (CPK), leukocytosis with a shift to the left, myoglobinuria (dead muscle tissues release myoglobin in urine), and acute renal failure. **Patients may die if treatment is delayed.**

In most cases, the symptoms develop within the first two weeks of medication treatment. The syndrome may occur with small doses of the medications. It can also develop after dosage increase, change to another drug, or after stopping an antiparkinsonian medication. Persons of any age can be affected, including children and adolescents.

Using lower average doses of a neuroleptic can prevent the development of NMS. Early diagnosis, immediate medication discontinuation, institution of intensive supportive care and medical monitoring in a critical care unit, and use of anticholinergic or dopaminergic medications (e.g., Symmetrel, L-dopa, and bromocriptine) and Dantrolene® (a muscle relaxant) have significantly reduced the fatality rate. If an individual requires antipsychotic drug treatment after recovery from NMS, the doctor should carefully consider reintroduction of drug therapy. The doctor must closely monitor the patient because NMS can recur.

Electrophysiological Side Effects

The administration of either lithium or Thorazine tends to yield a sudden increase of focal EEG abnormality as compared to baseline EEG. If lithium induces more focal abnormality of EEG, the behavior tends to worsen or show no change. However, if lithium causes a decrease of focal EEG abnormality, or if lithium produces changes such as diffuse slowing and slower alpha as compared to a normal baseline EEG, behavioral improvement tends to occur. This relationship between focal EEG abnormality and behavioral change also applies to Thorazine. If possible, lower the dose of the medication. Change to a medication of another class that has an equally therapeutic effect.

Convulsive Side Effects

Seizures are rare, but reports have shown serious side effects of a number of psychotherapeutic medications. Seizure side effects are more likely to be reported with newly marketed medications than with an older medication that has a known risk of seizure. Factors that increase the risk of medication-induced seizures include

- Present or past history of seizure

- Family history of epilepsy

- Simultaneous use of multiple psychotherapeutic drugs

- Postnatal brain damage

- Medications that have a higher risk of causing seizures than other drugs

- High doses or rapid upward titration

- Simultaneous use of multiple psychotherapeutic drugs

- Abrupt stop of the individual's benzodiazepines (anti-anxiety medications)

Individuals with poorly controlled epilepsy may have a higher risk of seizure secondary to psychotherapeutic medications. Doctors should prescribe more conservative dosing to these people. One should measure the anticonvulsant serum level and use low-risk medications (e.g., Mellaril) before beginning a psychotherapeutic medication.

If a patient on a psychotherapeutic medication has a seizure, the physician should screen him for medical or neurological disorders before assuming that the seizure is due to a medication. Such an approach avoids abrupt change of an effective therapy.

Cardiovascular Side Effects

Psychotherapeutic medications can produce abnormalities of blood pressure, pulse, and electrocardiogram (EKG), including cardiac conduction changes. Adults receiving psychotherapeutic medications may have pre-existing cardiovascular disease, which warrants particular caution.

Hypertension

Mild headache and/or palpitations manifest the mild form of this reaction. The severe form shows a sharp rise in blood pressure, often with systolic levels over 200 mm Hg and diastolic pressure levels over 120 mm Hg. High blood pressure may be accompanied by a severe, throbbing headache; flushing; sweating; palpitations; chest discomfort; a choking sensation; photophobia; nausea; and vomiting. If the patient does not receive treatment, he could have an intracranial hemorrhage, which can be fatal.

In mild cases with a hypertensive reaction, the treatment includes rest, reassurance, observation with blood pressure monitoring, and discontinuation of the medications. In severe cases the physician should consider medication therapy.

Orthostatic Hypotension (OH)

Historically known as postural hypotension, clinical OH is broadly defined as the change in blood pressure that occurs on rising from a supine to a vertical posture, resulting in symptoms of cerebral hypoperfusion (reduced blood supply to the brain). Although the absolute change in blood pressure levels necessary to produce clinical symptoms in an individual varies, one commonly used definition of OH is a fall in systolic blood pressure of greater than 20 mm Hg or a reduction in the diastolic blood pressure of greater than 10 mm Hg. Inadequate blood supply to the brain due to OH may cause lightheadedness and syncope (brief loss of consciousness). Dizziness is usually worse in the morning, occurs within minutes of standing, and is relieved by lying or sitting. The symptoms may be exacerbated by alcohol-induced vasodilatation (blood vessel dilatation) and by eating, due to increased blood flow to the liver and GI tract during digestion.

Prevention and Treatment of OH

Use a medication that has a lower rate of orthostatic hypotension. The incidence of OH is difficult to assess due to the lack of an exact definition and confounding factors like concomitant medications and disease states. Treatment success depends on the relief of symptoms with or without an increase in supine to standing blood pressure. The patient should try non-medical treatments. For example, sleep with the head in an elevated position, rise slowly from a seated position, avoid rapid change of posture; wear elastic garments; take small, frequent meals accompanied by coffee in the morning; ingest adequate sodium and fluid; and avoid hot weather, alcohol, and large meals that may cause vasodilatation. Physicians should prescribe medication only after non-medication therapies have failed or become intolerable to the patient.

Fludrocortisone is the drug of choice for OH, but is relatively contraindicated in individuals with congestive heart failure. Prostaglandin synthetase inhibitors (e.g., Indocin) are also used in individuals with OH of any cause, but have had limited success. Patients should only take the following sympathomimetic drugs under the supervision of a doctor:

- Phenylephrine
- Norepinephrine
- Phenylpropanolamine
- Tyramine
- Ephedrine
- Hydroxyamphetamine, with or without MAOIs like phenelzine and tranylcypromine
- Beta-adrenergic antagonists (e.g., Inderal)

The ergot alkaloids (e.g., ergotamine and dihydroergotamine) should only be administered to individuals with certain causes (etiologies) of OH and only under close supervision to check for the development of tolerance or adverse effects.

Conduction Delays

Generally, delays in cardiac conduction (transmission of impulses within the heart to maintain heart beats) are not clinically significant. However, the delays can be dangerous when they occur in individuals with pre-existing conduction disease. Change to medications that have a lower rate of such a risk.

Autonomic Nervous System Side Effects

Psychotherapeutic medications may cause side effects, including:

- Dry mouth
- Mydriasis (prolonged dilation of the eye's pupil)
- Blurred vision
- Failure of accommodation (inability of eyes to focus)
- Precipitation of acute glaucoma in individuals with narrow anterior chamber angles
- Urinary retention
- Sweating

- Nausea

- Vomiting

- Dysphagia (difficulty in swallowing)

- Paralytic ileus (loss of contraction in the intestine)

- Constipation

- Diarrhea

- Hypo- and hyperthermia.

If possible, change to medications that have a lower rate of developing the above side effects.

Gastrointestinal Side Effects

Xerostomia (Dry Mouth)

Most individuals experienced some improvement of xerostomia over time. Prolonged xerostomia may result in difficulties with chewing, swallowing, speaking, denture fit, increased risk of dental caries, candidiasis (fungus infection), or acute sialadenitis (inflammatory salivary gland disorder).

The physician should begin the treatment by eliminating medications known to induce xerostomia or substituting less anticholinergic drugs. Chewing sugarless gum or sucking on hard candies stimulates saliva production. Artificial saliva (e.g., Salivart®, Moi-Stir®) may help some individuals.

Dysphagia

This is the problem with swallowing. It can cause nasal or oral regurgitation or coughing while eating. Dysphagia could cause significant weight loss, aspiration, and asphyxiation. The doctor can substitute the medication with one that has a lower rate of the side effect.

Gastroesophageal Reflux

Gastric contents reflux into the esophagus causing regurgitation, a sour or bitter taste in the mouth, heartburn, chest pain, or aspiration with choking, wheezing, and coughing. Prolonged gastroesophageal reflux can cause ulcers in the esophagus and can lead to bleeding or narrowing of the esophagus.

If the reflux is mild, and the medication has to be continued, use an antacid or histamine H_2-receptor antagonists to reduce the acidity. Use metoclopramide to increase lower esophageal sphincter pressure and hasten gastric emptying. If the symptoms are severe, substitute the medication with one having a lower rate of risk.

Nausea, Anorexia, Increased Salivation, Vomiting, and Abdominal Pain

Withdrawal of psychotherapeutic medications can cause these symptoms. The withdrawal reactions are generally mild, and usually occur within the first week after discontinuation. They last for several days. Gradually tapering the dose may reduce the risk of such reactions.

Diarrhea

Medication-induced diarrhea occurs infrequently. It usually subsides after a short period. If the symptom continues, substitute a medication with a lower risk.

Other Gastrointestinal Side Effects

The side effects include constipation or abnormal distension resulting in paralytic ileus, megacolon, pseudo-obstruction, or actual mechanical obstruction. If the individual needs to take the offending medications for a prolonged period of time, he should also take bulk laxatives, stool softeners, or osmotic agents.

Endocrine and Metabolic Effects

Weight Gain

Weight gain is usually a result of increased food intake, often accompanied by craving sweets and other carbohydrates. When increased intake is combined with decreased activity, significant weight gain is likely. Drug-induced weight gain can distress patients and leads to non-compliance with medication. Steady weight gain may be detrimental to the course of many common health conditions, including hypertension, non-insulin-dependent diabetes mellitus (NIDDM), coronary heart disease, gallbladder disease, stroke, and breast cancer. Weight gain is also associated with impairment in physical functioning, quality of life, and mental health.

There is no satisfactory medical treatment for medication-induced weight gain, aside from substituting a different medication or discontinuing the medication. The doctor should switch the medication before the patient gains excessive weight. Occasionally, an anorectic agent (e.g., d-amphetamine) may help. The three basics of non-medical management of weight gain are exercise, diet/nutrition, and behavior modification. Regular exercise is the best predictor of weight loss, but individuals who are taking antipsychotics and feel somewhat sedated are unlikely to burn enough calories to lose weight. Patients with severe neurocognitive impairment are unlikely follow a diet and lose weight.

Decrease of Height and Weight

Stimulant drugs tend to suppress appetite. This produces slight-to-moderate growth suppression early in treatment, especially in the high-normal dose range. The drugs usually affect weight more than height; however, there is a significant decrease in both height and weight percentile on long-term stimulant administration.

Tolerance to stimulants develops, and eventually height and weight are not significantly affected. However, careful monitoring is especially advised for children who are small.

Hyperprolactinemia

Some psychotherapeutic medications can increase prolactin secretion from the pituitary gland, resulting in increased lactation (galactorrhea). Prolonged hyperprolactinemia can also lead to decrease of follicle-stimulating hormone (FSH) and luteinizing hormone (LH) released by the pituitary gland. Decreased FSH and LH can lead to diminution of ovarian function in females and testicular function in males. Men with hyperprolactinemia frequently develop impotence with loss of libido. Gynecomastia (enlargement of the breasts) sometimes occurs in men, but never galactorrhea. Women with hyperprolactinemia develop oligomenorrhea (decrease of menstruation) and amenorrhea (absence of menstruation), Galactorrhea is quite common.

Bromocriptine can be added for a short period of time in individuals whose medication has to be continued. Otherwise, the medication should be discontinued or replaced by a medication with a lower risk.

Hypothyroidism

This condition is caused by thyroid hormone deficiency, which results in a decrease in metabolism. If an individual develops hypothyroidism while responding positively to a psychotherapeutic medication treatment, the physician may add the thyroid hormone, Levothyroxine, in dosages that will maintain the normal thyroid stimulating hormone (TSH) levels.

Nephrogenic Diabetes Insipidus (NDI)

Most individuals with lithium-induced NDI tolerate the polyuria (excessive passage of urine) and require no intervention from a physician. The physician should stop the medication or replace it with another drug in individuals with severe NDI, where continued water intake caused by excessive thirst (polydipsia) cannot match the urine loses and leads to water intoxication. If the medication cannot be discontinued, diuretics can be used to treat the NDI.

Hypercalcemia

The increase of serum calcium level usually is mild. When the increase is more than 1.5 mg/dl or the individual becomes symptomatic (e.g., polyuria, myopathy, anorexia), the physician should discontinue the medication.

Decrease of Blood Sugar

If the medication cannot stop, consult an endocrinologist for recommendations. Otherwise substitute the medication with a drug with lower risk.

Decrease of Plasma Cortisol (Hydrocortisone) Level

Same as that for "decrease of blood sugar."

Hematologic Reactions

Aplastic Anemia

This is a condition of bone marrow failure and results in anemia, neutropenia (a decrease of neutrophils, which are a type of white blood cell), and thrombocytopenia (diminished number of platelets). Anemia leads to weakness, shortness of breath, palpitation, angina, and loss of energy. Neutropenia causes vulnerability to bacterial and fungal infection. Thrombocytopenia causes mucosal and skin bleeding. Aplastic anemia is the most serious of the medication-induced disorders because of its high rate of mortality.

If a patient has aplastic anemia, the physician should immediately discontinue the medication and promptly refer him for a bone marrow transplant.

Agranulocytosis

This is a condition with a severe decrease in the number of granulocytes (a type of white blood cell normally present in the blood). It may be asymptomatic at first, but later develops symptoms like a sore throat, fever, chills, and drenching sweats. If the offending medication continues, death from sepsis (bacteria-induced toxic condition) may occur.

If the total white count falls below 3500 and the granulocytes below 1500, the physician should discontinue the medication.

Eosinophilia

This is a major sign in a variety of medication-induced systemic disorders. It is a hematologic abnormality in skin rashes progressing to exfoliative dermatitis, but it may occur in other hypersensitivity states, such as vasculitis (inflammation of blood vessels), pulmonary infiltration, asthma, respiratory failure, pulmonary fibrosis, disseminated intravascular coagulation, purpura fulminans (skin infarction and/or gangrene), etc. Diagnosis is usually made after the symptoms promptly improve when the medication is discontinued but recur with resumption.

The physician should stop the medication or replace it with a medication from a different class with a lower risk of developing eosinophilia.

Thrombocytopenia

When platelets are significantly less than $20 \times 10^9/l$, severe hemorrhage from the mucous membrane or into the central nervous system may occur. With milder thrombocytopenia, trauma may cause bleeding at the sites of injuries in the form of small hemorrhages (petechiae, purpura, or ecchymoses).

The medication should be terminated or replaced by a medication from a different class and with a lower rate of developing thrombocytopenia.

Hepatic (Liver) Effects

Drug-induced hepatic injury is predominantly hepatocellular or cholestatic. The symptoms of liver cell toxicity are similar to acute viral hepatitis (i.e., nausea, fatigue, and anorexia). Hepatocellular degeneration, necrosis (cell death), or steatosis (accumulation of fat tissue) may result and could progress to death. Medication-induced cholestasis (retention of bile in the liver) may mimic obstructive jaundice.

Bone marrow depression and cholestatic jaundice rarely occur. They are sensitivity reactions, and they usually appear in the first two months of treatment. They subside on termination of the medication. There is cross-sensitivity among all of the phenothiazines, and the physician must use a drug from a different group when allergic reactions occur.

Genitourinary System Effects

Polyuria

This is primarily caused by the use of lithium. Individual education is an important aspect of managing lithium-induced polyuria.

Avoiding fluid restriction is the goal. Thiazide diuretics may reduce urine volume to a tolerable level. However, since thiazide may increase serum level, the doctor may have to reduce the lithium dosage. Should diuretics not work, or the patient cannot tolerate them, the doctor can prescribe Indocin.

Incontinence and Enuresis

If the physician can discontinue the medication or replace it with another, no treatment is necessary. Even with medication continuation, some individuals will spontaneously become continent. If problems persist, the physician can refer the patient to a urologist.

Other Urinary Problems

One problem is urinary retention with decreased frequency of urination, difficulty voiding, suprapubic discomfort, and reduced bladder sensation. Dosage reduction or discontinuation usually should reverse the problem. Should difficulties arise in individuals taking low-potency antipsychotics (e.g., Thorazine, Mellaril), either dosage reduction or changing to a less anticholinergic, higher potency medication (e.g., Haldol, Navane®) may be all that is necessary. However, switching to a high-potency neuroleptic drug may increase the risk of extrapyramidal side effects leading to the use of antiparkinsonian drugs (potent anticholinergics). The physician could use an alternate medication like Symmetrel. Acute episodes of retention may require catheter decompression of the bladder in a local emergency room.

There have been reports of acute renal failure following the overdose of a variety of psychotherapeutic medications. If an overdose occurs, go to a local emergency room as soon as possible. The doctor will start a high rate of urine flow with intravenous saline to reduce the risk of renal failure following the overdose.

Reproductive and Adverse Sexual Effects

Psychotherapeutic drugs may interfere with sexual physiology and response by a variety of mechanisms, including decreased or increased libido, decreased or increased erection and congestion, lubrication, decreased emission, and delayed or inhibited orgasm. The drugs may cause impotence, menstrual irregularities, absence of menstruation (amenorrhea), breast enlargement in males, breast enlargement or galactorrhea in females, and testicular swelling. Both antipsychotic and antidepressant medications inhibit sperm movement.

If the medication has to continue in females, consult a gynecologist for recommendations. Otherwise, the physician can substitute the medication with a drug with lower risk.

Skin Reactions and Photosensitivity

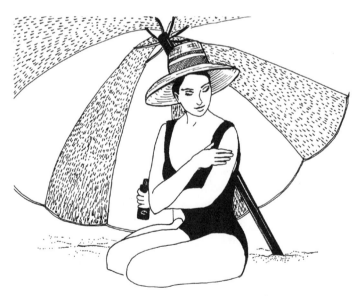

Physicians reported photosensitive skin reactions including skin rashes, as well as retinopathy (disorder of the retina) and hyperpigmentation, resulting from neuroleptics, especially Thorazine and Mellaril,® due to ultraviolet light breakdown in the skin causing a histamine reaction. A substitution of Thorazine and Mellaril is the best course to follow. Use sun blockers/lotions and hats and avoid sun exposure, especially at peak hours, to prevent the photosensitive reactions. Individuals on long-term medication should have periodic eye examinations.

Chapter 7

Development of New Medications

There are five goals in developing new medications and improving existing ones:

1. Widen the therapeutic index of existing medications.

2. Improve tolerability profiles of existing medications.

3. Improve treatment efficacy of existing medications.

4. Reduce the possible number of drug interactions of existing medications.

5. Develop new but safer and more effective medications to allow clinicians and patients to have more treatment options.

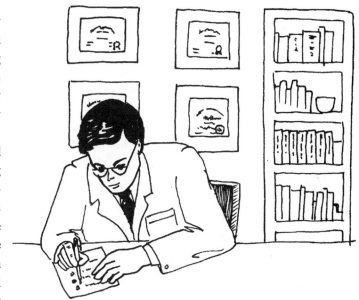

The first four goals apply to the new medications being developed based on knowledge learned from existing medications. The chemical structures and therapeutic profiles of the newly developed medications are usually similar to the existing medications. One example is the newly developed stimulant Concerta (a long-acting methylphenidate), which has chemical properties and therapeutic profiles very similar to that of Ritalin. The fifth goal, however, applies to the development of a new medication that has a very different chemical structure and profiles than that of the existing medications. One example is the newer antipsychotic, Seroquel (Quetiapine), which has a chemical structure and therapeutic profiles quite different than that of the traditional antipsychotic medications like Haldol.

The process used by the FDA to approve new medications includes estimating and maintaining the risk-to-benefit ratio of new medications This helps one realize the limitations of the data that support the efficacy and safety of an approved medication. Many practitioners tend to prescribe "new" medications. The information in this chapter will help you decide whether you want your child to take a new medication.

Role of the Food and Drug Administration

Congress established the Food and Drug Administration (FDA) in the 1930s to ensure the relative safety of food, cosmetics, and medications, as well as to regulate the marketing of such products.

The FDA and Development of New Medications

One focus of the FDA's activities is to ensure that drug companies do not market a new drug when the risk outweighs the benefit and that they do not promote medications for unapproved uses.

Before 1962, no proof of the effectiveness of medications was required, and drug companies commonly made extravagant claims for therapeutic benefits. New drugs could go from the laboratory to clinical testing without FDA's approval. Because efficacy was not rigorously defined, a number of therapeutic claims could not be supported by data. In addition, marketing companies seldom mentioned the risk-benefit ratio. Proof of efficacy of medications introduced after 1962 is required, as is documentation of relative safety in terms of the risk-benefit ratio for the disease to be treated.

Federal law requires sufficient pharmacological and toxicological research in animals before a medication can be tested in humans. This process takes from one-to-three years. The drug companies must submit research data to the FDA by an application for an investigational new drug (IND) before clinical studies can begin. Three phases of clinical testing/trials have evolved to provide the data that are used to support a new drug application (NDA). In general, the total time of drug development from the time of filing of an IND application to the final approval of NDA averages eight-to-nine years, and it may cost hundreds of millions of dollars.

There is increased tension between the FDA and drug companies, medical practitioners, and some consumer groups because of the lengthy process of new drug approval. The public, physicians, and pharmaceutical companies all agree that new drugs should be tested quickly, yet thoroughly, so that useful new medications can be available as soon as possible. Under public pressure and in response to the needs of individuals with life-threatening illnesses, the FDA has moved on several fronts. First, it has initiated new "treatment" IND regulations that allow individuals with life-threatening diseases (for which there is no satisfactory alternative treatment) to receive medications for therapy prior to final approval if there is some evidence of medication efficacy without unreasonable toxicity. Second, the FDA has established a priority system to expedite reviews for medications used to treat life-threatening diseases. Finally, the FDA is becoming more actively involved in drug development to facilitate the approval of drugs designed to treat life-threatening and severely debilitating diseases.

By working with the pharmaceutical industry throughout the period of clinical drug development, the FDA hopes to reduce the time from submission of an IND application to the approval of an NDA. Sufficient data should be available earlier in the development process to allow a risk-benefit analysis and possible approval. Coupled with this expedited development process is the requirement, when appropriate, for restricted distribution of the new drug to certain specialists or facilities to answer remaining issues of risks, benefits, and optimal uses of the drug. If these studies are inadequate or demonstrate a lack of safety or clinical benefit, the FDA may withdraw approval for the new drug.

Progress in accelerating the clinical trial process is already apparent. In the 1980s, it took approximately three years for the FDA to review the application and approve a new drug for clinical trials. Today, the average approval time is one year. For a medication that FDA deems a break-through drug, the review time drops to six months. Regarding the length of required clinical trials, a 1999 report from the Tufts Center for the Study of Drug Development showed that the average length of all clinical trials underway between 1996 and 1998 was 5.9 years—down from 7.2 years between 1993 and 1995.

There are critics who worry that the FDA has moved too quickly for consumer safety. As evidence, they pointed to several drugs that have been pulled from the market in the past three-to-four years. In fact, since 1980, there have been about 520 medicines approved by the FDA and about 12, or 2 percent, that the FDA has recalled because of safety concerns. Overall, it appears that the benefits of approved drugs outweigh the risks, and the current safety system is working.

Approved and Labeled Medications

A medication is "approved" for marketing if its database supports its benefit for a recognized condition, and its risks are sufficiently offset by the efficacy for a particular use. The term "labeling" refers to the uses (indications) that the drug company may promote for a new medication. Before a pharmaceutical company can market a new medication, it must prepare a package insert for physician use. The insert contains basic pharmacological information, as well as essential clinical information about approved indications, contraindications, precautions, warnings, adverse reactions, usual dosage, and available preparations. Promotional materials may not deviate from the information contained in the insert.

When a physician uses a medication for indications beyond those stated in the package insert, then he or she is prescribing an "approved" medication for an "*unlabeled*" or "*off-labeled*" use. The data supporting such uses typically come first from clinical experience with individual patients, then a series of case reports, and, finally, controlled studies. Some studies may be funded by government grants to researchers who have no commercial interest in the particular medication. Results from such studies are published in medical journals, but are generally not included in a new drug application to the FDA.

The FDA's Position on Unlabeled Medications

Even after the FDA decides that the efficacy of a new medication has been proven in the context of acceptable toxicity, the company cannot market that medication for unlabeled uses. Although the marketing company cannot promote such an unlabeled use, doctors are free to prescribe the medication for conditions if they are convinced that the medical literature and their clinical experience support such a use. The FDA takes the position that the individual physician may determine whether a medication could be helpful for an unlabeled use by a specific patient based on that physician's reading of the literature, as well as his experience. Otherwise, many people would not receive effective treatment because of insufficient commercial incentive to carry out the costly process needed to receive marketing approval for a specific indication (e.g., use the new medication in children or in a rare disease). Due to such economic considerations, there are many worthwhile uses of medication that remain "unlabeled."

Clinical Trial of a New Medication

When an investigator wishes to assess the safety, efficacy, and indications of a new medication, a systematic series of experiments (i.e., clinical trials) takes place. The results of the clinical trials form the basis for therapeutic decisions made by all physicians. It is therefore essential that physicians are involved and be able to critically evaluate the results and conclusions of such trials.

By the time a pharmaceutical company initiates an IND application and a new medication reaches the stage of testing in human beings, its pharmacokinetic, pharmacodynamic, and toxic properties have been evaluated in vitro and in several species of animals in accordance with FDA regulations and guidelines. Trials of medications in human beings in the United States are generally completed in three phases before a company can submit an NDA to the FDA for review and approval.

Understanding basic research methodology and important concerns involved in clinical trials of new medications will be helpful in learning about the trials.

Protection of Participating Volunteers

Most people know very little about the scientific basis and conduct of clinical trials for new medications. Therefore, they may unknowingly volunteer to risk their own health, and possibly their lives, to participate in a trial. To protect volunteers from potential abuses and address their concerns, clinical trial organizers incorporate many levels of oversight.

Doctors who participate in the clinical trial are ethically bound to provide patients with the best care possible, whether or not their patients are part of a trial. Physicians are never required to enroll people in an experimental study, and patients cannot be forced to join. When someone does decide to enroll, his doctor must provide a complete explanation, both orally and in writing, about the nature of the study and all available information about the potential risks and benefits of participating. If individuals or their responsible guardians agree to continue, they must do so in writing. This process is called "obtaining informed consent." Individuals always have the right to refuse to participate or to withdraw from a trial at any time.

Because no one can know in advance all possible side effects of an experimental medication, hospitals in the U.S. that run clinical trials operate an Institutional Review Board (IRB). This second level of oversight usually consists of a committee of caregivers, patient advocates, and other professionals (e.g., lawyers or members of the clergy). A general rule is that if there is any element of research involved (e.g., human subjects, systematic data collection, or intent to publish), the entire proposal must be submitted in writing for review by the IRB. The IRB must agree to a trial before it can begin at a site, and if the members become concerned about how a trial is progressing, they can stop the trial at their hospital or request changes in procedure.

As an additional layer of patient protection, each trial usually includes a Data Safety Monitoring Board (DSMB). This group of physicians and statisticians works independently of the sponsors of the drug trial and the scientific investigators. The group monitors the trial, continually checks safety, and periodically evaluates other aspects. If the DSMB finds that the treatment group is doing substantially better than the control group (or vice versa), the board can recommend that the trial be terminated.

Research Components of a Clinical Trial

To maximize the likelihood that useful information will result from an experiment, the experiment must define its objectives, select homogeneous populations of patients, find appropriate control groups, choose meaningful and sensitive indices of medication effects for observation, and convert the observations into data and then into valid conclusions. The following sections describe the major components of a clinical trial.

Pre-Experiment Research Planning

A clinical trial of a new medication requires careful planning. One should specify the questions that need answers. The questions should be few in number and precise. The trial should specify how it will achieve aims and what methods it will use. Basic decisions are necessary before attempting to fit the experimental question into a research design. Whether the treatment should be compared to a placebo or to a standard medication is one of those decisions.

Research Designs

There are two major categories of experimental designs: extensive (between groups) and intensive (within an individual).

Extensive Design

In the extensive design, the researchers analyze the medication across groups of patients. For example, the most common design randomly assigns one group of patients to an active medication and contrasts its effects with a group that receives a placebo (comparative or parallel design). The researchers compare the percentage of patients who improve in the medication group to the percentage in the placebo group.

Almost all diseases are highly variable in their progression. Remissions sometimes occur spontaneously. Researchers must be able to distinguish between a natural remission and one resulting from treatment. Inclusion of a control group, which receives either a placebo or the best currently available therapy, makes it possible to perform this comparison.

Similarly, having a control group enables doctors to assess the health problems unrelated to the new medication. For example, a medication being tested for treatment of a particular type of cancer might be suspected of causing nausea. But nausea can occur in just about anyone. Only if its incidence is significantly higher in the treatment group than in the control group is it considered a problem.

The research may use many different types of controls. Researchers have ethical considerations in deciding what controls to use in tests. For example, in therapeutic trials that involve life-threatening diseases for which there already is an effective therapy, the use of a placebo is unethical. Therefore, a new treatment must be compared to "standard" therapies.

The division of subjects into the test or control groups must occur randomly; otherwise, the final results will be skewed. If the leaders of the clinical trial consciously or unconsciously administered the test medication to healthier patients, it could appear to be more effective than a controlled group comprised of mostly patients who had failed all other medications (i.e., who were more likely to be among the sickest patients).

Ideally, neither the physicians nor the patients know who are in the treatment group or the control group; they are "blind" to the type of therapy they receive. The physician and the patients may have preconceived expectations from the treatment (i.e., placebo effect) that can confound the result of the study, particularly when the assessment of the treatment effect involves subjective responses. Therefore, double-blind, controlled studies are essential because about thirty percent of patients improve with a placebo (See Chapter 5). Furthermore, spontaneous improvement may occur. Double-blind and placebo-controlled procedures can control these variables.

To ensure success of the blinding procedure, investigators make the placebo pills look exactly like the tested medication. They treat the patients in either the medication group or placebo group in exactly the same way. Nonetheless, keeping a trial completely blind is simply impossible in some cases. For instance, if the medication being tested causes some kind of side effect, or if some patients chew the medication that has some unusual flavor, the patients will quickly figure out that they are in the treatment group.

Although the randomized, double-blind, controlled trial is the most effective design for avoiding bias and distributing unknown variables between the "treatment" and the "control" groups, it is not necessarily the best design for all studies. It may be impossible to use this design to study disorders that rarely occur or disorders that tend to be fatal.

Despite the above limits, the vast majority of the medical profession accepts randomized, controlled clinical trials as the required gold standard for deciding whether a treatment is useful. The methodology is still evolving, and some of the newer approaches to testing should be helpful.

Intensive Design

In the intensive design, researchers study the effect of the medication within individual patients. The most common procedure is to alternate between medication and placebo periods in a single patient. With intensive designs, changes in an individual's behavior during a waiting period or placebo period are compared with changes in that same patient after treatment. This design is particularly useful in assessing treatment effects in rare conditions because it circumvents the problem of obtaining an equivalent sample of patients for a control group.

The intensive design tests for true differential treatment effects in relation to the individual patient. The investigator is not restricted to group statistics when assessing medication efficacy. The intensive design also allows some estimate of trend effects within the patient.

A major problem with the intensive design is that it requires the behavior in question to be relatively stable over time. Thus, the natural history of the disease is essential. The investigator must be confident that the behavior/symptom is stable during the pre-medication phase (baseline period) and demonstrate that it changes abruptly when treatment begins.

A practical difficulty is that intensive designs take longer than extensive designs. If the patient is only available for a short period, intensive designs are usually ruled out. Another problem is that researchers cannot use intensive designs when the medication being tested has long-lasting, carry-over effects. If the effect of the medication is irreversible, the design cannot be used. If the carry-over effect is brief, the researcher must know its duration and allow for ample "washout."

Selection of Volunteers or Patients

Early planning stages must include a detailed description of healthy volunteers or patients in the study group. These include the diagnosis, inclusion and exclusion criteria, and a variety of demographic information. The sample has to be representative, and it should be as homogeneous as possible in respect to chronological age. Such an approach creates a narrow subgroup of patients for whom the new medication will be indicated once marketed.

Researchers should assess compliance with the experimental regimen before assigning volunteers to the experimental or control groups. Researchers should also assess the medication-taking behavior of the volunteers during the course of the trial. Noncompliance, even if randomly distributed between both groups, may cause falsely low estimates of the true potential benefits or toxicity of a particular treatment.

Sample Size

Researchers should estimate the sample size prior to beginning a clinical trial. This is to determine the power of the trial to detect a statistically significant effect if, in fact, one exists. Depending upon factors like the overall prognosis, the variability of the disease, the anticipated improvement, and variability in outcome or toxicity from the new treatment, the trial may need a very large number of subjects. Otherwise, the possibility of a false-negative result is high; that is, researchers will not find statistically significant differences between the two treatments even though differences actually exist.

Measures of Medication Effects

Researchers must measure the specific outcome of therapy that is clinically relevant and quantifiable. This should include both subjective and objective assessments that can determine whether a therapy improves the patient's well-being and quality of life. Wherever possible, researchers should use well-defined endpoints as measures rather than an intermediate point or a "surrogate marker." Endpoints describe unambiguous results that indicate exactly what the treatment can do. For instance, researchers' usual endpoint when screening a new antibiotic is whether a patient is free of infection after treatment. However, many ailments may not be so readily cured. Therefore, an alternative endpoint might be whether the progression of a depression has slowed or whether the rate of suicide attempts in the depressed subjects has fallen.

A "surrogate marker" is a clinical or laboratory test that correlates with the clinical outcome of a disease. Blood pressure, blood sugar, and premature ventricular complexes are examples of surrogate markers that are used as endpoints in clinical trials. Although surrogate markers can often reduce the length and sample size of a clinical trial, the results of such a trial may be misleading. For example, an individual's blood sugar may have improved and is within normal range, but he still may have symptoms of diabetes. The ultimate test of a medication's effectiveness must rest with actual clinical outcomes.

Baseline Measures

Baseline considerations are crucial to the proper design of the study. Since the symptoms may fluctuate from setting to setting, a stable baseline is needed before starting medication. This can usually be established within two weeks and should include at least two ratings while the subject receives a placebo.

A baseline placebo period serves more than one function. The period ensures "washout," helps the volunteers become used to taking the medication, and identifies placebo responders.

Phase I of Clinical Trial

In the first stage of a clinical trial, researchers gather information about whether a medication is safe to give to humans and, if so, how much they can tolerate. The investigators want to know what would be the maximum safe dose of the new medication. Phase I of the clinical trial requires about 10-100 volunteers, usually healthy people, to yield statistically meaningful conclusions. But if the possibility of extremely serious side effects exists, r esearchers conduct Phase I testing in patients having the condition that the new medication may treat. Potential harm then is balanced by potential benefit.

The initial dose is typically very low to minimize the possibility of a major reaction, but as doctors escalate the dose, the potential for problems increases. The trial team closely monitors the participants, constantly observing their behavior, and asking how they feel. The team encourages the participants to report any unusual feeling or changes in their physiological state. To spot problems early, the researchers regularly measure blood pressure, heart rate, and temperature; collect blood and urine samples; and monitor for any danger signs that animal studies have shown. The investigators also measure the level of medication in the bloodstream or tissues to determine how it is distributed in the body, how rapidly it reaches a therapeutic level, and how the body eliminates the compound. When combined, these data help determine the safe dosing regimen.

Assessment of risk or safety is a major objective of the Phase I trial. However, this is far more difficult to determine than whether or not a medication is efficacious (Phase II trial) for a selected clinical condition. The Phase I study lasts about one-to-two years and may cost up to ten million dollars.

Phase II of Clinical Trial

The main goal of Phase II is to find the experimental conditions that will allow the final phase of the trial to give a definitive result. In particular, researchers try to estimate the effective doses and duration of treatment and find who and how many people they should include in the final phase (Phase III) of the clinical trial. To gain statistically significant conclusions, Phase II needs about 50-to-500 patients with the targeted disease.

Researchers must immediately establish what will be the primary endpoint for determining the effectiveness of the new medication in a certain patient population. The Phase II trial usually employs the extensive (randomized and controlled) design described earlier. Selection of a proper control group is as critical to the eventual usefulness of an experiment as the selection of the experimental group. Researchers carefully review records of volunteers in both controlled and experimental groups during Phase II, and they constantly refine the dose and duration of treatment to be used in Phase III.

The Phase II study usually takes about two years to complete. The study could cost around twenty million dollars.

Phase III of Clinical Trial

The final stage of the clinical trial process, Phase III, is the most familiar to the general public. Usually about 1,000-to-3,000 (or more) carefully selected patients receive a new medication during phase III of clinical trials. By this point, the investigators running the trial have defined at least one group of patients that they expect to benefit, how the drugs benefit the patients, and the best way to administer treatment. The trial can confirm that a medication works.

If after careful statistical analysis the new medication proves to be significantly more effective than the control treatment, the trial is called "pivotal." Ordinarily, researchers must conduct two pivotal trials to prove to the FDA the value of a new therapy. But if the first result is sufficiently persuasive, one trial can be enough. If the trial convinces the FDA, the agency approves the medication for sale as a treatment for the particular disease.

Occasionally, the Phase III trial may show a trend in favor of the medication, but the effect will be too small to serve as statistically convincing proof. In such a case, statisticians have developed methods for pooling data from all the previous trials to conduct what they term "meta-analysis." Such evaluations remain controversial, however. The appeal of trying to salvage a valuable result from a collection of "near-misses" is strong, but questions remain about the validity of meta-analysis. The technique is subject to potential bias in terms of which studies were selected for inclusion and the comparability of those studies. The findings from a meta-analysis can be useful for interpreting a large amount of conflicting data, but the results are not generally consid ered definitive.

If the results of Phase III testing are ambiguous, leaders of a clinical trial usually try to extract some useful information out of their hard work. By observing the tremendous amount of collected data, the investigators might be able to discover a cluster of patients within the larger group who seem to respond positively. Researchers must then conduct another full-scale Phase III trial—this time with a more restricted set of patients—to prove whether the medication actually helped. In practice, initial

Phase III trials frequently fail to show adequate proof of a new medication's efficacy, and researchers must carry out several follow-up trials.

Phase III of the clinical trial usually takes about three-to-four years to complete, and it may cost forty million dollars or more. The rate at which a trial proceeds depends predominantly on the number of participating investigators and patients. The faster the researchers can collect the data, the sooner they can begin to interpret the information. This is particularly true for therapies that may offer important benefits to only a relatively small number of patients and for those that provide modest benefits for many people.

As a way to enroll as many patients as possible, as quickly as possible, trial leaders now run their studies at numerous sites around the world. More sites mean more patients. This also means a diverse group of people who are more representative of those who will one day be taking the medication or using the medical device. However, when involving more sites, the researchers may compromise the quality control of the trial (e.g., compliance with the research protocol and consistency of outcome measures).

Value of the Clinical Trial

With increasing cooperation among investigators and regulatory agencies around the world, we can expect that researchers will develop better treatments so that older and less effective medications will go by the wayside. The clinical trial process is the most objective method ever devised to assess the effectiveness of a treatment. The process is expensive and slow, and in need of constant refinement and oversight, but it is trustworthy.

Concerns about Clinical Trials

Because of the long-term nature of most psychiatric disorders, treatment with psychotherapeutic medications is best considered in terms of months or years of continuous or intermittent therapy, rather than just a few days or weeks. By contrast, the vast majority of the clinical trials involve short-term use. Thus, the current approach of clinical trials does not provide useful information on psychotherapeutic medications' long-term therapeutic and adverse effects. Even if a medication's effect is not seen in a clinical trial, it may still appear in the setting of clinical practice. In fact, about one-half or more of both useful and adverse effects of medications not recognized in the initial formal trials were later discovered and reported by practicing physicians.

Patients whose conditions are complicated by certain issues are potentially the most frequent recipients of medications, yet they are usually excluded from the clinical trials. Examples of these issues include the following: concomitant psychotherapeutic medications, serious medical conditions, concomitant (accompanying) substance abuse, central nervous system disease or trauma, age, etc. Thus, researchers cannot know whether the new medication would have the same effectiveness in these individuals as that shown in the clinical trial.

The majority of drugs prescribed for children have never been tested in youngsters to determine their safety and efficacy. Drug manufacturers have had no incentive to study children because doctors could legally prescribe adult products to youngsters. That changed two years ago when Congress granted manufacturers an extra six months of patent protection if they voluntarily test products pediatricians prescribe. Furthermore, since December of 2000, FDA regulations mandate that any new adult medication that could be used in children with the same disease must undergo pediatric study.

In recent years, human trials have become more than just a way to screen new medications. They have taken on an important role in the delivery of health care. Many patients view participation in a trial as the only way to obtain experimental medications that they consider potentially lifesaving, or the only way they can get expensive medications for free. If the patient selection includes too many such subjects, there could be a potential bias toward a positive response if extensive (randomized and controlled) design is not carefully implemented.

Because of the practice of randomization in clinical trials, patients often complain about being powerless "guinea pigs" for the far more powerful drug companies. These patients argue that those whose only hope could be the latest, cutting-edge treatments should have guaranteed access to them.

For many years, the pharmaceutical companies have done most of the work of clinical trials themselves. They hire physicians, data monitors, statisticians, and a variety of support people to carry out a massive endeavor. All of this is in addition to the local physicians and nurses who care for patients enrolled in the trial. The cost of this enterprise quickly becomes substantial, running into hundreds of millions of dollars. Although exact numbers remain elusive, the most widely quoted figure, from a 1993 study by the Boston Consulting Group, is about $500 million for each new medication that makes it to market. The estimate includes cancelled projects. As a result, drug companies want to recover their costs as expeditiously as possible. They also want to control the final decision regarding the announcement or publication of the testing results. Naturally, the drug companies would report results in only the most self-serving way.

Researchers involved in clinical trials have sometimes complained that sponsoring drug companies restrict what they can report to their colleagues and to the general public if a treatment appears not to work. On the other hand, in an attempt to minimize potential problems over financial conflicts, most medical societies and major journals now require researchers to submit a disclosure statement that describes how the test was financed, along with any other details relevant to conflicts of interest. The U.S. government requires a similar declaration from investigators who participate in government-sponsored trials or from consultants involved in grant or regulatory decisions at organizations such as the NIH or FDA.

The selection of patients for experimental trials usually eliminates those with co-existing diseases. Such trials usually assess the effect of only one or two medications, not the many that might be given to, or be taken by, the same patient under the care of a physician.

Clinical trials are usually performed with relatively small numbers of patients for periods of time that may be shorter than are necessary in practice, and compliance may be better controlled than it can be in practice.

The recent trend of testing new medications in foreign countries shows that these countries have less rigorous regulations than those in the United States. As some of the overseas clinical trial data have been used to get FDA approval, the effectiveness and safety of these new medications are uncertain.

Postmarketing Detection of Medication-Induced Adverse Reactions

Although Phase III of the trial may test hundreds or thousands of subjects, it may only treat a few hundred for more than three-to-six months, regardless of the likely duration of therapy that will be required in daily practice. It is obvious that a number of unanticipated adverse and beneficial effects of the new medications are detectable only after the medications have been on the market for several years and have been broadly used.

Researchers have developed strategies to detect adverse reactions after marketing a new medication. One approach for estimating the magnitude of an adverse drug effect is the "follow-up cohort" study of patients who are receiving a particular medication. Group studies can estimate the incidence of an adverse reaction, but they cannot, for practical reasons, discover rare events. To have any significant conclusion, a cohort study must follow at least several thousand patients who are receiving the new medication for a significant length of time. If the adverse event occurs spontaneously in the control population, substantially more patients and controls must be followed to establish that the new medication is the cause of the adverse event.

The other formal study is called the "case-control study." Researchers assess the potential for a new medication to cause a particular adverse event. Case-control studies can discover rare, drug-induced events. However, it may be difficult to establish the appropriate control group, and a case-control study cannot establish the frequency of an adverse drug effect.

Because of the shortcomings of cohort and case-control studies, researchers must use other approaches. Many countries, including the U.S., have established systematic methods for studying the effects of new medications after the FDA has approved them for distribution. The FDA may mandate specific *postmarketing surveillance programs* when a concern about the safety or efficacy of a new medication is suggested by either the pre-clinical or clinical database used for marketing approval.

In addition, spontaneous reporting of adverse reactions proves to be an effective way to provide an early warning signal that a new medication may be causing an adverse event. The researchers can then investigate the event by more formal techniques. The most important spontaneous reports are those that describe serious reactions, whether they have been described previously or not. It is the only practical way to detect rare events, events that occur after prolonged use of medication, adverse effects that are delayed in appearance, and many drug interactions. However, the system also monitors changes in the nature or frequency of adverse drug reactions due to the aging of the population, changes in the disease itself, or the introduction of new, concurrent therapies.

The primary sources for the reports are responsible, alert physicians. Other potentially useful sources are nurses and pharmacists. In addition, hospital-based pharmacies, treatment committees, and quality assurance committees frequently are charged with monitoring adverse drug reactions in hospitalized patients. Reports from these committees should be forwarded to the FDA.

The FDA encourages clinicians to send *adverse experience reporting* forms when a patient develops a problem during treatment. The simple forms for reporting are now readily available in the *Physicians' Desk Reference* and *AMA Drug Evaluations* and are mailed to all physicians at least once a year as part of the *FDA Drug Bulletin*. Additionally, health professionals may contact the pharmaceutical manufacturer, who is legally obligated to file reports with the FDA.

Find Latest Pharmaceutical News on FDA's Web Site

The FDA offers a comprehensive Web site, www.fda.gov, replete with up-to-date news of pharmaceutical product approvals, recalls, alerts and warnings. As with most government sites, fda.gov is well organized, with all links and information you will need to navigate the site right on the home page. If you decide that the benefits of participating in a clinical trial outweigh the risks, be sure to read the site's information on research and human subject protection.

Chapter 8

Psychotherapeutic Medications

This chapter introduces the classes of medications physicians frequently prescribe, or most likely will prescribe, for individuals with ASD. It includes information about drug nomenclature and classification. Each section discusses the basic actions and effects (psychopharmacology) of each class of medication. Appendix G has general information about these medications. Due to the scope of this book, some medical terminologies need further explanation. You should talk to your child's doctor about the risks, benefits, side effects, special precautions, and those difficult-to-understand medical terminologies relating to the prescribed drugs.

Names of Medications

Many medicines have several names, and this leads to confusion. The flood of new medications in recent years has added even more confusion.

If a new medication appears promising, and the manufacturer wishes to market it, the United States Adopted Name (USAN) Council selects a name. (The American Medical Association, American Pharmaceutical Association, and United States Pharmacopeial Convention, Inc. jointly sponsor the USAN Council.) This name is in addition to the medication's chemical name. The USAN Council's selection, the *nonproprietary* name, is often referred to as the *generic* name. A generic name is usually derived from the chemical structure of the medication. However, the USAN Council also assigns a *proprietary* name; that is, a brand name or trade name by the manufacturer (e.g., Ritalin for methylphenidate hydrochloride). The manufacturer usually chooses a brand or trade name that is euphonious, catchy, or emphasizes its main function (e.g., Allegra® for treatment of allergies, Lipitor® for controlling cholesterol, or Adderall® for management of attention deficit disorder).

A generic name is always lowercase. A trade or brand name starts with an initial uppercase letter and often carries the superscript ® for registered trade name (e.g. Prozac®). However, if more than one company markets the drug, or the patent on the compound has expired because of the lapse of seventeen years, any company can market the drug under its own brand name. Here are examples: lithium carbonate is Lithobid® by one manufacturer and Eskalith® by another, and fluoxetine HCl is Prozac and Sarafem®.

Once a successful new medication appears, other companies look for a competitive product. Mixtures of the medication with other agents are marketed, and each such mixture may have a separate brand name. An example is Dexedrine® (dextroam-

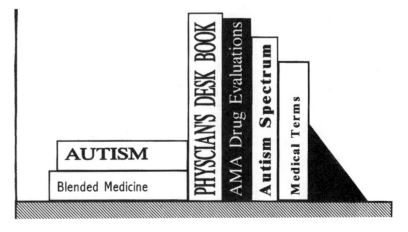

phetamine sulfate) and Adderall (dextroamphetamine sulfate, dextroamphetamine saccharate, amphetamine aspartate, amphetamine sulfate). Most of the look-alike medications are merely variations within a major class like serotonin reuptake inhibitors (e.g., Prozac and Paxil®) or within a chemical group such as methylphenidate (e.g., Ritalin and Concerta®). Most of the differences between the look-alike medications stem from pharmacokinetics (longer or shorter duration) and side effects rather than therapeutic effectiveness. While such differences may be valuable, they are extremely limited.

There is increasing worldwide adoption of the same name for each medication. For newer medications, other countries usually adopt the USAN for the generic name, but this is not true for older medications. International agreement on drug names is mediated through the World Health Organization and the pertinent health agencies of the cooperating countries.

When the medication is available under multiple brand names, and when the generic name more readily identifies the medication with its pharmacological class, physicians should use the generic name because it is less confusing. On the whole, however, physicians tend to use trade names despite the fact that only generic names appear in good journals or books that review their properties. The best argument for the use of a brand name is that more people can pronounce it and remember it because of advertising. For the same reason, I have used trade or brand names to describe medications. However, the brand names of the medications described in the rest of this chapter and in Chapter 13 are highlighted in uppercase (e.g., RITALIN, rather than Ritalin).

Classification of Psychotherapeutic Medications

Classifying medications is not easy. In most cases there are no sharp distinctions among them. Medications with almost identical chemical structures may cause entirely different effects. For example, both TOFRANIL (an antidepressant) and ANAFRANIL(an anti-obsessive-compulsive disorder medication) are tricyclics, while other medications whose chemical structures are quite different may cause almost identical results. Both LITHOBID® (lithium carbonate) and DEPAKOTE (valproic acid), for example, are anti-mania medications.

Some medications may have one effect at one dose and an entirely different action at another. A physician may prescribe TOFRANIL at a lower dosage for bed-wetting problems, but at a higher dosage for depressive disorder. A medication may have multiple effects, including both therapeutic and side effects, in a certain dose range. Depending on the population taking the medications, some of these effects may be desirable in one person and undesirable in another. The drowsiness side effect of CATAPRES is desirable for treating initial insomnia, but it is an undesirable effect for the treatment of ADHD. It is not surprising that different textbooks may classify drugs in a number of different ways.

Classification by Chemical Structure

One classification scheme that appears to be reasonable involves grouping medications according to their chemical structure. While this scheme may often group medications that have very similar behavioral effects, in many cases what appear to be relatively minor changes in the molecular structure of a medication can considerably change its basic activity in the body. There are many cases in which molecules that are identical, except for their being mirror images of each other, produce different results. Such molecules are called *optical isomers*. When one isomer binds, and the other does not, thereby inducing different effects, they are said to be stereospecific. For example, levo-morphine produces an analgesic effect, and detro-morphine, an inactive molecule, does not.

Classification by Action Mechanism

Another way that many researchers classify medications is according to the action mechanism. In this context, they describe medications as CNS *depressants* (e.g. MEBARAL) or *stimulants* (e.g., RITALIN). One might expect a depressant to decrease mood, motor activity, and the body's metabolic and physiological activities; reduce alertness and induce sleep; decrease brain activity and neurotransmitter turnover; and shift the EEG toward lower frequencies and higher amplitude waves. One might expect stimulants to do just the reverse. It is not that simple, however, because medications rarely do all of these things simultaneously. On the other hand, a medication may decrease the relative frequency of one set of behaviors while increasing the relative frequency of other sets. For example, RITALIN may decrease a child's activity level, but it may also increase a child's stereotyped behavior. Furthermore, lower doses of RITALIN may increase alertness, but at higher doses it may cause drowsiness. If one does not specify a particular set of behaviors or emotions and the dose of the medication, the terms "depressant" and "stimulant" mean little.

Classification by the Therapeutic Use

Most researchers in the field of psychiatry prefer to classify psychotherapeutic medications according to their predominant use. Unfortunately, this system is far from perfect because doctors may prescribe medications for different purposes, in different doses, and for different individuals. For example, PROZAC was originally developed for the treatment of depression and has been classified as an "antidepressant." However, doctors have widely used PROZAC in the treatment of obsessive-compulsive disorder.

Classification by Schedule—Controlled Drugs

The United States Congress passed the Controlled Substances Act of 1970 to improve the administration and regulation of manufacturing, distributing, and dispensing potentially dangerous medications. The act divides medications into five schedules:

- Schedule I drugs are those that have no currently accepted medical use in the United States. These are drugs having a high potential for abuse. Examples of such drugs are heroin, LSD, and mescaline.

- Schedule II drugs are those that have some currently accepted medical uses in the United States but have a high potential of abuse. Examples include amphetamines, cocaine, morphine, opium, and meperidine.

- Schedule III drugs are those with some currently accepted medical uses and less potential for abuse than Schedule I and Schedule II drugs. Examples of such drugs are compounds containing codeine; short-to-intermediate-duration barbiturates like amobarbital, pentobarbital, and secobarbital; and nonbarbiturate sedative-hypnotics like glutethimide (DORIDEN®).

- Schedule IV and Schedule V drugs are those with current medical uses and successively lower abuse potentials than those of Schedules I, II, and III. Included in Schedules IV and V are long-acting sedative-hypnotics, such as phenobarbital; anxiolytics (e.g., VALIUM); and low-potency narcotics, such as cough syrups with codeine.

Unlabeled Uses

When a medication has proved to be reasonably safe and effective for some specific symptoms or disorders, the FDA approves it for medical use, and it is officially labeled. This labeling includes the information that appears both on the outside of the medication container and on the package insert in the container. The FDA has final approval over what the manufacturer may recommend the medication for, and what it may say in its advertisements and marketing publications. However, the FDA does not have any authority over a physician's practice of medicine. There is also no federal law prohibiting physicians from prescribing an approved medication for anything they choose, although some states do place restrictions on what certain medications can be prescribed. Thus, many medications that have been approved for specific symptoms or disorders have been prescribed for entirely different purposes (i.e., unlabeled uses) than those stated by the manufacturer. For example, CATAPRES, approved as a medication for high blood pressure, has been prescribed for the treatment of ADHD and temper outbursts.

Investigational Drugs

An investigational drug is typically one that the FDA has not approved for marketing for human use. This designation may also refer to agents approved by the FDA for a specific indication but are being investigated for a non-labeled use. Examples of the latter include:

- A different preparation or formulation

- A higher than approved dosage

- Used by a different patient population

Problems with Classification of Medications

The first problem is that a medication may be used for several, widely disparate symptoms. For example, doctors can prescribe phenobarbital as an anticonvulsant, a sedative, or a hypnotic. Some antidepressants are increasingly being used in the treatment of pain, eating disorders, and phobias. Some anxiolytics appear equally effective in the treatment of certain types of depression.

The second problem is that some medications that seem to have the ideal properties for alleviating certain symptoms do not work in the long run. For example, amphetamine, which enhances mood in normal individuals, does not usually do so in depressed individuals. Even if it did, it would likely worsen depression shortly after these people stopped taking it. Third, in many cases, the qualitative effects of a medication are dependent upon dosage or on how long the patient has taken the medication. For these reasons, even authors who categorize drugs using the same basic rationale as that used in this book tend to have somewhat different classification schemes. Nonetheless, in this chapter, for the purpose of learning the general use of the commonly prescribed psychotherapeutic medications in the field of ASD, the medications are classified by their primary therapeutic use. I have assigned a medication to a class based on the usual use of the medication at the dose implicated in the drug action (e.g., at low doses, barbiturates are classed as hypnotics; at high doses, they are classified as anticonvulsants).

Sources of Medication Information

Among the available sources of information are pharmacology textbooks, leading medical journals, drug compendia, professional seminars and meetings, and advertising. Depending on their aims and scopes, pharmacology textbooks provide basic pharmacological principles, critical appraisal of useful categories of therapeutic medications, and detailed descriptions of individual medications that serve as standards of reference for assessing new medications.

The source of information most often used by physicians is an industry-supported *Physicians' Desk Reference (PDR)*. The information is identical to that contained in medication package inserts. There are, however, several inexpensive, unbiased sources of information on the clinical uses of medications that are preferable to the industry-supported PDR, and many are available on CD-ROM or diskette. The *United States Pharmacopeia Dispensing Information (USPDI)* comes in two volumes. The first volume, *Drug Information for the Health Care Professional*, consists of medication monographs that contain practical, clinically significant information aimed at minimizing the risks and enhancing the benefit of medications. USP staff develop monographs, and advisory panels and others review them. The *Advice for the Patient* volume reinforces, in lay language, the oral consultation provided by the therapist. The patient may receive this in written form.

AMA Drug Evaluations, compiled by the American Medical Association Department of Drugs in cooperation with the American Society for Clinical Pharmacology and Therapeutics, includes general information on the use of medications in special settings (e.g., pediatrics, geriatrics, cardiovascular, etc.) and reflects the consensus of a panel on the effective clinical use of therapeutic medications.

Facts and Comparison is organized by pharmacological classes and is updated monthly. This publication presents information in monographs in a standard format. It contains FDA-approved information and incorporates current data obtained from the biomedical literature. A useful feature is the comprehensive list of preparations with a "Cost Index," an index of the average wholesale price for equivalent quantities of similar or identical drugs.

Organizations in the United States publish over 1500 medical journals. Among those that are objective and are not supported by drug manufacturers include *Clinical Pharmacology and Therapeutics, Drugs, The New England Journal of Medicine, Annals of Internal Medicine, Journal of the American Medical Association, Archives of Internal Medicine, British Medical Journal, Lancet, and Postgraduate Medicine*. These journals contain original articles that timely evaluate and review the actions and effects of medications in human beings.

There are Internet sites that provide medication information. Some sites are free, but others require registration or subscription to enter the sites. The following are a few Web sites for medication information:

- www.webnd.com

- www.medscape.com

- www.micromedex.com

Your pharmacy may provide some basic pharmacological information about the medications that your child is taking. Make sure that you obtain this information each time you acquire the medications.

Classes of Psychotherapeutic Medications

The following sections briefly describe classes of psychotherapeutic medications and general information relevant to each class. However, details of each frequently used, or potentially used, medications are in alphabetical order in Appendix G. As this book is for parents and non-medical professionals, information relating to the injection form of medications is not included because injections are rarely used outside of hospital or clinic settings. Information on pregnancy and breast-feeding implications is not included because such conditions rarely happen to individuals with ASD.

Antipsychotics

Antipsychotic medications are a large group of psychotherapeutic medications mainly known for their antipsychotic clinical properties, although they are also effective in a variety of nonpsychotic disorders. Some authors often call them "major tranquilizers" because they calm highly excited individuals with schizophrenia or mania. However, the term may be inappropriate in certain cases. For example, they may also enhance the social interactions and increase the activity of catatonic (excessively inhibited) patients. Therefore, most practitioners prefer not to refer to these medications as major tranquilizers. Another term for these medications is *neuroleptics*. However, since this term technically means a medication capable of inducing severe neurological symptoms ("*lepsis*" is Greek for seizure), it is obviously inappropriate in the present classification context.

Antipsychotic medications selectively interact with the receptors of a variety of classes of neurotransmitters in the brains of humans. These include receptors of dopaminergic, serotonergic, a-adrenergic, histaminergic, and cholinergic systems, as well as calcium channels. Within the dopaminergic system, there are at least five types of receptors, and different antipsychotics have different affinities for these receptors, as they do for other types. With the possible exception of CLOZARIL, the most important variations in receptor action are in the adrenergic and cholinergic systems. This is because they influence side effects of the antipsychotic medications. Both the effectiveness and side effects of antipsychotics are related to their selective affinities and interactions with the receptors of the neurotransmitter systems.

Antipsychotic medications, as their name suggests, act against psychotic symptoms. These medications cannot "cure" the illnesses, but they can eliminate or reduce many of the symptoms. In some cases, they can also shorten the course of the illnesses.

A number of antipsychotic medications are available. They all work—the main differences are in the potency and side effects. If a person has to take a large amount of a "high-dose" (low-potency) antipsychotic medication, such as THORAZINE, to get the same effect as a small amount of a "low-dose" (high-potency) medication, such as HALDOL, why doesn't the doctor just prescribe "low-dose" medications? The main reason is the difference in their side effects. Some people have more trouble with certain side effects than other side effects.

A side effect is sometimes desirable. For example, the sedative effect of some antipsychotic medications is beneficial for patients who have trouble sleeping or become agitated during the day. In general, the high-potency antipsychotics are probably preferable to the low-potency drugs, mainly because they are less likely to cause sedation and adrenolytic actions like hypotension. Younger age groups seem more prone to dystonic reactions, which are intermittent or sustained muscular contraction or spasms that may produce an abnormal posture or involuntary movements.

Antipsychotic medications decrease specific symptoms in adults and adolescents, such as loose associations, delusions, hallucinations, and other bizarre and idiosyncratic thinking, but the medications do not dramatically affect primary symptoms of the childhood psychoses. Instead, the medications treat particular target symptoms in these serious disorders as an adjunct to other therapeutic efforts. The symptoms include:

- Severe withdrawal, excitability, anxiety, and cognitive disorganization of children with pervasive developmental disorders

- Hyperactivity and assaultiveness of retarded children with behavioral disturbances

- Severe hyperactivity of children with other developmental disorders that are not responsive to any other therapy

- Anxiety and agitation of acute confusional states, either functional or organically based

- Multiple tics of Tourette syndrome

There are no absolute indications for antipsychotic medications in individuals with ASD unless these people also have a psychiatric illness like schizophrenia or severe Tourette syndrome. However, there is a broad range of possible indications for medications when hyperactivity, aggression, self-injury, agitation, severe disorganization, or insomnia accompanies the ASD. Nevertheless, physicians should reserve antipsychotic medication for severe problems in which reasonable alternative treatments have failed. Short-term success with antipsychotics does not necessarily mean the patient will need these medications on a long-term basis. The physician must carefully re-evaluate the therapeutic benefits and monitor the patient for side effects.

Unlike some prescription medications, which must be taken several times during the day, patients can usually take antipsychotic medications just once a day. Thus, individuals can reduce daytime side effects by taking the medications once before bed. This is particularly appropriate in a case where the sedative effect of the drug is desired for nighttime sleep, thereby avoiding undesirable sedative effects during the day. Some antipsychotic medications can be injected once or twice a month. This ensures that the patient takes the medication on a reliable basis.

Just as people vary in their response to antipsychotic medications, they also vary in their speed of improvement. Some symptoms diminish in days, while others take weeks or months. For many individuals, we see substantial improvement by the sixth week of treatment, although this is not true in every case. If someone does not improve, the doctor may try a different type of medication. Medication treatment for a psychotic illness can continue for up to several months—sometimes longer.

Stimulants

Stimulants activate the level of activity, arousal, or alertness of the CNS to reduce fatigue and elevate mood in most people. Medications in this category include:

- Amphetamines (DEXEDRINE, ADDERALL)

- Methylphenidates (RITALIN, CONCERTA)

- Magnesium pemoline (CYLERT)

- Cocaine

- Caffeine

- Phenylpropanolamine (a common ingredient in over-the-counter appetite suppressors).

The amphetamines and methylphenidate are structurally similar to brain catecholamines and are called sympathomimetic compounds because they may mimic the actions of these brain neurotransmitters. The other (non-catecholaminergic) stimulants (e.g., caffeine) are not discussed in this book since they are not nearly as effective as the catecholaminergic stimulants and are not suitable for medical use.

Therapeutic Effects of Stimulants

Overall, about seventy-five percent of children without ASD see improvement in behaviors when treated with stimulants. Their improved "behaviors" are based on various measures. However, one should keep in mind that when some individuals respond poorly to one type of stimulant, they might respond to a different one. Therefore, the response of individuals to stimulants can be quite idiosyncratic and individualized.

Stimulants produce positive effects on sustained attention and persistence of effort to assigned tasks while reducing task-irrelevant restlessness and motor activity. These medications have also improved problems with aggression, impulsive behavior, noisiness, noncompliance, and disruptive behavior. Stimulants enhance performance on measures of vigilance, impulse control, fine-motor coordination, and reaction time. They may also enhance:

- Short-term memory

- Learning of paired verbal or nonverbal material

- Performance on both simple and complex learning paradigms

- Perceptual efficiency

- Speed of symbolic or verbal retrieval

However, stimulants do not change the functioning on more traditional measures of cognitive abilities (e.g., intelligence tests). The stimulant drugs allow individuals to show what they know but are unlikely to alter their knowledge of what needs to be done. Nevertheless, stimulants improve academic productivity and accuracy.

Stimulants increase ADHD children's compliance with parental and teacher commands. In turn, parents and teachers reduce their rate of commands and degree of supervision over these children, while increasing their praise and positive responsiveness to the children's behavior. Stimulants also enhance children's responsiveness to the interactions of others and improve their acceptance by peers.

Adults generally report elevations in mood and euphoria when taking stimulant medications. However, these effects are rarely seen in children. Some children do describe feeling "funny" or "different." Some children may have dysphoric reactions with sadness, fearfulness, or irritability. These mood changes occur later in the course of the dose response, typically as the medications are washing out of the body in late morning or late afternoon. Such reactions are frequently mild and dose-related, being more prevalent among children treated with higher dosages.

Potential Side Effects

Stimulants produce acute growth hormone release in both children and adults, which can lead to alterations in prolactin, cortisol, and b-endorphins. However, there is no evidence of long-term effects on the hypothalamic-pituitary-growth hormone axis. Despite some evidence of initial growth inhibition by stimulants, effects on eventual adult height are often insignificant. Effects on weight are also frequently minimal. Patients may lose one-to-two pounds during the initial year of treatment, showing a rebound in growth by the second or later years of treatment.

Stimulants may increase heart rate, as well as systolic and diastolic blood pressure. These effects appear to be small (e.g., about five-to-fifteen beats per minute) and are clearly dose-dependent. The cardiovascular effects of stimulants are subject to tremendous intra- and inter-individual variability. Black adolescents may have a greater risk for developing an incre ase in diastolic blood pressure.

Effects on sleep seem insignificant other than the mild insomnia experienced by the majority of children on stimulants. Some patients have headaches, anxiousness, irritability, or are prone to crying.

All of the stimulants seem to reduce appetite to some degree, although this is temporary and mainly limited to the time of peak effects. Some patients have stomachaches when taking stimulants, but these are usually of mild severity.

High doses of stimulants may adversely impact learning or other higher mental functions. High doses may produce an over-focusing or constriction of attention and, perhaps, even a mental equivalent of motor stereotypies, such as perseverative responding or diminished flexibility in problem solving. High doses of stimulants may also cause a child to appear too controlled or socially aloof. Typically, there is deterioration in behavior that occurs in the late afternoon and evening following daytime administrations of medication. About a third of the children taking stimulants may have rebound effects.

There are a number of cases of irreversible Tourette syndrome associated with stimulant treatment. Current evidence, however, implies that when Tourette syndrome emerges in association with stimulant treatment, it may simply be coincidental in that the children were likely to have developed the disorder independent of stimulant treatment. Research indicates that less than one percent of ADHD children treated with stimulants will develop a tic disorder, and that in about ten percent of the cases, stimulants may exacerbate pre-existing tics. Although the vast majority of such reactions subside once the stimulant is discontinued, there are a few cases where the tics apparently did not diminish in frequency and severity following termination of treatments.

Stimulants at higher doses can produce stereotyped behaviors, and these are occasionally seen in children. Stimulants may also increase choreiform (jerking) movements and self-directed behavior such as lip-licking, lip-biting, and light picking of the fingertips (not the nails). At very high doses, stimulants can produce temporary symptoms of psychosis:

- Thought disorganization

- Pressure to keep talking

- Tactile hallucinations

- Extreme anxiety

- Hyperacusis (painful sensitiveness to sounds)

Researchers have not focused on the side effects of using stimulants over several years with children and adolescents. Nevertheless, from current data, there is no reason to suggest that chronic stimulant use may cause any significant disadvantages.

Dosages and Administration

When physicians initially prescribe medication, they should use low, single, daily doses. They then can increase the dosage on a weekly basis and evaluate the clinical effectiveness and adverse effects. Although body weight is probably not related to drug response, using it as a rough guideline for determining a starting dose continues to have some merit.

Because many schools are reluctant to disperse prescription medications, doctors place many children on sustained-release forms of stimulants. The sustained-release forms have several benefits, such as making noontime medication administration at school unnecessary and affording greater confidentiality of treatment. However, the sustained-release Ritalin may be less effective than the standard preparation, especially during the first several hours after taking it. It does not remain a therapeutic dose throughout the school day, and this causes some children to experience peaks and valleys throughout the day. The use of the shorter-acting forms of these medications may be more ideal except in situations where in-school administration of the drugs is a significant problem. The problems include the lack of a school nurse and teasing or censure of the patient by peers.

The decision to give drug-free holidays (such as weekends and vacations) depends on the desired therapeutic effect and on the occurrence of adverse effects like anorexia, weight loss, or failure to gain appropriate weight or height. If the patient takes the medication primarily for classroom management, the physician can discontinue the medication on weekends, holidays, and summer vacations. If reinitiating the medication each Monday produces a renewal of side effects exhibited only at the start of each week, keeping the child on one-half or less of the regular dose during the weekend may solve the problem. If a child exhibits significant behavioral control difficulties at home as well as in school, he should take the medication seven days a week.

The patient could have to take stimulants for periods varying from months to many years. The need for stimulant medications does not necessarily cease when he reaches adolescence, and for some, the need may persist into adulthood.

Antidepressants

Physicians prescribe antidepressants for severe, unremitting cases of depression, generally for those depressions that have no clear causal events. Antidepressants, however, can also alleviate some milder depressions. Antidepressants take away or reduce the symptoms of depression. Doctors also prescribe antidepressants for disorders characterized principally by anxiety. They can block the symptoms of panic, including rapid heartbeat, terror, dizziness, chest pains, nausea, and breathing problems. They can treat some phobias and obsessive-compulsive symptoms.

There are a number of antidepressant medications available. They differ in their side effects and, to some extent, in their level of effectiveness. The oldest types are monoamine oxidase inhibitors (MAOIs) and tricyclic antidepressants (TCAs), which have a chemical structure with a three-ring nucleus. The TCAs include ELAVIL (amitriptyline), NORPRAMIN (desipramine), SINEQUAN® (doxepin), TOFRANIL (imipramine), PAMELOR® or AVENTYL® (nortriptyline), VIVACTIL® (protriptyline), and SURMONTIL® (trimipramine). There are a number of more recent antidepressants that have various nontricyclic configurations. These include the serotonin reuptake inhibitors (SRIs) such as PROZAC (fluoxetine), LUVOX (fluvoxamine), ZOLOFT (sertraline), PAXIL (paroxetine), CELEXA (citalopram), EFFEXOR (venlafaxine), and SERZONE (nefazodone). Also in the category of newer drugs are REMERON® (mirtazapine), WELLBUTRIN (bupropion) and DESYREL (trazodone). Bupropion and trazodone are not chemically related to TCAs or SRIs. The newer antidepressants are generally about as effective as the TCAs, although side effects and time of onset of action may differ.

MAOIs help depression that shows atypical features such as hypersomnia (excessive sleep) and overeating. However, physicians who treat ASD patients rarely prescribe MAOIs. This is because use of MAOIs imposes certain dietary restrictions.

The primary cellular actions of the antidepressants are on the monoamine neurotransmitter system. The monoamine neurotransmitters include acetylcholine, norepinephrine, serotonin, and dopamine. Generally, the antidepressants act by influencing the metabolism and/or reuptake of these neurotransmitters, which results in functionally increased levels of available neurotransmitters.

The selection of antidepressants depends on specific symptoms and side effects. If there is no dominant symptom, an SRI is a reasonable choice. If the dominant symptom is anxiety, the doctor may first consider PAXIL or LUVOX. For individuals with atypical depression characterized by excessive sleepiness and voracious appetite (but little agitation and marked signs of social withdrawal), PROZAC may be the initial drug of choice. If the patient does not respond to a given drug after an adequate trial, the physician must consider switching to a medication with a different neurotransmitter effect. The physician may rapidly decrease the dosage of the ineffective medication while adding the new medication in increasing doses and then continue the new medication for an adequate trial period.

Treatment effects of antidepressants generally will not begin to show immediately. With most of these medications, it takes from one-to-three weeks before changes begin to occur. Some symptoms diminish early in treatment, while others take more time. Early responses include relief of both anxiety and insomnia. Even though the patient may state that the depression has not lifted, there is usually increased energy and less preoccupation with somatic concerns in the first several weeks of therapy. Mood and sexual dysfunction are often the last problems to be relieved.

A relationship between dose and plasma level cannot be clearly defined due to possible genetic differences in metabolism. However, research finds a correlation between clinical response and plasma concentration in certain psychiatric disorders. Studies in children with behavioral disorders show that clinical response roughly parallels the plasma level. For example, TOFRANIL has the best clinical response if plasma levels are about 200-250 µg/mL.

Dosage of antidepressants varies, depending on the type of drug and the person's body chemistry, age, and, sometimes, body weight. Physicians usually start with low dosages and gradually raise them until reaching the desired response without the appearance of troublesome side effects. The lag in clinical response may be as much as several weeks, but the side effects of these medications limit the clinician's ability to rapidly increase the dosage. The lag time is apparently related to delays in achieving therapeutic blood levels and the interval required to affect neurotransmitter systems. The patient should take the drug for several weeks at maximum doses before the doctor considers the treatment a failure.

Except for some early adjustments, the patient does not have to use divided doses of antidepressants—a single dose at bedtime is adequate, particularly when the clinician takes advantage of the sedative side effects to help treat associated insomnia. The bedtime dose helps achieve compliance since people tend to take drugs at bedtime and not during the day. Maintenance dosages of tricyclic antidepressants are usually one-half to one-third the amount needed by the individual for treatment of an acute episode. The dosage is maintained for several months, and after that the prescription is for the lowest effective dose for as long as the depression continues. This involves a gradual downward adjustment of the dosage until the individual requires no medication. A process usually takes six or more months from the start of the depression. There are a number of possible side effects with antidepressants, depending on the medication. Appendix G describes the potential side effects.

Obsessive-Compulsive Disorder Medications

There are two groups of medications that are effective in the treatment of obsessive-compulsive disorder. They are tricyclic antiobsessional antidepressant (ANAFRANIL) and serotonin reuptake inhibitors (SRIs) like PROZAC, LUVOX, ZOLOFT, PAXIL, and CELEXA.

Antianxiety Medications (Anxiolytics)

Anxiolytics are drugs whose primary purpose is to relieve anxiety arising in normal life or in nonpsychotic psychiatric disorders such as those classified in DSM or ICD as anxiety, adjustment, somatoform (presence of physical symptoms) disorders. This somewhat arbitrary definition distinguishes anxiolytics from other medications, such as antipsychotics or antidepressants, which are also used in the treatment of anxiety, but were developed primarily for psychotic or severe mood disorders.

The term "minor tranquilizer" is sometimes used to describe the medications in this category. However, the word "minor" does not mean "mild." It actually means that physicians prescribe these medications to reduce less severe symptoms of psychological dysfunction. Many clinicians say "minor" is an inappropriate terms. Frequently prescribed anxiolytic medications (benzodiazepines) include:

- XANAX (alprazolam)

- LIBRIUM or LIBRAX (chlordiazepoxide)

- VALIUM (diazepam)

- ATIVAN (lorazepam)

- KLONOPIN (clonazepam)

- HALCION (triazolam)

- DALMANE (flurazepam)

The properties of these benzodiazepines (BZDs) are quite similar to those of the sedative-hypnotics. The various sedative effects differ mainly in milligram potency, dose-response curves, and onset and duration of action. All are general depressants of brain function and decrease anxiety, except HALCION and DALMANE, which are marketed for sleep problems. To varying degrees, all have the potential for dependency with tolerance and severe withdrawal symptoms. They are addictive and have cross-tolerance and cross-dependence.

On the whole, low-potency or long-acting medications like VALIUM are preferable because researchers have studied their adverse effects more closely. Also, the high-potency and/or short-acting medications tend to cause more problems of dependence, rebound, and withdrawals. In the case of sleep disturbances, however, a short-acting drug may be preferable, particularly if the patient will take it for only a very few days.

BZDs differ in duration of action in different individuals. Patients may take them two-to-three times a day or sometimes only once a day. Physicians generally start dosage at a low level and gradually increase it until symptoms decrease or cease entirely. The dosage varies, depending on the symptoms and the individual's body chemistry. Except in emergencies or anticipated short-term use, the dosage begins with a low amount (twenty-five percent) and then increases slowly over intervals of several days (five-to-seven) to allow time for accumulation in fat stores and production of active metabolites.

BZDs often may help for a time and then seem to wear off. The patient then needs an increased dose to achieve the same effect. However, patients should not take BZDs for more than four months, and shorter periods are desirable. The objective is to give the smallest therapeutic dose for the shortest time, but this is particularly important with anxiolytics since both duration and dose are correlated with adverse effects.

Researchers have not conducted many studies about anxiolytics in children and adolescents. Therefore, there is no established role or dosage. Since adolescents are often exposed to pressures to abuse drugs, and there are pharmacological similarities and cross-tolerance with alcohol, the anxiolytics, particularly BZDs, are not medications to be prescribed lightly.

A newer category of non-sedating, non-addictive anxiolytic drugs (e.g., BUSPAR) is now available. Its molecular structure is uniquely different from the rest of the anxiolytics. It also lacks their hypnotic, anticonvulsant, and muscle-relaxant properties. Therefore, it differs from the BZDs in that it does not impair motor skills. The new drugs do not appear to act synergistically with alcohol, and they are likely to possess a much lower potential for abuse, dependence, and withdrawal than the BZDs. Despite having no FDA-approved indications for use with persons younger than eighteen, the use of buspirone (BUSPAR) with children and adolescents is of great interest to child psychiatrists because of its minimal sedation and low potential for abuse.

Sedative-Hypnotics

Sedative-hypnotics (sometimes called depressants) sedate, calm, or relax most individuals at low doses and, at somewhat higher doses, induce sleep. The hypnotic effect of the medication-induced sleep is very different from the phenomena associated with hypnosis. The confusion is because we once believed that hypnosis induced a sleep-like trance. However, we now know that hypnotized people are very much awake. Many medications in this class, such as MEBARAL, are effective in reducing seizure activity and may be termed anticonvulsants. Physicians can also use these medications as muscle relaxants, although muscle relaxation is secondary to their effects on the CNS. Frequently used sedative-hypnotics are AQUACHLORAL® (chloral hydrate), ATARAX/VISTARIL (hydroxyzine), barbiturates (secobarbital, phenobarbital, and pentobarbital), BENADRYL® (diphenhydramine), and PHENERGAN® (promethazine).

The highly addicting medications with a narrow margin of safety, such as DORIDEN® (glutethimide), QUAALUDE® (methaqualone), and the barbiturates (with the exception of phenobarbital), should be avoided.

Anticholinergics

Anticholinergic drugs, such as COGENTIN (benztropine) and ARTANE (trihexyphenidyl), reverse the extrapyramidal side effects of the conventional antipsychotics. As such, the drug interaction is beneficial.

Opiate Blockers

There are medications with relatively pure, opiate-blocking properties that act by competitive binding at opioid (opiate-related) receptors. They can reduce the subjective effects of opiate narcotics and help reverse respiratory and cardiovascular depression caused by the overdose of opiates. Doctors use the opiate blockers to treat individuals with self-injury, social withdrawal, and ADHD. There are two frequently used opiate blockers: TREXAN (naltrexone) and NARCAN (naloxone).

Beta (β)-Adrenergic Blockers (β-Blockers or Beta Blockers)

Beta-adrenergic receptors are activated by adrenergic sympathetic nervous transmission and by endocrine catecholamines like noradrenaline. β-blockers can work on both β_1 and β_2 receptors. β_1 receptors are found mainly in the heart and brain, whereas the β_2 receptors are involved in the functioning of vascular, bronchial, and gastrointestinal organs. β_1-blockers tend to decrease heart rate, cardiac output, blood pressure, and maximum exercise tolerance. They also treat abnormal heartbeat (antiarrhythmic effect).

β_2-blockers block the action of sympathomimetic amines, leading to increase in airway resistance, which is potentially dangerous in asthma. INDERAL (propranolol) is the prototype of β-blockers. Psychiatrists use it to treat aggression and anxiety.

Alpha (α)-Adrenergic Agonists

The alpha-adrenergic receptor agonists stimulate presynaptic autoreceptors, leading to the release of noradrenaline, lowering of blood serotonin, and increase of dopamine turnover. They are primarily anti-hypertensive agents; however, they can help reduce over-excitability, over-stimulation, and impulsivity seen in patients with ADHD. They can also treat Tourettesyndrom, sleep problems, aggression, stuttering, and anxiety disorders. Two frequently used α-adrenergic agonists are CATAPRES (clonidine) and TENEX® (guanfacine).

Antimanics

Antimanics help in the treatment of manic symptoms, but they can also treat other symptoms that appear to be only tangentially related to mood. Since these medications decrease rapid mood swings, from mania to depression, physicians sometimes call them *mood stabilizers*. Although the antipsychotics effectively reduce manic symptoms and are often used for the initial treatment of mania, they are generally not used for chronic treatment in affective disorders because of their potentially severe side effects. There has not been a study of these medications in individuals with both ASD and mania because the latter disorder has rarely, if ever, been reported in individuals with ASD.

The medication of choice is generally a lithium salt, such as lithium carbonate (LITHOBID or ESKALITH). There are alternatives to lithium, including DEPAKOTE (divalproex sodium), DEPAKENE (valproic acid), TEGRETOL (carbamazepine), KLONOPIN (clonazepam), and CALAN® (verapamil).

Other Psychotherapeutic Medications

There are a few other medications that have been tried in individuals with ASD: PONDIMIN (fenfluramine), synthetic ACTH analog, ORG 2766, and SECRETIN. See Appendix G for information.

Chapter 9

Generic Drugs

In 1950s, legislatures in the United States passed anti-substitution laws to curb the marketing of counterfeit drugs. These laws require pharmacists to dispense only the brand of drug that the physician prescribes. To encourage original research and new drug development, brand-name drug firms can have at least five years of exclusive marketing after New Drug Application (NDA) approval. After the patent of the brand-name drug expires, other companies can submit an Abbreviated New Drug Application (ANDA) to produce "generic drugs."

During the 1970s, states began to repeal their anti-substitution laws in the belief that consumers could save money through the availability of generic drugs. The repeal of anti-substitution laws or the enactment of drug product selection acts allowed replacement of brand-name pharmaceuticals with generically equivalent drug products. The laws vary from state to state, but their underlying purpose is the same: reducing prescription drug costs. Cost reductions result from the availability of lower cost generics and from price competition between brand-name and generic drugs.

In 1984, Congress passed the Drug Price Competition and Patent Term Restoration Act in order to provide an expedited approval process and reduce the cost of generic drugs. This act enticed many pharmaceutical companies to enter the billion-dollar, generic-drug market. Generic manufacturers, as well as brand-name manufacturers, produce generic drugs. Additionally, many brand-name manufacturers distribute, under their own names, products manufactured by generic companies. Brand-name manufacturers account for seventy-to-eighty percent of the generic drug market.

According to the law of many states, when a pharmacist receives a prescription for a brand-name drug, he or she may dispense (or the individual may request) a generically equivalent drug. However, the pharmacist cannot dispense a generically equivalent drug that is more expensive than the brand-name drug. If the dispensed drug is not the prescribed brand, the pharmacist must indicate on the prescription label both the brand prescribed and the brand dispensed.

Additional impetus for being cost-conscious comes from Medicaid and third-party insurance carriers who have regulations that stipulate the maximum dollar amount that they will reimburse for a given quantity of a given drug. This amount (frequently called maximum allowable cost or MAC) is usually determined by the cost of generically equivalent drugs.

Any savings from dispensing a generically equivalent drug must be passed on to the individual or the third-party payment source. Because of various factors, including the frequency of drug use, availability from only one manufacturer, the cost of filling a prescription, and the mark-up of the pharmacist, the average savings of prescribing the least expensive generic drugs is about five percent. Of course, savings in individual situations can be very much greater. On the other hand, the lower wholesale cost of the generic drugs is sometimes not fully reflected in the retail prices of those drugs.

What Is a Generic Drug?

A generic drug is basically a copy of a brand-name drug. It is a product that may have a different color, flavor, or shape, but it contains the same active ingredients and is identical in strength or concentration, dosage form, and route of administration as the brand-name drug. The drug companies formulate the product to meet the same or comparable standards of quality, purity, identity, and bioavailability. (Bioavailability is the rate and extent to which the active drug ingredient is absorbed into the body and becomes available to its site of action.) The drug companies must adequately label the generic and manufacture it in compliance with the same Current Good Manufacturing Practice regulations as the brand-name drug. However, manufacturers of generic drugs approved by the ANDA process do not have to resubmit documentation of the drug's safety and efficacy. Legal standards for purity, quality, strength, labeling, and packaging for drugs marketed are listed in the *United States Pharmacopeia (USP)*. This official book provides detailed identification and assay techniques, as well as dissolution standards for drugs.

The FDA sets the standards and reviews all drugs before they are marketed. Although generic drugs in general are "chemically equivalent," they are not necessarily "therapeutically equivalent" to brand-name drugs. The FDA lists drugs that are therapeutically equivalent in the annual *Approved Drug Products with Therapeutic Equivalence Evaluations (Approved Drug Products),* which is also known as the "orange book." Over eighty percent of the 8000-plus products listed in *Approved Drug Products* have been determined to be therapeutically equivalent. The FDA only recommends substitution among products that are listed as therapeutically equivalent in this publication. About half of all current prescription medications have a generic version.

Controversy over Generic and Brand-Name Drugs

The Food and Drug Administration says consumers can have confidence in the purity and efficacy of those generic drugs it has declared equivalent to a brand-name drug. The FDA says approved generic substitutes should render the same therapeutic benefit. But as more and more manufacturers enter the billion-dollar generic drug market, the potential for lost profits has prompted brand-name pharmaceutical manufacturers to campaign against generic drugs and publicize the merits of brand-name products. Some consumers also insist that they can tell the difference between generic and brand-name drugs.

There has been an increase in reports concerning lack of efficacy and safety of generic drugs. During a nine-month period in 1997, doctors reported to the FDA's MedWatch program more than 400 "adverse events" that occurred after substituting generics for brand-name drugs.

Some Physicians Are Skeptical About Generic Drugs

Not all doctors are comfortable recommending a generic alternative, even though the FDA determines that a generic is therapeutically equivalent to its brand-name counterpart before approving it for marketing. A recent survey of consumers showed that only fifty percent said their physicians had ever mentioned generic drugs to them. Failure to raise the subject could be due, in part, to a doctor's mixed feelings about generic alternatives. For more than a decade, use of generic drugs has remained at about forty percent of the prescriptions written, far below the estimated potential of seventy-five percent.

Laws in some states allow doctors to prohibit the filling of prescriptions with generic equivalents by writing the prescription with the notation, "dispense only as written" or similar language.

A major area of concern for physicians is the generic substitution for certain categories of medications, known as narrow therapeutic index or critical dose drugs. Questions about this small category of drugs have muddied the water and made physicians more leery about going the generic route. Among the groups of drugs that some pharmacists and physicians believe could have a narrow therapeutic window are certain anticoagulants, estrogen products, psychotherapeutic medications, antiarrhythmic drugs, anti-rejection medications, and cancer chemotherapeutic agents.

What Is a Preferred Drug List?

To hold down costs, managed-care health plans and pharmacies are pushing drug substitutions. They are switching patients from brand-name to generic drugs, from one generic version to another, or from one brand to another. Some health plans have developed a Preferred Drug List, which includes both generic and brand-name prescription medications that the FDA has approved. The physicians affiliated with these health care plans are "encouraged" to prescribe medications that are on the list. Cost is an important factor in a health care providers' selection of the "preferred drugs." A physician who has carefully adjusted the dose of a drug to a patient's individual requirements for chronic therapy could be reluctant to surrender control over the source of the drug that the patient receives.

A member's (patient's) prescription drug benefit program determines coverage of preferred or non-preferred medications. Some members may not have coverage for non-preferred products, while others could have to pay a higher copayment for non-preferred medications. If a member uses a participating pharmacy, and the prescribed drug is on the preferred list, the pharmacy will fill and dispense the prescription. If the prescribed drug is not on the Preferred Drug List, the pharmacist will usually make a reasonable effort to contact the member's doctor and ask if a preferred alternative is appropriate.

Be more aware and concerned about the growing tendency of pharmacies to switch a prescription to a drug with a different chemical composition based on the Preferred Drug List.

What Can a Consumer Do?

Generic drugs are thirty-to-sixty percent less expensive than their brand-name counterparts. By using generic drugs, one can save money but lose the power in making drug choices and risk treatment effectiveness. As mentioned earlier, state laws allow substitution of brand-name drugs with generic drugs. Some state laws require substitution unless the prescribing physician specifies otherwise. However, the FDA has not recognized all generic drugs as equivalent to the brand-name counterparts. If your child's physician prescribes generic drugs, ask the physician or the pharmacist whether the prescribed generic drugs are in the FDA's "orange book." You can also obtain the information on the agency's website at www.fda.gov/cder/drug.htm.

If you insist that your child be given brand-name medications, you can request that doctors write "dispense as written" or "DAW" on the prescriptions. However, keep in mind that "DAW" should not be used unnecessarily because generic drugs can provide significant cost savings.

Regarding the practice of adhering to the Preferred Drug List, you should support or work with consumer advocate groups or organizations to make states pass a law that would stipulate the drug formularies—or preferred lists of covered drugs—allow for exceptions when medically necessary.

Chapter 10

Selecting Medications for Neuropsychiatric Disorders

This chapter provides information on clinical features of co-existing neuropsychiatric disorders or conditions frequently seen in individuals with ASD, as well as recommendations for choosing effective medications for each disorder or condition. However, this chapter is not a substitute for an informed discussion between you and your child's physician about the diagnosis and the selection of appropriate medications. **You must always discuss treatments with the doctor because this chapter is neither medical advice, nor is it in any way a substitute for a physician's expertise**.

This chapter describes a decision-making process that incorporates a growing database for the optimum use of medication therapies in clinical practice. When sufficient research data are lacking, I offer suggestions based on my own clinical and research experience. The goal is to provide an understandable, logical, treatment strategy so that you will be able to discuss your child's treatment with a doctor who is not familiar with ASD.

Clinical Indications for Medication Therapy

There are two main classes of indication for psychopharmacotherapy: the disorder and the behavior or symptom. While this distinction can be rather artificial at times, at other times it is very real. For example, if a child has a clear diagnosis of ADHD (disorder indication) and also exhibits severe self-injurious behavior for no apparent reason (behavioral/symptomatic indication), he would need medications that treat both a disorder and a symptom.

There are relatively high frequencies of comorbid (co-existing) neuropsychiatric disorders or conditions in ASD if the DSM-IV or ICD-10 diagnostic criteria are modified for use in the ASD population. For example, The DSM-IV and ICD-10 diagnostic criteria for OCD requires the presence of ego-dystonic obsession (intrusive thoughts that are beyond one's control). However, the diagnosis of OCD may be considered in lower-functioning and non-verbal individuals if they show repetitive behaviors that appear to be controlled by some thoughts. Another example is making a diagnosis of major depression in non-verbal and/or lower-functioning individuals, even in the absence of subjectively reported depressed mood, worry, guilty feeling, and suicidal ideation as required by the DSM-IV and ICD-10.

To be more relevant to people with ASD, this chapter does not list the "diagnostic criteria" for various psychiatric disorders, as specified by the DSM-IV and ICD-10. Instead, it describes core features of various neuropsychiatric disorders and symptom clusters as indications for considering medication therapy.

Obsessive-Compulsive Disorder (OCD)

Approximately seventy-five percent of children with autistic disorder have difficulty in adapting to new situations, are disturbed by changes in the familiar environment, and show a resistance to learning or practicing a new activity. About fifty-to-eighty percent of these children have unusual preoccupations:

- Attachments to unusual objects, rituals or compulsions (such as insisting on certain foods)

- Repeating dialogue from radio and television

- Spending a great deal of time memorizing weather information, state capitals, or birth dates of family members

- Continually talking about and playing with a single toy

- Repetitively writing or drawing numbers, words, pictures, or maps

About fifty percent of children with autistic disorder have unusual sensory interests. In high-functioning adults with autistic disorder, about eighty-five percent continue to demonstrate stereotyped, compulsive behaviors, including arranging objects.

Due to difficulties in communicating with other people, as well as showing appropriate affect, individuals with ASD do not seem to resist their compulsions, complain about the compulsive acts, or manifest distress. This raises the possibility that clinicians may hesitate to diagnose superimposed OCD in persons with ASD. However, some of these obsessive and/or compulsive symptoms have obvious similarities to those seen in OCD. In some higher-functioning individuals with ASD, the symptoms and behaviors described above could possibly be features of a co-existing OCD but were never recognized. Several investigators have reported cases with both ASD and OCD.

Obsessions

These are persistent, anxiety-provoking, unwanted ideas, thoughts, images, or impulses that repeatedly well up in the mind of the person with OCD. Impulses or images include aggressive or horrific impulses and sexual imagery. These thoughts, impulses, and images are intrusive (ego-dystonic), unpleasant, and produce a high degree of anxiety. Unwanted ideas or thoughts include:

- Persistent fears that harm may come to oneself or a loved one

- A belief that one has a terrible illness

- Repeated thoughts about contamination

- Repeated doubts

- Religious scrupulousness

- An excessive need for symmetry or exactness, or an excessive need to do things perfectly or in an exact order

Compulsions

Compulsions are repetitive behaviors in response to obsessions (i.e., intended to ward off harm to the person with OCD). Some people with OCD have regimented rituals, while others have rituals that are complex and changing. The compulsions include:

- Washing

- Checking

- Counting

- Repeating words silently

- Hoarding

- Endlessly rearranging objects in an effort to keep them in precise alignment.

Other Characteristics

Most of the time, people with OCD know that their obsessive thoughts are senseless and that their compulsions are not really necessary. Most people with OCD struggle to banish their unwanted, obsessive thoughts and keep themselves from engaging in compulsive behaviors.

- People with OCD often attempt to hide their disorder rather than seek help. They are often successful in concealing their obsessive-compulsive symptoms from friends and co-workers.

- OCD tends to last for years, even decades. The symptoms may become less severe from time to time, but they are usually chronic.

- People with OCD struggle against their compulsions. They often develop a dysphoric mood and become irritable, tense, and depressed.

Medication Treatment for OCD

Treatment of OCD with mild symptoms:

- Start with behavioral therapy

- If response is insufficient, add an SRI or ANAFRANIL (as the last choice in individuals prone to seizure disorders)

- If response is still insufficient, sequential trials of other SRIs (e.g., PROZAC, then LUVOX, PAXIL, ZOLOFT, CELEXA, etc.)

Treatment of OCD with moderate-to-severe symptoms

- Start with an SRI plus behavioral therapy

- If the response is insufficient, use sequential trials of other SRIs or ANAFRANIL (as the last choice in individuals with history of seizures, or current seizure disorder)

- If response is still insufficient, add BUSPAR or KLONOPIN

Maintenance Medication Therapy for OCD

Clear clinical evidence indicates that most individuals relapse if SRIs are discontinued

- Continue the medication for six months, then taper the dose gradually until symptoms re-emerge

- Revert to the dose used immediately prior to the symptoms' re-emergence, with indefinite length of therapy and follow up with the prescribing physician every two-to-three months

Quasi-Obsessive-Compulsive Disorder

In individuals with ASD and the above unusual behaviors, such as resistance to change, ritualistic/compulsive behaviors, and unusual attachment, that severely interfere with their daily functioning, they may not receive a full diagnosis of OCD based on DSM-IV/ICD-10 criteria. However, their clinical manifestations can be considered variants of OCD, and they should be treated in a similar fashion.

Tic Disorders

Many individuals with ASD, particularly with autistic disorder, display tic-like symptoms like grimacing, hand flapping or twisting, toe walking, lunging, jumping, darting or pacing, body rocking and swaying, and head rolling or banging. In some cases the symptoms appear intermittently, whereas in other cases they are continuously present. They are usually interrupted by episodes of immobility and odd posturing with head bowed and arms flexed at the elbow. Some of these symptoms have obvious similarities to those seen in tic disorders.

Studies report that about seventy percent of people with autistic disorder had stereotyped hand-finger mannerisms and/or stereotyped utterances. Twenty-five to forty percent had self-injury and about ten percent had tics. There are some recent studies describing the development of Tourette syndrome in individuals with autistic disorder. It is unclear, however, how frequently the two disorders might occur coincidentally. It is also uncertain how this finding might be linked to the etiology of the two disorders.

What Are Tics?

A tic is a sudden, involuntary, rapid, recurrent, non-rhythmic, stereotyped motor movement or pattern of vocalization.

- The motor tics most commonly involve the head, but could involve the torso and limbs.

- Coprolalia (uncontrolled shouting of obscenities), is the phonic tic in thirty percent of cases.

- Tics are experienced as irresistible, but can be suppressed for varying lengths of time.

- Tics are exacerbated by stress and decreased during absorbing activities.

- Sleep greatly reduces symptoms.

- Tics wax and wane over weeks to months.

- Diagnostically, tic disorders can be sub-classified based on duration and variety of tics.

- Transient tic disorder includes motor or vocal tics lasting for at least four weeks, but for no longer than twelve consecutive months.

- Tourette syndrome and chronic motor or vocal disorder can have a duration of more than twelve months. Tourette syndrome differs from the others in that diagnosis requires multiple motor tics and at least one vocal tic.

- Common simple motor tics include eye blinking, neck jerking, shoulder shrugging, and facial grimacing.

- Common simple vocal tics include throat clearing, grunting, sniffing, snorting, coughing, and barking.

- Common complex motor tics include facial gestures, grooming behaviors, jumping, touching, stamping, and smelling an object.

- Common complex vocal tics include repeating words or phrases out of context, corpolalia (use of socially unacceptable words, frequently obscene), palilalia (repeating one's own sounds or words), and echolalia (repeating other people's words).

- Rare complications of severe tic disorders include self-injurious behaviors (head banging, striking oneself, picking skin) and orthopedic problems (from knee bending, neck jerking, or head turning).

Medication Treatment of Tic Disorders

Severity of symptoms varies between individuals, and only children and adults whose relationships, performance, and self-esteem are impaired should be considered for medication treatment.

- Start with HALDOL

- If response is insufficient, switch to ORAP

- If response is insufficient with either HALDOL or ORAP, switch to CATAPRES

- If response is still insufficient, use one of the above medications and add an SRI or serial trials of SRIs

- If all the above medications have failed to show significant efficacy, consider either RISPERDAL or calcium channel blockers like CALAN and ADALAT

Trichotillomania

A symptom of trichotillomania is the impulse to pull out one's hair, often involving multiple sites. Some clinicians think that this condition is a variant of OCD, based on similarities in symptoms, family history, and response to treatment.

Medication Treatment of Trichotillomania

- Start with HALDOL

- If the response is insufficient, switch to a drug like ORAP or lithium

- If the above medications do not produce a sufficient response, choose the one with the best response and add an SRI or sequential trials of SRIs

Attention Deficit Hyperactivity Disorder

Many young children with ASD are markedly overactive. The literature reports that about fifty percent of children with autistic disorder were hyperactive, impulsive, and had poor attention and concentration. A significant number of children with ASD may conceivably have co-existing attention deficit hyperactivity disorder (ADHD).

Two core symptom clusters characterize the essential features of ADHD: inattention and hyperactivity/impulsivity in two or more settings (home, school, physician's office, etc.). The classic presentation involving both symptom clusters is called ADHD, combined type. Individuals with prominent symptoms from only one cluster may have the diagnoses of ADHD, predominately inattentive type, or ADHD, predominately hyperactive type.

Symptoms of ADHD

Symptoms of Inattention

- Failure to give close attention to detail

- Careless mistakes in schoolwork, homework, etc.

- Difficulty in sustaining attention in tasks or at play

- Failure to listen when spoken to directly

- Failure to follow through on instruction

- Failure to complete schoolwork, chores, or job duties

- Difficulty in organizing tasks and activities

- Reluctance to engage in tasks that require sustained mental effort (or avoiding tasks altogether)

- Losing things necessary for tasks or activities

- Easily distracted by extraneous stimuli

- Forgetfulness in daily activities.

Symptoms of Hyperactivity

- Excessively fidgeting with hands or feet

- Squirming in seat or leaving seat in classroom or in other situations where remaining seated is expected

- Running about or climbing excessively

- Difficulty in playing or engaging in leisure activities quietly

- On the go as if driven by a motor; excessive talking

Symptoms of Impulsivity

- Blurting out answers before hearing the entire questions

- Difficulty in waiting for a turn in games

- Often interrupting or intruding on others

Problems persist into adolescence and adulthood in approximately 30-to70% percent of patients.

Medication Treatment of ADHD

In low- or middle-functioning individuals with ASD or higher-functioning individuals with other neurological disorders such as seizure disorders, Tourette syndrome, etc., the following may be necessary:

- Begin sequential monotherapy trials with CATAPRES, TENEX, and HALDOL for hyperactivity and impulsiveness, or

- Begin sequential monotherapy trials with TCAs (TOFRANIL, NORPRAMIN, PAMELOR), WELLBUTRIN, PROZAC, and NALTREXONE for inattention, impulsiveness, and other hyperactivity problems

In higher-functioning individuals without other neurological disorders:

- Monotherapy begins with RITALIN or DEXEDRINE

- If no response or insufficient response, sequential monotherapy trials with RITALIN or DEXEDRINE (the one that has not yet been used), ADDERALL, or CONCERTA begin

- If no response or insufficient response, monotherapy with CYLERT begins

- If the response is still insufficient with all of the above stimulants, the physician can conduct sequential trials with TCAs, WELLBUTRIN, NALTREXONE, PROZAC, CATAPRES, and TENEX

Disturbances in Mood and Affect, Including Depression and Bi-Polar Disorder

All forms of mood and affective disorder occur in persons with ASD who are less likely to seek or be referred for help for subjective dysphoria. In the absence of problematic behavior, caregivers often ignore depression and social withdrawal. For those affectively disordered who have disruptive symptoms, there is a tendency to focus on the problem behaviors without sufficient attention to the underlying affective disturbance.

The affective (emotional) expression of persons with ASD may be flattened, excessive, or inappropriate to the situation. Their mood is often unstable; sobbing, crying, or screaming episodes may be unexplained or inconsolable. Periodic laughing and giggling may occur for no obvious reason. Major depression may occur during adolescence and adult life. Major depressive disorder can also occur in children as young as six years-of-age, based on the same diagnostic criteria used for adults.

Depression may develop when a person realizes, at least partially, that he has a handicap. This is more likely in those with higher levels of ability. However, depression can also occur in lower-functioning individuals. One study reported that about ten percent of children with autistic disorder had depressive mood, about forty percent had irritability or agitation, about thirty percent showed inappropriate affect, and ten percent had sleep problems. Investigators have reported cases with both autistic disorder and unipolar or bipolar affective disorders.

The essential features of depressive disorders include the following symptoms:

- Depressed mood as indicated by either subjective report or other people's observation (in children and adolescents this can be irritable mood, sad expression, sad tone of voice, or fearfulness)

- Diminished interest or pleasure in all, or almost all, activities, including a change in responding to behavioral "rewards"

- Significant weight loss when not dieting, weight gain, or decrease or increase in appetite

- Insomnia or hypersomnia

- Psychomotor agitation or retardation

- Fatigue or loss of energy

- Somatic complaints such as headaches or gastrointestinal distress

- Feeling of worthlessness or inappropriate guilt

- Diminished ability to think or concentrate

- Indecisiveness

- Inability to perform usual activities of daily living or prevocational tasks

- Deterioration in self-care (poor hygiene)

- Increased self-injurious behaviors and stereotypies

- Recurrent thoughts of death, recurrent suicidal ideation without a specific plan, a suicide attempt, or a specific plan of committing suicide

- Psychotic features, including mood-related or unrelated delusions, and hallucinations, although these occur infrequently

Types of Depressive Disorders

Major Depressive Disorder, Bipolar Versus Unipolar

The crucial element of both bipolar and unipolar disorders is the occurrence of an affective episode. The very important distinction is that a bipolar disorder includes hypomanic, manic, depressive, and mixed episodes, whereas a unipolar disorder includes only depressive episodes.

In bipolar disorder, a continuum of severity in both the manic and the depressive phases can range from non-psychotic to psychotic, to delirious or stupor. The interplay between mania and depression is integral to understanding bipolar disorder. Thus, depression may:

- Precede an episode of hypomania or mania

- Intermingle with manic symptoms during an acute exacerbation (e.g., mixed episodes)

- Succeed a hypomanic or manic phase

- Occur as a distinct episode in an intermittent and irregularly alternating pattern with hypomanic or manic episodes

These clinical presentations have important implications for management because drug treatment of the depressive phase may precipitate a manic swing or a more virulent course of the illness. Therefore, if bipolar disorder exists or is suspected, individuals in the depressed phase are best managed by using a combination of a mood stabilizer and an antidepressant.

Melancholia (Classic Depression)

This subtype of major depressive disorder (MDD) has features that distinguish it from other subtypes of MDD. These features include:

- A profoundly depressed mood and appearance

- Anhedonia (loss of capacity to experience pleasure)

- Accompanying feelings of helplessness, hopelessness, worthlessness, and guilt over imagined "sins"

- Problems with initial, middle, and terminal insomnia

- Significant anorexia, often with appreciable weight loss

- Obvious psychomotor retardation or agitation

- An absence of mood reactivity

- A diurnal variation in the severity of symptoms

- Age of onset in the mid-forties

Atypical (Non-Classic Depression)

Clinical presentations of this MDD subtype include:

- Hypersomnia

- Hyperphagia (ingestion of a greater than optimal quantity of food)

- Psychomotor agitation

- Anxious or irritable mood

- Rejection hypersensitivity

- Age of onset in the mid-twenties

Psychotic or Delusional Depression

Psychotic depression is often characterized by the presence of mood-congruent (the symptom is consistent with the mood state) delusions or hallucinations. Examples include the false belief that:

- Others have malicious intent toward him because he is perceived as "too smart"

- One is being unfairly punished because of having "Asperger Syndrome"

The presence of delusions may lead to an erroneous diagnosis of schizophrenia in younger patients or dementia with paranoia in the elderly.

Dysthymia

Dysthymia represents a chronic, but less severe, form of depression. Depressed mood and partial neurovegetative symptoms are typically present for sustained periods, sometimes years.

Dual Depression

Individuals who meet criteria for both MDD and dysthymia have a "double" or "dual" depression.

Seasonal Affective Disorder

Seasonal affective disorder (SAD) is a recurrent depressive illness that regularly coincides with particular seasons. The two predominant presentations have bimodal peaks of depression onset, either in the spring or in the fall. There appears to be a correlation with age, such that the mean age of onset is in the mid-twenties.

Mixed Anxiety and Depression

The most frequent combinations of anxiety and mood disorders include:

- Panic disorder and major depression

- Panic attacks and major depression

- Obsessive-compulsive disorder and major depression

- Generalized anxiety and major depression

- Agoraphobia and major depression

Depression Associated with Medical Disorders

Physical problems that may complicate or underlie a depressive condition include:

- Subclinical hypothyroidism

- Malabsorption due to various gastrointestinal conditions (e.g., Crohn's disease)

- Unrecognized malignancies

- Neurological diseases (e.g., Parkinson and Huntington)

- Chronic renal failure

- Co-existing dementia

- Autoimmune disorders

Premenstrual Dysphoric Disorder

Premenstrual dysphoric disorder (PMDD) affects three-to-eight percent of women in their reproductive years. Unlike the much milder and more prevalent premenstrual syndrome (PMS), PMDD's symptoms can include persistent irritability or marked anger, mood changes, tension, marked anxiety, dysphoria, hopelessness, self-deprecation, fatigue, decreased energy, dyssomnia, appetite fluctuations, and feeling out of control.

Drug-Induced Depression

Conditions mimicking MDD can occur secondary to a wide variety of prescribed drugs like RESERPINE, METHYLDOPA or alcohol abuse and dependence.

Treatment-Resistant Depression

This is persistence of a significant depression for at least six weeks despite appropriate treatment, such as a course of treatment with an SRI antidepressant at the minimal effective dose or a TCA at therapeutic plasma concentrations. The most common causes for no response to antidepressants are:

- Incorrect diagnosis

- Noncompliance with the medication regimen

- Subtherapeutic doses

- Insufficient time on treatment

- Not addressed and ameliorated significant psychosocial stressors

Medication Treatment of Depression

When selecting an antidepressant (AD), always consider the following:

- If the individual (or a family member) has had a previous positive response to a particular drug, consider it a first choice

- Number and quality of controlled trials, including data on effectiveness for severe, as well as milder, episodes

- Years and characteristics of patients treated in terms of age, health status, and concurrent medications

- Safety and tolerability, keeping in mind that these are different concepts (i.e., a treatment may be safe but poorly tolerated, whereas another treatment is well-tolerated but with a low margin of safety)

- Likelihood of pharmacokinetic or pharmacodynamic interactions, with the goal of minimizing adverse interactions with other drugs or medical conditions

- Ease of taking the AD to maximize the likelihood of treating the patient with the optimal dose and facilitating patient compliance

If individuals have predominant symptoms of insomnia or psychomotor agitation, a more sedating drug (e.g., amitriptyline, doxepin, or DESYREL) may initially benefit, but could later cause problems in therapy.

Individuals with cardiovascular disorders, or those predisposed to anticholergenic adverse effects (e.g., elderly or diabetic patients), do best on drugs low in these effects (e.g., NORPRAMIN, DESYREL, WELLBUTRIN, SRIs, EFFEXOR, and SERZONE). Patients with an eating disorder (anorexia or bulimia) or a history of seizures should not take WELLBUTRIN because there is an increased risk of seizures.

Highly suicidal individuals should only take medications posing less risk of death with an overdose and less risk of interacting with other drugs taken in an attempt to overdose (e.g., ZOLOFT and EFFEXOR).

When a patient has psychotic symptoms, the doctor should prescribe a combination of an AD plus antipsychotic (AP). As an alternative, the doctor can institute a trial with electric shock treatment (ECT).

Advantages of many of the newer ADs are simplicity of use and freedom from some of the more dangerous adverse effects of the TCAs.

There are no compelling data to support the overall efficacy of one SRI over another. Patients who do not respond well to one SRI will respond to a second trial with another SRI. Therefore, it may be more prudent to switch to a class of ADs with a different mechanism of action.

Administration of Antidepressants

Standard doses of ADs, especially in the earliest phases of therapy, can heighten anxiety, irritability, and restlessness. As a result, the physician should start with low doses and use a gradual upward dosage adjustment (titration), as tolerated. A slower titration in the earliest phases of treatment or the judicious addition of an anxiolytic helps.

Most ADs have a delayed onset of action, and individuals may not experience substantial relief for two or more weeks. Therefore, additional medications may be appropriate during the early phase of treatment to provide more rapid relief. One common example is the concurrent use of benzodiazepines (BZDs) to relieve associated insomnia or severe anxiety.

The patient's psychomotor agitation or retardation often improves first, followed by concentration and increased capacity for interpersonal contact. Subjective sense of depression, anhedonia, and hopelessness may not improve until the fourth-to-sixth week of treatment.

An adequate AD trial involves an adequate dose for an adequate period of time. If the depressive episode does not stop after this trial, sequential trials with alternate ADs (usually from a different class) or use of an augmenting agent are the most common strategies.

Treatment Phases

MDD is frequently a recurrent illness. Therefore; treatment is divided into three phases:

- Acute therapy to induce a remission

- Maintenance therapy to prevent a relapse into the current episode

- Prophylactic therapy to prevent recurrence of MDDafter at least six months of full remission from a prior episode.

Medication Treatment of an Acute Depressive Episode

Major Depressive Disorder (Mild to Moderate, Single or Recurrent)

There are three ways to initiate treatment. The physician could start with an SRI, EFFEXOR, or SERZONE. If a previous AD was effective in the patient or a family member, he may prescribe it. The third medication treatment is using a heterocyclic AD such as NORPRAMIN. If its side effects are tolerated, a secondary amine TCA could be chosen.

- If response is partial, combine with lithium or a thyroid supplement or PINDOLOL

- If the response is insufficient, use two different ADs concurrently (e.g., slowly add an SRI to a TCA)

- If psychosis emerges, add an antipsychotic (e.g., HALDOL or RISPERDAL)

- If the response is still insufficient, add ECT

Major Depressive Disorder with Marked Anxiety, Panic Attacks, or Agitation

- Start with BZD or DESYREL, plus an AD (not with SERZONE)

- If the response is insufficient, switch the AD class [e.g., NORPRAMIN (a heterocyclic AD) to PAXIL (an SRI)]

- If response is insufficient, add an AD of another class (e.g., WELLBUTRIN, an aminoketone)

- If response is insufficient, add a mood stabilizer such as DEPAKOTE

- If psychosis emerges, add an antipsychotic (e.g., HALDOL or RISPERDAL)

- If response is still insufficient, add ECT

Bipolar Depressive Disorder

- Start with an AD plus a mood stabilizer

- If response is partial, combine with lithium or a thyroid supplement or PINDOLOL

- If the response is still insufficient, use two different ADs concurrently (e.g., slowly add an SRI to a TCA)

- If psychosis emerges, add an antipsychotic (e.g., HALDOL or RISPERDAL)

- If response is still insufficient, add ECT

Atypical Depressive Disorder

- Start with an MAOI

- If response is partial, combine with lithium or a thyroid supplement or PINDOLOL

- If the response is insufficient, slowly add a TCA (do not add an SRI, SERZONE, or EFFEXOR)

- If psychosis emerges, add an antipsychotic (e.g., HALDOL or RISPERDAL)

- If response is still insufficient, add ECT

Psychotic Depression

- Start with an AD plus antipsychotic

- If response is insufficient, add ECT

Depression with Serious Suicidal Risk, Rapid Physical Deterioration, or Prior History of Non-Response to Medication or Good Response to ECT

Treat with ECT

Cyclothymia

- Start with lithium or another mood stabilizer

- If depressive episodes recur, add a cyclic antidepressant or an MAOI

Seasonal Affective Disorder

Phototherapy may be an effective treatment for seasonal affective disorder

Premenstrual Dysphoric Disorder

- Start with PROZAC

- If the response is insufficient, conduct sequential trials with other SRIs, SERZONE, EFFEXOR, ANAFRANIL, and BZDs

Drug-Induced Depressions

Treatment of these disorders is first directed at the causative agent (e.g., reserpine, α-methyldopa). Withdrawing the offending compound and providing supportive care may be all that is required, with the symptoms dissipating in days or weeks. If the measure is not effective, initiate an AD.

Treatment-Resistant Depression

There are three major options available when treatment results in no response. When there has been no benefit, stop the current AD and start a trial with an unrelated agent (e.g., switch from a cyclic antidepressant to an SRI, EFFEXOR, SERZONE, or MAOI). When there has been a partial response, increase the effects of the current agent with lithium, thyroid hormone, or an anticonvulsant. If the above methods do not work, concurrently use two different classes of ADs (e.g., a cyclic antidepressant plus MAOI).

Maintenance and Prophylactic Therapy of Depressive Disorders

Maintenance therapy refers to preventing a relapse. It is mandatory following a successful remission. Continue the therapy six-to-twelve months after an acute depressive episode. After twelve months, medications can usually be tapered over a period of several weeks to avoid autonomic rebound or SRI discontinuation syndrome. If symptoms reemerge, the physician should start the medication again and maintain it for an additional three-to-six months before attempting to taper the medication again.

Prophylaxis refers to the prevention of recurrent episodes. Prophylaxis involves the indefinite continuation of medication, usually over many years, particularly if the episodes have early indications of an attack or develop insidiously. In individuals with recurrent, severe, unipolar depressions and high risk of suicide, indefinite prophylactic ADs with the least adverse effects may be required.

Major Depressive Disorder after Remission of First Episode

Continue on the AD that produced a good response for six-to-twelve months with follow-up by the prescribing physician every two-to-three months.

Major Depressive Disorder, after Remission of First Episode and on Maintenance Therapy

If symptoms reemerge after discontinuation of the AD, reinstate the same AD for an indefinite length of therapy with follow-up by the prescribing physician every-two-to-three months.

Major Depressive Disorder with Multiple Episodes, after Remission of the Current Episode

Continue on the AD that produced a good response for an indefinite length of therapy, with follow-up by the prescribing physician every two-to-three months

Atypical Depressive Disorder, after Remission of First Episode

Continue on the MAOI that produced a good response for six-to-twelve months, with follow-up by the prescribing physician every two-to-three months.

Atypical Depressive Disorder, after Remission of First Episode and on Maintenance Therapy

If the symptoms re-emerge after stopping the MAOI, reinstate the same MAOI with an indefinite time and follow it up with the prescribing physician every two-to-three months.

Atypical Depressive Disorder with Multiple Episodes, after Remission of the Current Episode

Continue on the MAOI that showed a good response for an indefinite length of therapy and follow it up with the prescribing physician every two-to-three months.

Bipolar Depressive Disorder, after Remission of First Episode

Continue on the AD and mood stabilizer with a good response for six-to-twelve months and follow it up with the prescribing physician every two-to-three months. If symptoms reemerge after discontinuation of the AD plus the mood stabilizer, reinstate the same AD plus mood stabilizer with an indefinite length of therapy, followed up by the prescribing physician every two-to-three months.

Bipolar Depressive Disorder with Recurrent Episodes, after Remission from Current Episode

Continue on the AD plus a mood stabilizer with a good response for an indefinite time, followed up by the prescribing physician every two-to-three months. If depressive symptoms re-emerge, add another AD from another class. If psychosis emerges, add an antipsychotic (AP). If depressive symptoms re-emerge and psychosis emerges, add an AD of a different class and an AP.

Major Depressive Disorders with Psychotic Features, after Remission of the Current Episode

On the AD plus an AP with a good response for six-to-twelve months, followed up by the prescribing physician every two-to-three months

If symptoms re-emerge after discontinuation of the AD plus an AP, reinstate the same AD plus AP for an indefinite length of therapy, followed up by the prescribing physician every two-to-three months

Major Depressive Disorders with Psychotic Features, Recurrent Episodes or Chronic, after Remission from the Current Episode

Continue on the combination of AD, AP, and a mood stabilizer with a good response for an indefinite length of therapy, followed up by the prescribing physician every two-to-three months

Premenstrual Dysphoric Disorder

Continue with the medication that showed previous effectiveness throughout the menstrual cycle. Periodically re-evaluate the need for the medication

Mania and Hypomania

It is very rare that young children with ASD develop hypomania or mania. However, their hyperactivity, impulsivity, mood swing with irritability and periodic laughing, and grandiose talks (particularly in individuals with Asperger Syndrome) sometimes may be diagnosed as symptoms of hypomanic or manic episodes by clinicians who are not familiar with ASD. On the other hand, because of an increased rate of bipolar mood disorders in family members of persons with Asperger Syndrome, it is conceivable that some individuals with ASD, particularly those with Asperger Syndrome, may develop hypomania or mania in late adolescence or adulthood as co-morbid conditions. Therefore, it is important that you know the features of hypomania, mania, and other mood disorders.

Symptoms of Mania

The essential features of mania include:

- A distinct period of an elevated, expansive, or irritable mood

- Inflated self-esteem, ranging from uncritical self-confidence to marked grandiosity, often reaching delusional proportions

- Decreased need for sleep

- Hyperactivity

- Hypersexuality

- More talkative than usual or pressure to keep talking—at times so pronounced that it becomes almost incomprehensible

- Flight of ideas or subjective experience that thoughts are racing

- Distractibility

- A significant increase in pleasurable but risk-taking activities (e.g., overspending) that have a high potential for painful consequences

- Change of affect characterized by rapid shifts from euphoria to anger

- Increased psychomotor agitation, irritability, aggressiveness, or self-injurious behavior when the goal-directed behavior is thwarted

- Florid psychotic features; for example, delusions and hallucinations (infrequent)

Symptoms of Hypomania

Hypomania is a less severe form of its manic counterpart, and typically does not have many of the consequences experienced during an acute, full-blown episode. Subtle indicators of hypomania include:

- A transition period in and out of depression

- Increased productivity

- Heightened perceptions

- Symptom overlap and fluctuation

- An altered view of spouse, friends, and others.

Bipolar I disorder is characterized by a history of one or more manic episodes and one or more mixed or major depressive episodes. This category can be further sub-classified as manic, hypomanic, mixed, or depressed in presentation.

Bipolar II disorder is defined by the presence or history of at least one hypomanic episode and at least one major depressive episode, but never presenting with a full manic or mixed episode (see below).

Mixed Manic States

Mixed manic states are the simultaneous presence of both significant depressive and manic symptoms without meeting full criteria for either or both mood syndromes. This may be a relatively common occurrence. Aggression and anxiety may be important components, in addition to dysphoria, in defining mixed states.

Cyclothymia

Cyclothymia is a milder version of the classic bipolar disorder. It has a chronic course (i.e., two years or more), with swings between mild depressive and hypomanic symptoms that never reach the severity of a full manic or depressive episode.

Rapid Cyclers

Rapid cyclers represent a more severe, treatment-resistant subgroup characterized by a minimum of four episodes (i.e., hypomanic, manic, depressive, o r mixed) within a period of twelve-months.

Medication Treatment of Acute Manic Episode

Manic Episode with Mild-to-Moderate Symptoms

- Start with lithium (with blood level ranges of 0.8 to 1.2 mEq/L) or DEPAKOTE (with blood level ranges of 50 to 125 µg/mL)

- If response is insufficient and with marked agitation, add a Benzodiazepine (BZD)

- Add thyroid supplement if TSH elevated

- If the response is still insufficient, add an AP

- If response is still insufficient and with immediate danger, add ECT after discontinuing lithium

Manic Episode with Moderate to Severe Symptoms and/or Psychotic Symptoms

- Start with an AP plus lithium or DEPAKOTE

- If response is insufficient, add a BZD; add thyroid supplement if TSH is elevated

- If response is still insufficient and with immediate danger, add ECT after discontinuing lithium

Manic Episode in Rapid Cycler, or Mixed States, or Prior Non-Response with lithium

- Start with DEPAKOTE with/without BZD/AP

- If response is insufficient, switch DEPAKOTE to TEGRETOL with/without BZD/AP

- If response is still insufficient, use TEGRETOL plus DEPAKOTE with/without BZD/AP

- If response is still insufficient and with immediate danger, add ECT

Maintenance and Prophylaxis Therapies for Manic Episodes

The majority of bipolar individuals who have a manic or depressed episode will have one or more recurrence. Therefore, development of effective and safe long-term treatments is critical.

Lithium or DEPAKOTE Responders, after Remission of First Acute Episode or a Recurrent Episode

- If lithium (blood level 0.8-1.2 mEq/L) or DEPAKOTE (blood level 50-150 μg/mL) is effective, continues the drug for one-to-two years, have a follow-up by the prescribing physician every two-to-three months

- Then slowly taper lithium or DEPAKOTE over several weeks

- If relapse occurs, check blood level or resume lithium or DEPAKOTE for an indefinite time, followed up by the prescribing physician every two-to-three months

- Add thyroid supplementation if TSH is elevated

Patient noncompliance may be significantly high within the first year of treatment, particularly in individuals with Asperger Syndrome and manic episode. The following may play a role in noncompliance:

- Sensitivity to somatic adverse effects (especially memory problems, impaired coordination, weight gain, and tremor)

- Cognitive and psychological adverse effects on long-term lithium treatment without relapse

- The positive reaction to early euphoria and/or hypomania

- Severity of illness

At the beginning of medication treatment, you and other caretakers must work out a plan with your child to ensure compliance.

Unusual Nervousness and Anxious Behaviors

Among the individuals with autistic disorder, about twenty-to-sixty percent had fears, and about seventy-five percent had separation anxieties. Some of these subjects might indeed have general anxiety disorder (GAD) or panic attacks. However, due to clinicians' lack of experience working with persons with ASD, the possibility of co-existing GAD or panic attacks may have been misdiagnosed and mistreated.

Anxiety is characterized by fear and apprehension that may or may not be associated with a clearly identifiable stimulus. Anxiety is a common reaction to significant life stress seen in conjunction with almost every psychiatric disorder and is also a common component of numerous organic disorders.

Individuals with ASD may have difficulty verbalizing subjective anxiety. The physician can observe and measure physiological symptoms such as hyperventilation, cardiovascular changes such as elevated blood pressure and heart rate, and excessive perspiration (diaphoresis).

Panic reactions, phobias, and performance anxiety may all quickly lead to self-injurious or aggressive outbursts, or stereotypic motor behaviors. These anxiety-discharge behaviors tend to decrease by removing the provoking agent.

The avoidant behavior tends to generalize to a wider arena, resulting in a pattern of phobic avoidance with recurrent panic attacks. This pattern of reinforced anxiety-discharge behaviors may result in a pattern of severe behavioral outbursts resembling a psychotic disorder. In this fashion, anxiety disorder may lead to behavior disturbances equivalent in severity and generalization to affective disorder and schizophrenia.

Symptoms of Generalized Anxiety Disorder (GAD)

The essential features of GAD are persistent anxiety and worry associated with some of the following symptoms occurring more days than not for at least six months or longer:

Motor Tension—Shakiness, jitteriness, jumpiness, trembling, tension, muscle aches, fatigue, inability to relax, eyelid twitch, furrowed brow, strained face, fidgeting, restlessness, and being easily startled

Autonomic Hyperactivity—Sweating; heart pounding or racing; rapid or irregular heartbeat; cold, clammy hands; dry mouth; dizziness; lightheadedness; paresthesias (tingling in hands or feet); upset stomach; hot or cold spells; frequent urination; diarrhea; nausea; discomfort in the pit of the stomach; lump in the throat; flushing; pallor; high resting pulse; high respiration rate, or breathing problem, etc.

Apprehensive Expectation—Anxiety, uneasiness, feeling of apprehension, worry, fear, rumination, and anticipation of misfortune to self or others

Vigilance and Scanning—Hyper-attentive behavior resulting in distractibility, difficulty in concentrating or mind going blank, insomnia, feeling "on edge," irritability, and/or impatience

Medication Treatment Plan for GAD

The preferred medication for most anxiety disorders is Buspirone (BUSPAR) or tricyclic antidepressants. The benzodiazepines such as alprazolam (XANAX), diazepam (VALIUM), chlordiazepoxide (LIBRIUM or LIBRAX) and lorazepam (ATIVAN) are the second line of drugs of choice because there is a potential for developing tolerance and dependence, as well as the possibility of abuse and withdrawal reactions. When the doctor prescribes benzodiazepines, the patient should use them for brief periods.

Treatment of Acute Anxiety

Ideally, for treatment of acute anxiety, the chosen medication should be with the lowest possible dose for the shortest possible time. Dosages should be flexible rather than arbitrary. The patient should take them intermittently at a time of increased symptoms rather than on a fixed daily schedule. In general, one-to-seven days of medication treatment is recommended for a reaction to an acute situational stress, although one-to-six weeks of treatment may be needed for short-term anxiety due to specific life events.

Mild Acute Anxiety Episode

- Start with cognitive behavior therapy in higher-functioning, older adolescents and adults; if there is no response or insufficient response, add a BZD

- Start with a BZD in lower-functioning individuals

- If no response or insufficient response, add BUSPAR

Moderate-to-Severe Acute Anxiety Episode,

- Start with a BZD plus cognitive behavior therapy in higher-functioning , older adolescents and adults
- If there is no response or insufficient response, add BUSPAR

Treatment of Chronic Anxiety

Chronic Anxiety with Prior BZD Treatment

- Add BUSPAR, then taper BZD

Chronic Anxiety without Prior BZD

- Start with BUSPAR
- If there is no response or insufficient response, add a BZD
- If still no response or insufficient response, taper BZD and add an AD (TCA, SRI, MAOI) or taper BUSPAR and add an AD

Chronic Anxiety with Panic Attacks or Depressive Symptoms

- Start with an AD with/without BZD or BUSPAR

Maintenance and Prophylaxis Therapies for Generalized Anxiety Disorder

Clinical judgment plays a major role in the decision to continue anxiolytic treatment beyond four-to-six weeks. Although long-term administration may maintain initial improvement, it is unlikely to result in further gains. However, the chronic nature of anxiety disorders and the frequency of eventual relapse after treatment discontinuation suggest that in some individuals, long-term treatment is necessary.

Periodic reassessment of the efficacy, safety, and necessity of long-term, anxiolytic therapy is necessary. The high rate of comorbidity for GAD with other psychiatric disorders suggests that an alternate approach (such as adding an antidepressant while tapering off an anxiolytic medication) may be more appropriate in certain individuals.

Panic Disorder

Panic disorder is characterized by recurrent, unexpected, panic attacks with a distinct period of intense fear, heightened arousal, or anticipatory anxiety that is accompanied by some of the following somatic or cognitive symptoms without apparent cause:

- Palpitations, pounding heart, or accelerated heart rate
- Sweating
- Flushing
- Trembling or shaking
- Sensation of shortness of breath or smothering (dyspnea)
- Feeling of choking
- Chest pain or discomfort

- Nausea or abdominal distress (butterflies in the stomach)
- Feeling dizzy, unsteady, lightheaded, or faint
- Feeling of unreality or depersonalization (being detached from oneself)
- Despair or fear of losing control, or going crazy
- Sense of catastrophic fear of dying
- Paresthesia (numbness or tingling sensations)
- Chills or hot flushes

Most individuals will have many of the symptoms during an attack, but not necessarily every possible symptom. There is also a group that has these attacks without the subjective sense of anxiety or that do not experience sufficient symptoms to meet diagnostic criteria (i.e., limited symptom attacks). Individuals may develop three distinct disorders:

- The panic attack itself
- A secondary, anticipatory anxiety that they will have another episode in certain places
- A phobic avoidance of the feared situation

These symptoms typically occur in public places, such as supermarkets, restaurants, elevators, and crowded stores.

Medication Treatment of Panic Disorder

Mild Panic Attacks

- Start with behavioral therapy
- If response is insufficient, add an SRI or a TCA
- If response is still insufficient, add ALPRAZOLAM or CLONAZEPAM

Moderate Panic Attacks

- Start with a TCA or an SRI plus behavioral therapy
- If response is insufficient, add ALPRAZOLAM or CLONAZEPAM
- If response is still insufficient, add MAOI

Severe Panic Attacks

- Start with a TCA or an SRI plus ALPRAZOLAM or CLONAZEPAM and behavioral therapy
- If response is insufficient, add MAOI
- If response is still insufficient, add DEPAKOTE, with or without a BZD

Phobic Disorders

All phobic disorders are characterized by disabling anxiety (at times also associated with panic attacks) and avoidance because of:

- Exposure to places or situations from which one cannot escape

- A specific, feared object or situation (e.g., heights)
- Certain types of social or performance situations

Agoraphobia

Agoraphobia is the dread of being in places or situations from which escape might be difficult. It also includes worry about suddenly developing embarrassing or incapacitating panic-like symptoms (e.g., loss of bladder control or dizziness) for which help might not be available. The agoraphobic individual often restricts travel, needs a companion when away from home, and endures intense anxiety when confronted with a feared situation. Agoraphobia may be associated with or without panic disorder.

Medication Treatment of Agoraphobia

Mild Agoraphobia

- Start with behavioral therapy
- If response is insufficient, add an SRI or a TCA
- If response is still insufficient, add ALPRAZOLAM or CLONAZEPAM

Moderate Agoraphobia

- Start with a TCA or an SRI, plus behavioral therapy
- If response is insufficient, add ALPRAZOLAM or CLONAZEPAM
- If response is still insufficient, add MAOI

Severe Agoraphobia

- Start with a TCA or an SRI, plus ALPRAZOLAM or CLONAZEPAM and behavioral therapy
- If response is insufficient, add MAOI
- If response is still insufficient, add DEPAKOTE with or without a BZD

Social Phobia

Social phobia is the persistent fear of being judged by others and/or embarrassing oneself in public (e.g., fear of being unable to answer questions in social situations or choking when eating in front of others). Exposure to the feared situation provokes an immediate anxiety response. As a result, the individual prefers to avoid the phobic situation or endures it with intense anxiety.

Medication Treatment of Social Phobia

- Start with behavioral therapy
- If response is insufficient, add an SRI
- If response is still insufficient, add ALPRAZOLAM or CATAPRES or an MAOI (must wait at least two weeks after discontinuation of the SRI—longer for PROZAC—before starting MAOI)

Specific Phobia

Formerly called simple phobia, specific phobia is a marked, excessive, or unreasonable and persistent fear of a specific object or situation such as snakes, heights, or thunderstorms.

Medication Treatment of Specific Phobia

- Start with behavioral therapy (systematic desensitization)

- If response is insufficient, add PROPRANOLOL

- If response is still insufficient, add an MAOI (e.g., PHENELZINE)

Disturbances of Thought

Many individuals with ASD show symptoms of social isolation, impairment in role functioning or grooming, and inappropriate affect. These symptoms resemble the prodromal or residual symptoms of schizophrenia. Many higher-functioning people with autistic disorder or Asperger Syndrome exhibit illogical thinking, incoherence, and poverty in content of speech. Some individuals with ASD have inappropriate laughing or weeping due to the inability to comprehend the meaning of events. Some higher-functioning, verbal persons with autistic disorder or individuals with Asperger Syndrome have strange beliefs, interests, or sensory dysfunction. Examples: they believe there is no air in other states, so they do not want to travel to other states; have idiosyncratic interests such as spending an enormous amount of time studying dinosaurs; or have sensory experiences such as seeing other people's faces in the air when alone in the room.

These symptoms border on delusions or hallucinations. Clinicians unfamiliar with ASD frequently see the symptoms as clinical manifestations of schizophrenia and other psychotic disorders, leading to misdiagnoses. Nonetheless, a minority of individuals with ASD can also develop schizophrenia or other psychotic disorders.

Schizophrenia

Schizophrenia is characterized by a history of deterioration from a higher level of function, and symptoms of hallucinations, cognitive disturbances such as illogical or tangential thinking, paranoia, delusions; bizarre rituals and behavior; withdrawal, and blunting of affect. Examples of delusions and hallucinations include the following.

- Audible thoughts (i.e., voices speak the patient's thoughts out loud)

- Voices arguing (e.g., two or more voices argue or discuss issues, sometimes referring to the patient in the third person)

- Voices commenting on the patient's behavior

- Somatic passivity believed to be imposed by outside forces

- Thought withdrawal by outside forces, leaving the patient feeling as if his or her mind is empty

- Thought insertions by outside forces

- Thought broadcasting (i.e., thoughts escape from the patient's mind and are overheard by others)

- Impulsive volitional acts, or feelings that are not one's own but are imposed by outside forces

- Delusional perceptions (i.e., the individual attributes delusional meaning to normal perceptions).

Medication Treatment of Schizophrenia

While there were trends at times favoring one conventional antipsychotic (AP) over another (e.g., HALDOL over THORAZINE), an inspection of the data finds none is consistently superior to another. All conventional APs produced consistent changes in the same symptoms. If all conventional APs are equally effective, how does one choose the best drug for a given individual? Because their action is related to structural similarities shared by most compounds in this class, there is no reason to expect a given individual to respond differently to a particular drug. So the critical consideration usually involves differences in adverse effects.

The introduction of atypical and novel APs, such as CLOZARIL, RISPERDAL, ZYPREXA, and SEROQUEL, has dramatically affected the decision-making process in choosing an AP. These new agents both minimize neurological adverse effects and qualitatively improve at least some psychotic symptoms to a greater degree.

There is no evidence that combining two APs is superior to bioequivalent amounts of a single agent. One exception may be the combined use of a conventional neuroleptic with a novel AP such as HALDOL plus ZYPREXA, or, alternatively, the combination of two novel agents (e.g., CLOZARIL plus RISPERDAL). This is because these novel APs may be sufficiently different that, when combined with each other or with conventional APs, some patients may gain a better overall effect.

Antipsychotic Dosing Strategies

Because the onset of improvement is approximately one-to-two weeks with most APs, one should start with a low-to-moderate dose (i.e., HALDOL, 4-12 mg/day; MELLARIL, 300-400 mg/day; RISPERDAL, 2-4 mg/day) that is maintained for that period. While the doctor can adjust the dosage more frequently to control adverse effects, he or she should not adjust it daily on the basis of therapeutic effect because of the length of these agents' half-lives.

<u>Mild-to-Moderately Severe Acute Schizophrenic (Psychotic) Episode</u>

- Start with an AP and adjust the dosage to the maximum recommended

- If response is insufficient, sequential trials of APs of different classes (e.g., HALDOL, RISPERDAL, ZYPREXA, SEROQUEL, CLOZARIL) are indicated

- If response is still insufficient, the doctor may consider co-administration of two atypical APs (e.g., RISPERDAL plus CLOZARIL)

<u>Acute schizophrenic (psychotic) episode, with marked agitation or catatonia</u>

- Start with an AP and a higher potency BZD, such as ATIVAN or clonazepam.

- If response is insufficient, switch to an AP of a different class

- If response is still insufficient and poses an immediate danger, add ECT

Schizophreniform Disorder

Individuals with this condition manifest the symptoms of an acute exacerbation of schizophrenia, but they make a complete recovery. The early-onset, active, and residual phases last no more than six months.

Medication Treatment of Schizophreniform Disorder

The treatment is the same as that described under the medication treatment of schizophrenia. In some individuals, if all the APs fail to show treatment effect, the physician may consider lithium.

Brief Psychotic Disorder

Brief psychotic disorder is an acute psychotic response to a severe stressor that generally subsides in one day to one month. We frequently see this phenomenon in adolescents or young adulthood without early-onset symptoms or lasting impairment.

Medication Treatment of Brief Psychotic Disorder

The treatment is the same as that described under the medication treatment of schizophrenia

Delusional Disorder

This disorder is characterized by one or more delusions of at least one month's duration. Delusions may be excessive sexual desire (erotomania), grandiose, jealous, persecutory, somatic, mixed, or non-specified.

Medication Treatment of Delusional Disorder

The treatment is the same as that described under the medication treatment of schizophrenia

Schizoaffective Disorder

Schizoaffective disorder (SA) has both psychotic and mood symptoms. Individuals do not clearly meet the diagnostic criteria for either schizophrenia or a major mood disorder. SA can be divided into SA bipolar or SA depression subtypes.

Medication Treatment of Schizoaffective Disorder

- Start with an AP plus lithium, DEPAKOTE, or TEGRETOL for SA bipolar subtype; or start with an AP plus an AD for SA depression subtype

- If response is insufficient, switch to an AP and/or an AD of a different class

- If response is still insufficient, add ECT

Chronic Antipsychotic Refractory Psychosis

Medication Treatment

- Sequential trials of novel APs

- If response is insufficient, add lithium, DEPAKOTE, TEGRETOL, or an AD

- If response is still insufficient, add ECT

Maintenance and Prophylaxis Therapy for Schizophrenia and Other Psychotic Disorders

Because the majority of schizophrenic individuals have a chronic disorder, the issue of maintenance therapy becomes critical. In the past, many individuals with schizophrenia quickly relapsed when physicians withdrew their medications. Therefore, doctors recommend maintenance medication therapy to prevent such relapses.

People who have had many episodes but make a good recovery from the acute exacerbation, benefit the most from maintenance medication. There may be exceptions, however, to the general rule of maintenance therapy. For example, a brief reactive psychosis in response to a severe stressor may occur only once, making long-term drug maintenance unnecessary. Doctors must look at maintenance therapy in the context of the long-term consequences in order to minimize more serious adverse effects.

Low-Dose Maintenance Strategy

The low-dose strategy is to maintain individuals on a continuous lower dose of AP that would increase only when early-onset signs occur. There are two major concerns with such a strategy.

1. With too low a dose, individuals are at risk of developing a more frequent increase in the severity of the disorder. This usually requires increased doses and may contribute to the development of a more severe form of the disorder not amenable to future drug intervention.

2. It increases the risk of tardive dyskinesia (TD). Ideally, it is one of the atypical APs that has shown positive treatment response and is used for maintenance therapy. The risk of TD would be significantly reduced.

On low-to-moderate doses of an AP, the treatment is effective for preventing acute episodes for one-to-two years. If a relapse occurs, the physician should increase the AP dosage. If the response is still insufficient, the doctor may prescribe a different AP.

With a positive response for six months, the prescribing physician may continue the AP for an indefinite time but decrease the dose, with follow-up every two-to-three months

Targeted Treatment Strategy

An alternate strategy to low-dose maintenance is targeted treatment. The patient only receives medication therapy when prodromal symptoms are apparent. These symptoms include increased anxiety, dysphoria, lability of mood, loss of interest, reduced energy, discouragement about the future, reduced attention, increased internal preoccupation, increased illusions, racing thoughts, vague digressive speech, eccentric behavior, nightmares or insomnia, and deterioration of personal care. A targeted treatment strategy uses these symptoms as cues to restart drug therapy, thus avoiding continual AP exposure.

- As soon as the prodromal symptoms are confirmed, the physician should start the AP found previously effective

- If response is insufficient, switch to a different AP

- With positive response on the AP for six months, taper off the AP and follow-up by the prescribing physician every two-to-three months

Long-Acting, Antipsychotic Treatment Strategy

In individuals who have poor oral absorption, or in those who have clear problems with compliance, depot (long-acting) AP is a possibility. The goal is to establish the lowest, effective maintenance dose, mindful that too low a dose may increase the risk of relapse. Conversely, too high a dose may expose the individual to unnecessary adverse effects and increase noncompliance.

When initiating depot AP, choose a conservative dose, realizing that it may take several months to establish steady-state levels. It may also be necessary to supplement treatment with oral AP during this early phase until the required maintenance level is ascertained.

If the depot dose is too high, as evidenced by the appearance of persistent adverse effects, the physician should treat the side effects immediately. Reduce the dose of the depot AP at the next scheduled injection, or extend the injection intervals until adverse effects are controlled.

If psychotic symptoms re-emerge before the next scheduled depot AP injection, an oral AP can be used to control the symptoms. The depot dosage should be increased at the next scheduled injection.

Self-Injurious Behaviors

Self-injurious behavior (SIB), such as head-banging; finger-, hand-, or wrist-biting; or scratching of the face or extremities may occur in lower-functioning individuals with ASD. SIB may be constant (compulsive SIB) or intermittent (paroxysmal SIB) or occasional (episodic SIB). Some SIB may relate to other neuropsychiatric disorders like Tourette syndrome. Other SIB may relate to frustrations. However, much of the SIB does not have a clear reason due to communication difficulties of individuals with ASD. This behavior affects the persons with ASD as much as their caregivers.

The only established treatment is behavioral intervention, which requires an extraordinary investment in time and professional effort. However, there are only a few intensive and effective treatment programs in this country; therefore, only a minority of people with severe SIB have received intensive behavior treatment. For most individuals with ASD and severe SIB, physical restraint with a helmet, handcuffs, or leather straps are the usual treatment. Studies of medication treatment of SIB in ASD have been quite limited.

Medication Treatment of Self-Injurious Behaviors

Self-Injurious Behaviors as a Clinical Feature of Tourette Syndrome

The same as that described for Tourette syndrome

Self-Injurious Behaviors Without Readily Identifiable Causes

Use sequential trials of NALTREXONE, PROZAC, and DESYREL

Agitation and Aggressive Behaviors

Some individuals with ASD may become agitated and physically attack other people or destroy objects or properties. Some of the aggressive and destructive behaviors may relate to frustrations of these individuals due to inability to cope with task demands, difficult/challenging games and toys, or dysfunctional/broken toys. They may react to being stopped from doing things they like or may be reacting to caregivers' attempts at using physical control. The aggressive and/or destructive behaviors are impulsive and thoughtless, driven by powerful and unanticipated emotions like anger or fear.

Drastic mood change due to a mood disorder causes some aggressive or destructive behaviors. Other aggressive and/or destructive behaviors may be executed with a purpose in mind. This type of aggression is called predatory aggression. It tends to show up in individuals with Asperger Syndrome. There are, however, some behaviors that do not seem to have any clear causes but are being mostly driven by powerful and unanticipated emotions. Impulsive and mood disorder-related aggressive or destructive behaviors may respond to drugs. Predatory aggression does not respond to drugs, except to the extent that they produce sleep and apathy.

Medication Treatment of Agitation with Aggressive and Destructive Behaviors

Behaviors Due to Inabilities to Cope with Task Demands, Challenging Games and Toys, or Broken Toys

- Start with behavioral therapy

- If response is insufficient, add CATAPRES

- If response is still insufficient, switch to PROZAC or PAXIL (as low a dose as possible)

Behaviors Due to Being Stopped from Doing Things

- Start with low dose of an SRI plus behavioral therapy
- If response is insufficient, conduct sequential trials of other SRIs
- If response is still insufficient, add a small dose of RISPERDAL

Behaviors Due to Mood Disorder

- Start with lithium or DEPAKOTE
- If response is insufficient, add a BZD; add thyroid supplement if TSH is elevated
- If the response is insufficient, add an AP
- If response is still insufficient and the patient is in immediate danger, add ECT after discontinuation of lithium

Behaviors for No Apparent Reason

- Start with CATAPRES plus behavioral therapy
- If response is insufficient, add an SRI
- If response is insufficient, conduct sequential trials of other SRIs
- If response is still insufficient, add HALDOL, RISPERDAL, DESYREL, DEPAKOTE, INDERAL, BZD, or lithium (sequential trials)

Behaviors Associated with ADHD

- Start with lithium
- If response is insufficient, add HALDOL, RISPERDAL, DESYREL, DEPAKOTE, or INDERAL (sequential trials)

Sleep Problems

Unusual Sleeping Patterns

A significant number of individuals with ASD experience sleep-related problems. Some individuals develop completely reversed sleep patterns—they sleep during the day and wake during the night. Some individuals seem to need much more time to settle down to sleep. Some individuals tend to wake up at about one or two in the morning and stay awake for a few hours. Others seem to need less sleep than most people, and they tend to go bed late and wake up early in the morning. These individuals can keep the entire family awake every night because of their unusual sleep patterns.

There are many reasons for having sleep disturbances, and there are several different types of sleep disturbances (disorders): primary sleep disorders, sleep disorders related to another mental disorder, sleep disorders related to a general medical disorder, and sleep disorders that are substance induced.

Primary sleep disorders can be divided into three major groups:

1. **Dyssomnias**—the predominant disturbance is the amount, quality, or timing of sleep

2. **Hypersomnias**—disorders of excessive sleepiness

3. **Parasomnias**—the predominant disturbance involves pathological, behavioral, or psychological events that occur with sleep, specific sleep stages, or sleep-wake transitions

Dyssomnias

Primary Insomnia

Primary insomnia is the difficulty initiating or maintaining sleep or by not feeling rested after an apparently adequate amount of sleep. These characteristics last at least one month. Further, the insomnia causes significant stress or impairment in various areas of functioning. This condition may represent a lifelong pattern of poor sleep habits, or it may develop as a result of distressing events but then persists after the stressor resolves. It is characterized by daytime worry about being able to fall or stay asleep.

Circadian Rhythm Sleep Disorder

This disorder occurs when there is a mismatch between the normal rest period schedule for a person's environment and the person's circadian sleep-wake pattern. It usually improves when the person is able to resume a normal sleep-wake pattern. There are four subtypes: delayed sleep phase type, jet lag type, shift work type, and unspecified.

Hypersomnias

Hypersomnia is characterized by excessive daytime sleepiness for at least one month. The daytime sleepiness (falling asleep easily and unintentionally) is not accounted for by an inadequate amount of nighttime sleep. Another criteria is the presence of hypersomnia nearly every day for at least one month or episodically for longer periods of time, resulting in occupational or social impairment.

Narcolepsy

Narcolepsy may be either of an unknown cause or, more rarely, secondary to organic brain damage. Its characteristics include irresistible attacks of sleep lasting from thirty seconds to twenty minutes and the accelerated appearance of rapid eye movement (REM) sleep, usually within ten minutes of going to sleep. Additional symptoms may include brief weakness in isolated muscle groups or paralysis of almost all skeletal muscles (cataplexy) triggered by intense emotion, with or without a concurrent sleep attack; sleep paralysis, and hallucination preceding sleep (hypnagogic) or partially awakening from sleep (hypnopompic).

Breathing-Related Sleep Disorder

Breathing-related sleep disorder is a potentially life-threatening, abnormal respiratory condition. It includes cessation of both nasal and oral air flow (apnea), which in some individuals may last up to two minutes. The most prominent sign is loud snoring. Typical complications include insomnia and excessive daytime sleepiness due to frequent nighttime awakenings. There are three forms of breathing-related sleep disorders:

1. Obstructive sleep apnea, involving blockage of the oropharynx

2. Central sleep apnea, involving lack of diaphragmatic effort

3. Central alveolar hypoventilation, which most commonly occurs in very overweight individuals.

Parasomnias

This group of disorders is characterized by the occurrence of an abnormal event during sleep, specific sleep stages, or the threshold between sleep and wakefulness. These conditions usually involve complaints focused on the abnormal occurrence itself rather than any effect it might have on sleep. Parasomnias include: nightmare disorder, sleep terror disorder, and sleepwalking disorder.

Nightmare Disorder

Formerly known as dream anxiety disorder, this condition involves vivid dreams, often characterized by recurring themes of threats to survival, security, or self-esteem. Because the dreams are most likely to occur during REM sleep, involuntary agitation is minimal during the dream but may occur upon awakening. If the dreams are caused by a known organic factor, such as a medication or general medical condition, there is no nightmare disorder.

Sleep Terror Disorder

This disorder (also known as pavor nocturnus) has recurrent episodes of abrupt awakening from sleep in the first third of the major sleep episode, usually during nonrapid eye movement (NREM) periods. The episode can be dramatic and is likely to begin with a panicky scream. The person often sits up in bed, exhibiting signs of intense anxiety and involuntary arousal (e.g., rapid heart rate, rapid breathing and pulse, dilated pupils, sweating, etc.). He or she may be confused, disoriented, and unresponsive to comforting gestures. Individuals may describe a sense of terror and fragmentary images, but they usually cannot recall a complete dream.

Sleepwalking Disorder

Sleepwalking disorder (or somnambulism) is characterized by episodes of complex behaviors that initially include sitting up and performing perseverative movements (e.g., picking at the sheet). This usually occurs during NREM sleep. Sleepwalking disorder often proceeds to such activities as leaving the bed, walking, dressing, and opening or closing windows and doors.

Sleep Disorders Related to Another Mental Disorder

- Insomnia related to another mental disorder, but is sufficiently severe to warrant independent clinical attention.

- Hypersomnia related to another mental disorder, but is sufficiently severe to warrant independent clinical attention.

Sleep Disorders Due to a General Medical Disorder

- Insomnia due to a general medical disorder, but sufficiently severe to warrant clinical attention.

- Hypersomnia due to a medical disorder but sufficiently severe to warrant clinical attention.

- Parasomnia due to a medical disorder but sufficiently severe to warrant clinical attention

Sleep Disorders Due to Substance Abuse

- Insomnia due to substance abuse but is sufficiently severe to warrant clinical attention.

- Hypersomnia due to substance abuse but is sufficiently severe to warrant clinical attention.

- Parasomnia due to substance abuse but is sufficiently severe to warrant clinical attention

Medication Treatment of Sleep Disorders

Primary Insomnia Due to Poor Sleep Habits

- Start with sleep hygiene techniques

- Restrict sleep to a minimum to no afternoon/evening nap and insist on appropriate bedtime

- Control stimulations—ban watching TV in the evening, control lighting and sound of the bedroom, limit fluid intake in the evening, etc.

- Use relaxation techniques such as appropriate reading or music, bedtime muscle relaxation exercises, etc.

- If response is insufficient, add small dose of CATAPRES or MELATONIN for initial insomnia (inability to sleep), or MELATONIN, DESYREL, short-to intermediate-acting BZD (e.g., PROSOM) (sequential trials) for waking up after two-to-three hours of sleep or waking up early in the morning. If using a BZD, use should be at the lowest possible dose for the shortest possible time, and on an intermittent, rather than a regular, basis

- If effective, discontinue the medication after one-to-two months and re-evaluate the need for a sleep medication

- If response is still insufficient (this rarely happens), use a sedative-hypnotics (e.g., AMBIEN) for not more than three weeks

Primary Insomnia Due to Other Mental or General Medical Disorders

- Treat the mental disorder or general medical disorder

- Start with the sleep techniques described under *Primary Insomnia Due to Poor Sleep Habits*

- If response is insufficient, add a small dose of CATAPRES, MELATONIN, or BENADRYL for initial insomnia (difficulty in falling asleep). Use MELATONIN, DESYREL, short-to intermediate-acting BZD like PROSOM (sequential trials) for initial insomnia, waking up after two-to-three hours of sleep, or waking up early in the morning. If using a BZD, use the lowest possible dose for the shortest possible time, and on an intermittent rather than a regular basis

- If response is sufficient, discontinue the medication after one-to-two months and re-evaluate the need for a sleep medication

- If response is still insufficient (this rarely happens), use a sedative-hypnotics (e.g., AMBIEN) for not more than three weeks

Other Insomnias Due to Prescribed Medications

- Switch to a different medication with equal effectiveness but without the side effect of insomnia

- Start with the sleep techniques previously described under *Due to Poor Sleep Habits*

- If response is insufficient, add small dose of CATAPRES, MELATONIN, or BENADRYL for initial insomnia (difficulty in falling asleep). Use MELATONIN, DESYREL, short-to intermediate-acting BZD (e.g., PROSOM) (sequential trials) for initial insomnia and/or waking up after two to three hours of sleep, or waking up early in the morning. If a BZD is used it should be prescribed at the lowest possible dose for the shortest possible time, and on an intermittent rather than a regular basis

- If response is sufficient, discontinue the medication after one-to-two months and re-evaluate the need for a medication

- If response is still insufficient (this rarely happens), use a sedative-hypnotic (e.g., AMBIEN) for not more than three weeks

Insomnias Due to Substance Abuse

- Treat substance abuse and discontinue the non-prescribed drugs

- Start with the sleep techniques previously described under *Primary Insomnia Due to Poor Sleep Habits*

- If response is insufficient, add small dose of CATAPRES, MELATONIN, or BENADRYL for initial insomnia (difficulty in falling asleep). Use MELATONIN, DESYREL, short-to-intermediate-acting BZD like PROSOM (sequential trials) for initial insomnia or waking up after two-to-three hours of sleep, or waking up early in the morning. If prescribing a BZD, the doctor should prescribe it at the lowest possible dose for the shortest possible time, and on an intermittent rather than a regular basis

- If response is sufficient, discontinue the medication after one-to-two months and re-evaluate the need for a sleep medication

- If response is still insufficient (this rarely happens), use a sedative-hypnotics (e.g., AMBIEN) for not more than three weeks and monitor the patient closely to prevent abuse

Sleep Terror Disorder and Sleepwalking Disorder

These two disorders are much more distressing to the parent than to the child. These are unpredictable and infrequent (usually not more than once a week), which hardly justifies keeping a child under constant medication with its consequent risks. Furthermore, there is strong evidence that children will outgrow these disorders. However, if after a thorough assessment, and the physician determines that medication treatment is appropriate (e.g., sleepwalking becomes potentially dangerous), start with a BZD such as VALIUM or a TCA such as ELAVIL. The doctor should prescribe the BZD at the lowest possible dose for the shortest possible time, and on an intermittent rather than a regular basis. The need to continue the BZD or TCA should be re-evaluated after one-to-two months of good response.

Narcolepsy

Narcolepsy is managed by daily administration of a stimulant such as RITALIN, 10 mg in the morning, with increased dosage as necessary.

Breathing-Related Sleep Disorder

Weight reduction is one treatment for sleep apnea. Another is the continuous pressure of air through the nasal passage while the patient sleeps. DIAMOX (acetazolamide, an AED) may help.

Problems with Toilet Training

Some children with ASD may have difficulty with toilet training. They may continue to have problems with unintentional urination (enuresis) beyond the usual age of toilet training.

Nocturnal Enuresis

According to studies in the US, UK, Israel, and African countries, about 10% of six-year-olds suffer from nocturnal enuresis (bed-wetting) There is a spontaneous remission rate of 15% per year thereafter. Nocturnal enuresis does not have an identifiable organic cause in 97-99% of the cases (primary enuresis). The organic causes of nocturnal enuresis are diabetes mellitus, diabetes insipidus, sleep apnea, urinary tract infection, neurogenic bladder, etc. Among the most commonly accepted factors associated with nocturnal enuresis are: smaller than normal bladder capacity, bladder-sphincter dysfunction, and impaired arousal from deep or delta sleep.

Medication Treatment of Enuresis

- Start with non-medical treatment

- If medication treatment is decided upon, use DDAVP or DITROPAN in children under seven, and use DDAVP, DITROPAN, DETROL, TOFRANIL (sequential trials) in children older than seven years. When TOFRANIL is used, taper it after three-to-six months, taper DITROPAN after two months, and taper DDAVP after two months to evaluate the further need of medication.

Problems with Social Withdrawal

Some individuals with ASD become socially withdrawn due to lack of interest in other people or social activities, having a depressive disorder, or becoming nervous about socializing with people because of personality or years of unpleasant experiences.

Medication Treatment of Social Withdrawal

- In individuals who are not interested in other people or social activities, the physician could prescribe REVIA or a small amount of PROZAC

- In individuals whose social withdrawal is related to depressive or anxiety disorder, start with an SRI (as low dose as possible). If response is insufficient, use sequential trials with other SRIs and BUSPAR

Eating Problems

It is not infrequent that individuals with ASD have problems eating. Many of them have a problem with "picky eating," while others are hungry all the time. The reasons for these eating problems are not always clear. In some individuals, sensitive or obsessive-compulsive to the taste, smell, color, or texture of foods or drinks may be the reason for picky eating. In other individuals, boredom, depressive disorder, anxiety, or side effects of medications may be the cause for "hungry all the time." The role of medication treatment in these individuals has yet to be defined. Individuals with ASD usually do not develop other eating disorders like anorexia nervosa or bulimia nervosa, although there are such case reports in some literature.

Anorexia Nervosa

The characteristics of this disorder are a relentless pursuit of thinness and a morbid fear of being "too fat." Most experts consider the patient's distortion of body image central to the diagnosis. Anorexia nervosa is also characterized by the refusal to maintain a normal body weight and the obsession with dieting or fasting to the point of losing too much weight. Some individuals lose weight through excessive exercise. Individuals with anorexia nervosa often suffer from complications such as hypotension, hypothermia, and abnormal ECGs.

Bulimia Nervosa

Binging and purging, disturbances of mood, and neuroendocrine abnormalities characterize this disorder. Binges range from two-to-twenty times per week, with fifty percent occurring daily and one-third occurring several times a day. Up to one-third of bulimics have a history of anorexia nervosa, and approximately one third also use laxatives. Depression, self-criticism, and self-induced vomiting may follow each binge.

Medication Treatment of Eating Problems or Disorders

<u>Picky Eating</u>

- Comprehensive treatment including nutritional counseling, behavior modification techniques, and individual, group, and family therapy (especially for those older and higher-functioning individuals)

- If the response is insufficient, use sequential trials with SRIs

- If the response is still insufficient, the physician may add an AP (ZYPREXA, SEROQUEL or RISPERDAL) that tends to increase appetite

<u>Hungry All the Time</u>

In individuals with boredom:

- Begin behavior modification techniques

- If the response is insufficient, employ sequential trials with stimulants

In individuals who are on prescriptions

- Switch to another medication that causes less severe side effects of increased appetite

- If the response is insufficient, use sequential trials with stimulants

In individuals with depressive disorders, see *Medication Treatment of Depression*.

<u>Anorexia Nervosa</u>

- Comprehensive treatment including nutritional counseling, behavior modification techniques, and individual, group, and family therapy, plus an SRI

- If the response is insufficient, use sequential trials with other SRIs

- If the response is still insufficient (especially when complicated by psychotic symptoms), the physician may prescribe an AP (ZYPREXA, SEROQUEL or RISPERDAL)

<u>Bulimia Nervosa</u>

- Comprehensive treatment including nutritional counseling, behavior modification techniques, and individual, group, and family therapy plus PROZAC

- If the response is insufficient, the doctor may prescribe sequential trials with other SRIs, DESYREL, and WELLBUTRIN

Treatment of Two or More Simultaneously Existing Disorders or Conditions

<u>ADHD plus Tic Disorders</u>

Treat ADHD first, then treat tics.

<u>ADHD</u>

In low- or middle-functioning individuals, begin monotherapy with a TCA. If no response or insufficient response, use sequential trials with other TCAs, WELLBUTRIN, and REVIA for inattention, impulsiveness, and hyperactivity, or sequential trials with CATAPRES, TENEX and HALDOL for hyperactivity and impulsiveness

In higher-functioning individuals, begin monotherapy with a TCA. If there is insufficient response, sequential trials with other TCAs, WELLBUTRIN, and REVIA for inattention, impulsiveness, and hyperactivity, or sequential trials with CATAPRES, TENEX and HALDOL for hyperactivity. If there is no response or insufficient response to above medications, sequential trials with RITALIN, DEXEDRINE, ADDERALL, and CYLERT are indicated.

Tics

- If the tics do not respond to the above medications or the above medications increase tics, and HALDOL has not been tried, add HALDOL

- If there is an insufficient response, switch to ORAP

- If the response is insufficient response, switch to CATAPRES if it has not been used for ADHD

- If all the above medications have failed to show significant efficacy for treatment of tics, consider either RISPERDAL or calcium channel blockers like CALAN and ADALAT

ADHD Plus Obsessive-Compulsive Symptoms

In low- or middle-functioning individuals with ADHD and obsessive-compulsive symptoms, simultaneously treat ADHD and symptoms of OCD. For ADHD, begin with a TCA. If response is insufficient, sequentially try other TCAs, WELLBUTRIN, and NALTREXONE for inattention, impulsiveness, and hyperactivity, or sequential trials of CATAPRES, TENEX and HALDOL for hyperactivity and impulsiveness.

For mild OCD or OC symptoms, start with behavior therapy, if is no response or insufficient response, add PROZAC. For moderate-to-severe symptoms, start with PROZAC plus behavior therapy. If no response or insufficient response, use sequential trials with other SRIs. If there is still no response or an insufficient response, consider ANAFRANIL in individuals without history of, or current, seizure disorder. If response is still insufficient, add BUSPAR or KLONOPIN.

In high-functioning individuals with ADHD and obsessive-compulsive symptoms or disorder but without other neurological disorders (e.g., seizure disorder), simultaneously treat ADHD and OCD or symptoms. For ADHD, begin with RITALIN or DEXEDRINE. If response is insufficient, use sequential trials with either RITALIN or DEXEDRINE (the one that has not yet been used), ADDERALL, and CYLERT. If response is still insufficient with all of the above stimulants, try sequential trials with TCAs, WELLBUTRIN, REVIA, CATAPRES, and TENEX.

For mild OCD or OC symptoms, start with behavior therapy in children and young adolescents or cognitive behavior therapy in older adolescents and adults. If the response is insufficient, add PROZAC. For moderate to severe symptoms, start with PROZAC plus behavior therapy in children and young adolescents, or cognitive behavior therapy in older adolescents and adults.

- If no response or insufficient response, use sequential trials with other SRIs

- If still no response or insufficient response, consider ANAFRANIL

- If still no response or insufficient response, add BUSPAR or KLONOPIN

In high-functioning individuals with other neurological disorders (e.g., seizure disorder), ADHD, and obsessive-compulsive symptoms or disorder, simultaneously treat ADHD and OCD symptoms. For ADHD, begin with a TCA. If the response is insufficient, use sequential trials with other TCAs, WELLBUTRIN, or REVIA for inattention, impulsiveness, and hyperactivity, or sequential trials with

CATAPRES, TENEX and HALDOL for hyperactivity. If the response to these medications is insufficient, sequentially try RITALIN, DEXEDRINE, ADDERALL, and CYLERT (monitoring liver function regularly for patients taking CYLERT).

For mild OCD or OC symptoms, start with behavior therapy in children and young adolescents or cognitive behavior therapy in older adolescents and adults; if the response is insufficient, add PROZAC. For moderate-to-severe symptoms, start with PROZAC plus behavior therapy in children and young adolescents or cognitive behavior therapy in older adolescents and adults.

- If no response or insufficient response, use sequential trials with other SRIs

- If still no response or insufficient response, add BUSPAR or KLONOPIN

ADHD Plus Anxiety Disorders

In low- or middle-functioning individuals, treat ADHD and anxiety disorders simultaneously. For ADHD, begin with a TCA; if response is not sufficient, use sequential trials with other TCAs, WELLBUTRIN, and NALTREXONE, for inattention, impulsiveness, and hyperactivity, or CATAPRES, TENEX and HALDOL for hyperactivity and impulsiveness

For anxiety disorders, begin treatment of an acute anxiety episode with a BZD, adding BUSPAR if the response is insufficient. For chronic anxiety disorder, and the patient is already on a BZD, add BUSPAR, then taper BZD. If the patient is without prior BZD, start with BUSPAR and add a BZD if the response is insufficient, then taper BUSPAR. If the response is still insufficient, taper BZD or BUSPAR and use sequential trials with SRIs

Simultaneous treatment of ADHD and anxiety disorders is also recommended in higher-functioning individuals. Treat ADHD in individuals with other neurological disorders (e.g., seizure disorder) beginning with a TCA. If response is not sufficient, use sequential trials with other TCAs, WELLBUTRIN, and REVIA, for inattention, impulsiveness, and hyperactivity, or sequential trials with CATAPRES, TENEX and HALDOL for hyperactivity. If the patient does not respond sufficiently to these medications, use sequential trials with RITALIN, DEXEDRINE, ADDERALL, and CYLERT. Monitor liver function regularly when using CYLERT.

In higher-functioning individuals without other neurological disorders, begin simultaneous treatment of ADHD and anxiety disorders with RITALIN or DEXEDRINE. If the response is not sufficient, use sequential trials with either RITALIN or DEXEDRINE (the one that has not yet been used), ADDERALL, or CONCERTA and CYLERT. If none of these stimulants provide a satisfactory result, use sequential trials with TCAs, WELLBUTRIN, NALTREXONE, CATAPRES, and TENEX.

Begin treatment with psychotherapy for older adolescents and adults who experience a mild acute anxiety episode. If the response to psychotherapy is not sufficient, add a BZD, then add BUSPAR if necessary. For treatment of moderate-to-severe acute anxiety in older adolescents and adults, begin with a BZD plus psychotherapy, adding BUSPAR if the response is not satisfactory.

Begin treatment of chronic anxiety disorder with BUSPAR in patients who are without prior BZD, adding a BZD and then tapering BUSPAR if response is insufficient. If the patient is already on a BZD, first add BUSPAR and then taper BZD. If response is still insufficient, taper BZD or BUSPAR and use sequential trials with SRIs.

ADHD Plus Depression

For ADHD with mild depression in low- or middle-functioning individuals or in high-functioning individuals with other neurological disorders, treat ADHD first, then treat depression.

Begin ADHD treatment with a TCA. If the response is insufficient, use sequential trials with other TCAs, WELLBUTRIN, and REVIA, for inattention, impulsiveness, and hyperactivity, or sequential trials with CATAPRES, TENEX and HALDOL for hyperactivity and impulsiveness. If ADHD symptoms and depression persist, switch to an SRI. Use sequential trials with other SRIs if the response is insufficient. If ADHD responds to one of the TCAs or WELLBUTRIN, but depression persist, add an SRIs to treat depression. If the response to the SRI is not sufficient, use sequential trials with other SRIs

For ADHD with moderate-to-severe depression in low- or middle-functioning individuals or in high- functioning individuals with other neurological disorders, simultaneously treat ADHD and depression. Begin treatment of ADHD with a TCA. If the response is insufficient, sequentially try other TCAs, WELLBUTRIN, and REVIA, for inattention, impulsiveness, and hyperactivity, or CATAPRES, TENEX and HALDOL for hyperactivity and impulsiveness.

Begin treatment of depression with a TCA that is being used to treat ADHD. If the TCA provides and insufficient response, add an SRI while ADHD is being treated with other medication. If response remains insufficient, sequentially try other SRIs. If response continues to be insufficient, switch from the SRI to WELLBUTRIN if it has not been used for ADHD

In high-functioning individuals, without other neurological disorders, suffering from ADHD with mild depression, treat the ADHD first, then treat the depression. Begin treatment of ADHD with RITALIN or DEXEDRINE. If no response or insufficient response, use sequential trials with either RITALIN or DEXEDRINE (the one that has not yet been used), ADDERALL, or CYLERT (monitor liver function closely). If still no response or insufficient response with all of the above stimulants, use sequential trials with TCAs, WELLBUTRIN, REVIA, CATAPRES, and TENEX. If ADHD symptoms and depression persist, switch to an SRI, followed by sequential trials with other SRIs until a sufficient response is obtained.

If ADHD responds to one of the stimulants or TCAs, or WELLBUTRIN, but depression persists, add an SRI while the ADHD is being treated with an effective stimulant or TCAs. If still no response or insufficient response, use sequential trials with other SRIs

For ADHD with moderate-to-severe depression in high-functioning individuals without other neurological disorders, simultaneously treat ADHD and depression. Begin with RITALIN or DEXEDRINE to treat ADHD. If response is not sufficient, use sequential trials with either RITALIN or DEXEDRINE (the one that has not yet been used), ADDERALL, or CONCERTA, and CYLERT. Closely monitor liver function in patients taking CYLERT.

If still no response or insufficient response with all of the above stimulants, use sequential trials with TCAs, WELLBUTRIN, REVIA, CATAPRES, and TENEX. If ADHD symptoms and depression persist, switch to an SRI if it has not been used for depression. If still no response or insufficient response, use sequential trials with other SRIs.

Begin treatment of depression with an SRI while ADHD is being treated with other medication. If no response or insufficient response, use sequential trials with other SRIs. If still no response or insufficient response, switch to a TCA or WELLBUTRIN if they have not been used for ADHD.

ADHD Plus Hypomania or Mania

For patients with ADHD plus hypomania or mania, treat the hypomania or mania first, then treat ADHD. Start treatment of hypomania or mania with lithium or DEPAKOTE. If TSH is elevated, add a thyroid supplement. If the response is insufficient and there is marked agitation, add a BZD. If still no response or insufficient response, add an AP. If response is still none or insufficient, and the patient is in imminent danger, add ECT after discontinuing lithium.

If hypomania or mania responds to above treatment, but ADHD symptoms are persistent, add CATAPRES, switching to TENEX if the response is not satisfactory. If response remains insufficient, use sequential trials with RITALIN, DEXEDRINE, ADDERALL, and CYLERT. Closely monitor liver function in patients taking CYLERT.

If the patient has ADHD plus hypomania or mania with psychotic symptoms, treat hypomania or mania and psychotic symptoms first, then treat ADHD. Begin treatment of hypomania or mania with psychotic symptoms with an AP and lithium or DEPAKOTE. If the response is insufficient, and the patient has marked agitation, add a BZD. Add a thyroid supplement if TSH is elevated. If response is still insufficient, and the patient is in imminent danger, discontinue lithium and add ECT.

If hypomania or mania responds to above treatment, but ADHD symptoms persist, add CATAPRES, switching to TENEX if response is insufficient. If the response continues to be unsatisfactory, use sequential trials with RITALIN, DEXEDRINE, ADDERALL or CYLERT.

ADHD plus Agitation with Aggressive and Destructive Disorder

In low- or middle-functioning individuals or in higher- functioning individuals with other neurological disorders, simultaneously treat ADHD and agitation when the patient has aggressive or destructive behaviors due to inabilities to cope with task demands, difficult games and toys, or broken toys.

Begin treatment of ADHD with CATAPRES, continuing to sequential trials with TENEX and HALDOL for hyperactivity and impulsiveness if response to CATAPRES is not sufficient. If response to TENEX and HALDOL is insufficient, use sequential trials with TCAs, WELLBUTRIN, and REVIA. Begin treatment of agitation with behavior therapy while the patient is being treated for ADHD. If ADHD does not respond to CATAPRES, switch to the minimum possible dose of PROZAC or PAXIL.

For aggressive or destructive behaviors due to inabilities to cope with task demands, difficult games and toys, or broken toys in higher-functioning individuals without other neurological disorders, simultaneously treat ADHD and agitation

Begin treating ADHD with RITALIN or DEXEDRINE. If the response is insufficient, use sequential trials with RITALIN or DEXEDRINE (the one that has not yet been used), ADDERALL, and CYLERT (monitor liver function closely). If still no response or insufficient response with all of the above stimulants, sequentially try TCAs, WELLBUTRIN, and REVIA. Begin treatment of agitation with behavior therapy while the patient is being treated for ADHD. If ADHD does not respond to CATAPRES, switch to the minimum possible dose of PROZAC or PAXIL.

Chapter 11

Diagnosis and Treatment of Seizure Disorders

Individuals with ASD, particularly autistic disorder, are especially vulnerable to the development of seizure disorders (also called epilepsy). During the first decade of life, the incidence of epilepsy in children with autistic disorder is higher than that in the general population. Overall, seizure disorders have been noted in between one-fourth and one-third of people with autistic disorder. Individuals with ASD and with both a severe mental deficit and a motor handicap are at the greatest risk of seizure disorder. While the majority of individuals with ASD had seizure onset before the age of one, seizures may begin in early childhood or early adolescence. Although the most common type of seizure is the generalized tonic-clonic seizure, other seizure disorders can occur in individuals with ASD. Features of different seizure disorders may be difficult to separate from features of ASD or other neuropsychiatric disorders, so you must learn about clinical features and management of various seizure disorders. You may see several seizures your child has and not even know what they are. Even when you recognize a seizure, you might not know that a temporary medical condition has caused it. Lack of knowledge might lead you to take actions that you and your child might later regret.

Depending on the kind of seizures an individual has, and how successful treatment is in preventing them, epilepsy can be anything from a relatively mild, self-limiting disorder with few long-lasting effects, to a persistent, devastating condition that affects almost everything the individual does.

This chapter briefly describes the clinical manifestations of the more frequently observed seizure disorders and their effect on the cognitive and behavioral functions of patients. You will learn the characteristics of the commonly used anticonvulsant medications and the general medical treatments for seizure disorders.

I do not mean this to be a comprehensive guide for the assessment, diagnosis, and treatment of seizure disorders. This should certainly be left to specialists in the area (i.e., neurologists specialized in seizure disorders). Rather, the chapter is to help you learn to recognize an epileptic seizure when it happens and how to give basic first aid. It will also show you how to work with your child's doctor when anti-seizure drugs, also called anticonvulsants and antiepileptic drugs (AEDs), are necessary.

What Is Seizure Disorder?

Seizure disorder is a common neurological condition. It takes the form of brief, temporary changes in the normal functioning of the brain's electrical system. Normally, nerve cells discharge their tiny bursts of electrical energy independently, on and then off. With epilepsy, groups of cells begin to discharge all at the same time, and more than the usual amount of electrical energy passes between cells. This sudden overload may stay in just one small area of the brain, or it may swamp the entire system. Although one cannot see what is happening inside a person's brain during a seizure attack, one can see the unusual body movements, the effects on consciousness, and the changed behaviors that the malfunctioning cells produce. These changes are called epileptic seizures.

Classification of Seizure Disorders

Individual seizures are either focal/partial or generalized, depending on the initial abnormality seen on EEG recordings of the seizure event. Partial seizures arise from a particular brain region, often identifiable on cerebral imaging studies such as an MRI. Although focal/partial seizures may remain localized until they cease, it is not uncommon for them to become generalized seizures. Many become generalized so quickly that the caregivers usually do not notice the initial focal manifestations of the seizures. However, other focal seizures become generalized after an appreciable time has elapsed.

Generalized seizures begin with a widespread, bilateral, and synchronous hemispheric involvement. Epileptic seizures may be convulsive or non-convulsive in nature, depending on where in the brain the malfunction occurs and how much of the total brain area is involved. The following information is based on the 1981 International Classification of Seizure Disorders.

Simple Partial Seizures

In simple partial seizures, the individual does not lose consciousness and can interact normally within the environment (except for those limitations on specific functions caused by the seizure). The seizures may not be obvious to onlookers, other than the individual's preoccupied or blank expression. These seizures are often mistaken for acting out, bizarre behavior, hysteria, mental illness, psychosomatic illness, or parapsychological or mystical experiences. Simple partial seizures can be classified according to symptoms.

Seizures with Motor Signs

- Focal motor without march is where the seizures remain localized until they cease

- Focal motor with march, also called Jacksonian seizure, has several characteristics. Body parts are often initially involved distally, and then more proximal portions are involved. Jerking begins in the fingers or toes and may proceed to involve the hands, then the arms, and sometimes spreads to the whole body, and becoming a convulsive seizure

- Postural signs include turning the eyes and head turn to one side; at times the individual gazes at the hand on that side

- Phonatory (vocalization or arrest of speech)

Seizures with Somatosensory Symptoms

- Tingling

- Pins and needles sensation

- Experiencing a distorted environment with visual light-flashing taking the forms of zigzag lines, circumscribed circles, squares, stars, or animals that appear smaller than actual size

- Auditory-buzzing, loud swishing noises, and other easily recognized, complex auditory and visual hallucinations

- Olfactory fit, experiencing odd smells; gustatory and vertiginous-tornado fits

Seizures with Autonomic Symptoms or Signs

- Epigastric sensation

- Nausea

- A generally "funny" feeling in the stomach

- Recurrent abdominal discomfort and vomiting

- Pallor, sweating, and flushing

- Salivation

- Piloerection (bristling of body hairs)

- Pupillary dilation

Seizures with Psychic Symptoms

- Dysmnesic (impaired memory) symptoms, including distortion of memory or time, flashback experiences, deja vu, or occasionally experiencing a rapid recollection of episodes from life

- Cognitive disturbances, including dreamy states, sensations of extreme pleasure or joy, displeasure involving feelings of unexplained fear and intense depression, and rarely with anger or rage, distortions of time sense

- Illusions with objects appearing deformed in size, shape or structure

- Hallucinations with sounds of voices or music or scenes

Complex Partial Seizures

When the individual has impaired consciousness, the seizure is a complex partial seizure. This type of seizure is also called a psychomotor or temporal lobe seizure. Impairment of consciousness may be the first clinical sign of complex partial seizures. However, in some cases, complex partial seizures may evolve from *simple partial seizures*.

The main features of the complex partial seizures vary, but they usually include impairment or alteration of consciousness (occurring either near the beginning or during the seizure attack), unresponsiveness, and automatisms, including repetitive complex motor activities that are purposeless, undirected, and inappropriate to the situation. Examples of automatism include:

- Lip smacking, repetitious swallowing or chewing

- Fidgeting movements of the fingers or hands

- Gestural movements such as clapping or scratching

- Picking up objects, fumbling with or picking at clothing, trying to disrobe

- Walking or riding a bicycle with an appearance of either goal-directed or completely disorganized, appearing unaware of surroundings or dazed

- Stereotyped verbal response to stimulation, or repetitive utterance or mumbling

Psycho-illusory phenomena may occur at the onset of an attack, including a sense of detachment or depersonalization, forced thinking, visual distortions and formed hallucinations, visceral sensations, and a feeling of intense emotion such as fear, loneliness, depression, sadness, anger, joy, or ecstasy. At times, fear during a seizure may lead to running away. Once a pattern of complex partial seizure attack is established, the same set of actions usually occur with each seizure attack that lasts a few minutes.

Immediately after the seizure attack, individuals are confused and recover full consciousness slowly. During a time of incomplete awareness, they may resist restraint and react aggressively or angrily to objects and persons in their way. However, rage attacks or temper tantrums do not occur as manifestations of epilepsy. The individuals do not have any memory of what happened during the seizure. Complex partial seizures are often mistaken for drunkenness, intoxication on drugs, mental illness, indecent exposure, or disorderly conduct.

Tonic-Clonic (*Grand Mal*) Seizures

A tonic-clonic seizure (also called a *grand mal* seizure) is a generalized seizure. Its characteristics include abrupt onset with immediate loss or alteration of consciousness and an abrupt fall. During the tonic phase the body becomes rigid. There is forced exhalation against a partially closed space in the vocal cords that often leads to a hoarse cry. There are massive, sustained contractions of the entire musculature with limb extension and back arching (a stiffening of the whole body), lockjaw (trismus), shallow breathing or temporarily suspended breathing, and upward deviation of the eyes. There are marked autonomic phenomena, including dilatation of pupils, salivation, perspiration (diaphoresis), and dramatic rises in blood pressure and heart rate to two-to three-times normal levels. Often there is urinary incontinence, and sometimes there is fecal incontinence as well. This tonic phase lasts from several seconds to several minutes, and a bluish discoloration of the skin (cyanosis) develops.

The tonic phase is followed by the clonic phase. There is uncontrolled jerking with the head bent backwards. The arms are usually flexed, and the lower extremities are extended. The clonic phase can continue for minutes, waxing and waning. In most instances the clonic phase gradually subsides as the jerks decrease in frequency.

After the clonic phase, the patient slowly regains full consciousness and is typically confused and excessively drowsy (somnolent) for minutes to hours after an attack. When fully awake, the patient may complain of a headache and muscle pain, but is otherwise unaware (amnesic) of what happened. Tonic-clonic (grand mal) seizures are sometimes mistaken for a heart attack, stroke, or an unknown, but life-threatening, emergency.

Absence (*Petit Mal*) Seizures

Absence seizures (also known as *petit mal* seizures) manifest as momentary lapses in awareness (amnesia). They begin and end abruptly, rarely lasting more than a few seconds. There is no warning or post-seizure attack period. Sometimes attacks are so brief that they escape detection. The individual having the seizure is unaware of what is going on during the seizure, but quickly returns to full awareness once it has stopped.

In a typical absence seizure attack, the patient abruptly loses consciousness, ongoing activity ceases without significant alteration in postural tone, and the individual's eyes stare vacantly straight ahead or may roll upward. There is no movement except possibly some subtle fluttering of the eyelids or eye blinking, twitching of the mouth muscles, or some chewing movement of the mouth. Other common features are autonomic phenomena such as dilatation of the eyes' pupils, change in skin color, rapid heart rate (tachycardia) and bristling of hairs (piloerection) and automatisms (aberrations of behavior). At the end of the seizure, the individual suddenly resumes his previous activity as if nothing had happened, without any post-seizure confusion or drowsiness. Dozens to hundreds of seizures may occur in a single day.

Some children with absence seizures may have attacks when exposed to flashing or flickering lights, black and white patterns that strobe, and certain intense flashing effects in videogames. Absence seizure is one of the benign forms of childhood seizure that usually responds well to treatment with AEDs and may disappear at adolescence. These petit mal seizures are often mistaken for daydreaming, lack of attention, or deliberate ignoring of adult instructions.

Atonic Seizures (Drop Attacks)

The legs of a child between two-and-five years-of-age suddenly collapse under him, and he falls. After ten seconds to a minute, he recovers, regains consciousness, and can stand and walk again. Atonic seizures are often mistaken for clumsiness, lack of good walking skills, or a normal childhood "stage."

Myoclonic Seizures

Myoclonic seizures are often mistaken for clumsiness or poor coordination. These seizures manifest as sudden, brief, massive muscle jerks that may involve the whole body or parts of the body. They may cause a person to spill what he was holding or fall off a chair. Sometimes these become generalized tonic-clonic seizures. Adolescence may be a time when this type of seizure disorder (called juvenile myoclonic epilepsy) begins. Juvenile myoclonic epilepsy responds well to treatment, but the seizures usually return when the medication is discontinued.

Other Seizure Disorders

Infantile Spasms

Infantile spasms are a rare form of epilepsy that affects children in a narrow age range, starting between three and twelve months and stopping at age two-to-four. These children may experience developmental delay and go on to have other types of seizures. About one in ten also develops Lennox-Gastaut syndrome.

Lennox-Gastaut Syndrome

Lennox-Gastaut syndrome typically begins between the ages of one and six and has mixed seizures, including convulsions, myoclonic seizures, and drop attacks (atonic seizures). Children with drop attacks may have to wear helmets to protect their faces and heads from the effects of these frequent falls. Children with Lennox-Gastaut may have developmental delays as well as other neurological challenges.

Differential Diagnosis of Seizure Disorders

Recognition of epileptic seizure (ES) is important because it is very easy to mistake epilepsy for some of the other conditions briefly mentioned above. A convulsive seizure may look like a heart attack, and cardiac-pulmonary-resuscitation (CPR) techniques may be used when they are not necessary. A period of automatic behavior may be interpreted as public drunkenness, being drunk and disorderly, or being high on illegal drugs.

On the other hand, many neurological or psychiatric conditions, as well as behaviors in infants and children, can mimic an epileptic event. These episodes are non-epileptic seizures (NES), and they can resemble almost any seizure phenotype, but are behavioral and emotional manifestations of psychological distress, conflict, or trauma that have no identifiable EEG or neurological correlate.

Common NES include the following.

- Syncope, which is a brief loss of consciousness due to lack of oxygen to the brain

- Breath-holding spells

- Parasomnias (disorders related to sleep)

- Gastrointestinal reflux (stomach contents flow back up into the throat)

- Movement disorders like paroxysmal choreoathetosis (extreme range of motion, jerky involuntary movements, and fluctuation in muscle tone from floppy to overly tight)

Historically, many terms have been used to label NES. Clinicians use terms like pseudoseizures, pseudoepileptic seizures, nonepileptic events, nonelectrical seizures, hysterical seizures, and nonepileptic attacks. This causes much confusion.

Despite technological advances and the accumulation of clinical experience with epilepsy and its imitators, experts often find it difficult to differentiate epileptic from nonepileptic events. Overlap between the appearance of ES and NES is considerable. Investigations designed to separate or otherwise classify NES patients according to neuropsychological and personality profiles have yielded mixed results. Adding to the complexity of differential diagnosis is the fact that a significant number of individuals with NES have concomitant histories of neurological trauma, including seizures and other nonspecific EEG abnormalities. Accurate diagnosis often requires considerable gathering and sorting of data by an interdisciplinary team from neurology, neurophysiology, neuroradiology, psychiatry, and neuropsychology.

Prevalence of Seizure Disorders

More than two million Americans have epilepsy, which is about one person in one hundred. Approximately 300,000 American children under the age of fourteen have seizures that recur unexpectedly from time to time. While seizures can begin at any time of life, three-out-of -four new cases begin in childhood, and fifty percent of all cases begin before the age of twenty-five. Between two and five percent of all children between the ages of six months and five years experience a convulsion when they have a fever with a childhood illness. Individuals with ASD have even higher risks of having seizure disorders.

Causes of Seizure Disorders

There are many different reasons why some people develop seizure disorders. Pinpointing the causes is difficult at any age. At present, about seventy percent of seizure disorders do not have clear causes, a condition described as idiopathic. Some possible causes:

- Problems with brain development before birth

- Lack of oxygen during or following birth

- Brain injury during or following birth that leaves a scar in the brain

- Unusual structures within the brain

- Tumors

- Prolonged seizure with fever

- The after-effects of severe brain infections like meningitis or encephalitis

- Chromosomal disorders like tuberous sclerosis

Epilepsy in adults may be the result of a head injury, often from auto accidents, or may date from their childhood years. Sometimes there is a family history of seizures, including feverish (febrile) seizures, epilepsy, and seizures in childhood that later went into remission. Absence seizures, juvenile myoclonic epilepsy, and familial neonatal seizures (seizures in the newborn) are three types of epilepsy that tend to run in families and may have a genetic basis.

Frequency of Seizures

In the North Carolina Autism Society survey among the individuals with autistic disorder, the numbers given for different seizure frequencies were as follows:

- More than one seizure a month, about 19%

- More than three per year, but less than one a month, about 12.0%

- Less than three per year, about 15%

- None in the last year, about 9%

- None in the last two years, about 5%

- None in the last three years, about 32%

- No seizures observed, about 8%

Effects of Seizure Disorders

The type of seizure, age of seizure onset, seizure duration, and seizure severity impact the intellectual and emotional functioning of individuals with epilepsy. In general, more severe and chronic types of epilepsy tend to have high associations with mental retardation, while in less severe seizure disorders, evidence for cognitive and behavioral dysfunction is more difficult to demonstrate scientifically. However, researchers have not thoroughly studied the relative contributions of anti-seizure drugs, psychosocial factors, and underlying causes of the seizures to mental retardation.

On average, many children with epilepsy test within the same range as other children, but their achievement at school is often lower. There are several possible reasons for this, including side effects from the medication, absences from school for medical tests or doctor visits, and anxiety about having seizures at school. Seizures may also affect memory or attention. After a seizure, a child may be unable to remember anything that happened the previous day or immediately afterward. Chronic seizure disorders may also indirectly lead to chronic cognitive deterioration.

Seizures may directly lead to disturbed behavior in the form of organic mental disorders. Intractable epilepsy can be a disabling disorder that drastically affects individuals' emotional well-being. Seizure disorders may cause loss of independence, alter an individual's sense of self-efficacy, and produce excess disability in terms of financial and social burden.

Parents of children with seizure disorders often watch their children closely for fear of not being able to catch the next attack. Parents can become overprotective. They can potentially upset normal family relationships by developing abnormal attachments to the children. This could cause the children to develop abnormal attachments to them. Parents usually prevent their child from interacting in a normal manner with peers because of their overprotection. This interferes with the child's overall developmental progress.

Parents may set lower standards for their child. Lower standards for one child in a family can result in that child's academic underachievement, or it might engender feelings of jealousy or sibling rivalry. The child may also become self-conscious, feel vulnerable, or believe that he is in some way flawed and unable to compete with peers. The interplay between these biopsychosocial factors can adversely affect the child's behavioral and emotional functioning through causes that are independent of the seizure disorder.

Assessment and Diagnosis of Seizure Disorders

What You Can Do to Facilitate Diagnosis

You could miss the more subtle signs of the condition in your child, so you could also miss the opportunity for early diagnosis and treatment. The symptoms listed below are not necessarily indicators of a seizure disorder; they may be caused by some other, unrelated conditions. However, if you see one or more of the following symptoms in your child, you should seek a medical evaluation.

- Episodes of staring or short attention blackouts that look like daydreaming

- Episodes of head nodding, rapid eye blinking, or chewing at inappropriate times

- Brief periods when there is no response from the child to questions or instructions

- Episodes of dazed and confused behavior

- Sudden falls for no apparent reason

- Stomach pain followed by confusion and sleepiness.

- "Fainting spells" with lost control of bladder or bowel, followed by extreme fatigue.

- Periods of blackout or confused memory

- Involuntary movements such as muscle jerks

- Excessive thrashing around while asleep, or waking with a bitten tongue or unexplained bruises

- Unusual sleepiness and/or irritability when wakened in the morning

- A convulsion, with or without fever

- Complaints of odd sounds, distorted vision, episodes of fear, or short-lived "funny" feelings or feelings of impending disaster

Seizure Disorders Diagnosed by Physicians

Physicians make a diagnosis based on the description of the events given by the individuals who have seizures and their family members or caregivers. A child, especially an older child, may remember and be able to describe what happens to him physically and mentally before and after a seizure. It is essential that you can provide a thorough and accurate history including:

- A description of the characteristics of the attacks, including age of onset, date and circumstances of the first attack, one or more than one seizure type, manifestations of seizure attacks and immediately after seizure attacks, any change of seizure pattern, any recognizable precipitating or associated factors, frequency of attacks, and longest seizure-free interval

- A pertinent past history, including details of birth, postnatal and early development, serious illness, trauma, ingestions or toxic exposures, reactions to immunizations, and school performance

- A relevant family history (e.g., other family members with a seizure history)

The majority of the time, the above information is enough to make an accurate diagnosis. On occasion, however, the information may simply not provide enough insight for an accurate diagnosis. Under these circumstances, the physician may require further testing.

Neurophysiological Testing of Epilepsy

An EEG examination can provide useful information to support the clinician's initial diagnostic suspicion. In EEG examinations, the technician places electrodes over the patient's scalp to detect the brain's electrical signals. This is a painless test, but if an individual is afraid, if may be helpful to administer a mild sedative.

In individuals with epilepsy, abnormalities in EEG printouts can often help the physician in making a diagnosis. The most common and characteristic abnormality is that of a "spike discharge." This discharge resembles a spike in the line of brain waves. The point on the EEG where the spike occurs helps determine the location in the brain that is the seizure's focus. However, nonspecific EEG abnormalities are not uncommon in individuals without a seizure disorder.

The most definitive diagnostic information is obtained if a seizure is actually witnessed during the EEG test. Since most routine office EEGs last less than one hour, the chance of a seizure occurring during the test is unlikely unless the seizure events are very frequent. When a diagnosis remains elusive, other procedures could be required to increase the likelihood of recording a seizure. These procedures are induction or provocative testing and video-EEG monitoring.

Placebo Induction or Provocative Testing

Physicians frequently use placebo induction or provocative testing procedures to aid in the differential diagnosis of seizure disorders. The goal of the following techniques is to induce a spell identical to the individual's spontaneous episodes.

- Photic stimulation

- Hyperventilation

- Tactile compression

- Injection of normal saline or other chemical placebos

- Placement of epidural patches soaked in alcohol

- Hypnotic suggestion

Spells elicited by these techniques are very similar to typical events and support the diagnosis of seizure disorder. Videotapes made during the induction test to record the seizure events are particularly valuable in assessing the extent to which an induced spell resembles previous events.

When an induction is appropriate, the doctor must obtain permission from your child and you for trying a procedure that may produce a clinical spell similar to those occurring spontaneously. Consent allows you and your child to actively participate rather than just being a bystander or subject of the diagnostic process.

Video-EEG Monitoring

This is a more advanced test for the diagnosis and classification of seizures. The patient comes to a hospital room that has been equipped for the test. The doctors, nurses, and technologists are specially trained in treating seizures. Preparations are similar to a routine EEG, but the patient can do different things, similar to those he would do at home. This test takes place over a longer period of time than a routine EEG. People with infrequent seizures may need monitoring for several days to increase the probability that a seizure event is recorded.

Cameras positioned in the room record all of the person's actions, and the EEG records electrical data. In the event of a seizure, the electrical activity of the brain during the episode can be compared to the simultaneous camera recording made before, during, and after the seizure.

Management and Treatment of Seizure Disorders

Once the diagnosis is established, treatment requires active interactions between multiple factors including the individual with epilepsy, his family, medical professionals, other caregivers, and the environment. This means that some individuals with seizure disorders will need specialized planning, with goals and objectives carefully spelled out, and a partnership between the parents and the school or employers. Part of that planning is to ensure that the individual is included in regular school or job activities and is not excluded because of having epilepsy. The goal for your child is a normal and active life without frequent crises and emergency room visits. Seizures may make that goal more difficult, but with a supportive family, a good medical team, new medications and procedures, accepting teachers or employers, and a lot of love, it can be done.

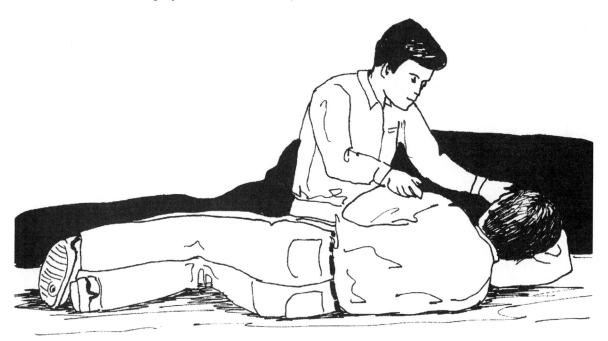

In general, the management and treatment of seizure disorders in individuals with ASD is very similar to that in epileptic patients without ASD. Since seizure types are so different, some require different kinds of action, and others require no action at all.

Emergency Treatment

An uncomplicated convulsive seizure is not always a medical emergency, even though it looks like one. It stops naturally after a few minutes without ill effects. The average individual is able to continue about his business after a rest period and may need only limited assistance, or no assistance at all.

However, if your child has a seizure caused by known medical conditions, such as encephalitis, meningitis, heat exhaustion, poisoning, hypoglycemia, high fever, and head injury, he needs immediate medical attention. You should always call an ambulance when your child has a convulsive seizure in any of the following situations:

- The seizure has occurred in water

- The seizure continues for more than ten minutes

- There are signs of injury

First Aid for Your Child

Seizures can occur at any time without warning. You need to know first aid techniques that can help you safely manage your child's attacks. For example, if your child has a convulsive seizure, do not put hard implements in his mouth. This is dangerous. Turning the child on one side is a much better way to prevent choking and keep the airway clear. Other techniques for helping a person having a seizure are described below.

Simple Partial Seizure

No action is needed other than reassurance and emotional support unless the seizure becomes convulsive. If that happens, apply first aid as described below under generalized tonic-clonic seizure.

Complex Partial Seizure

Speak calmly and reassuringly to your child and others. Guide the child gently away from obvious hazards. Stay with him until he becomes completely aware of the environment. Do not grab and hold him unless a sudden danger threatens his safety. Do not try to restrain the child and do not shout. Do not expect your child to respond to verbal instructions.

Generalized Tonic-Clonic (*Grand Mal*) Seizure

Protect the child from nearby hazards. Loosen his tie or shirt collar. Place a folded jacket under his head. Turn the child on side to keep the airway clear. Reassure the child when he regains consciousness. If multiple seizures occur, or if one seizure lasts longer than ten minutes, take the child to the emergency room. Do not put any hard implement in the mouth or hold the tongue. Do not give liquids during or just after a seizure. Use oxygen only if there are symptoms of a heart attack. Do not use artificial respiration unless breathing is absent after muscle jerks subside, or unless the child has inhaled water. Do not restrain the child.

Atonic Seizure (Drop Attack)

No first aid is needed unless your child hurt himself as he fell, but he should be given a thorough medical evaluation if a fall might cause serious injuries.

Absence (*Petit Mal*) and Myoclonic Seizures

No first aid is needed.

First Aid for Special Circumstances

Seizure in Water

Support your child in the water with the head tilted so his face and head stay above the surface. Move the child out of the water as quickly as possible with the head in the tilted position. Once on dry land, begin artificial respiration at once if the child is not breathing. Call an ambulance immediately, even if he appears to be fully recovered.

Seizure in a Plane, Bus, Train, or Car

Quickly manage to have enough space to lay your child across two or more seats with head and body turned on one side. Once he has fully regained consciousness, you can help him into a resting position in a single seat. He can be turned gently while in the seat so that he is leaning toward one side.

Pillows or blankets can be arranged so that the head does not hit unpadded areas of the plane, bus, or train. However, take care that the angle at which your child is sitting is such that the airway stays clear and breathing is unobstructed. When a seizure happens in the car while you are driving, immediately find a safe place to park and then follow the above steps.

Medication Treatment of Seizure Disorders

In the past, if a child had a seizure, the physician immediately prescribed medication. The general consensus among physicians was that letting the child have additional seizures was very harmful. We now know that such a concern is essentially unwarranted. Physician are now better able to advise families concerning the risks and benefits involved in refraining from medication treatment for the child who has had a seizure. Studies show that individuals may have a single seizure and never have a recurrence. The chronic use of potentially toxic medication to prevent something that may never happen is unwarranted.

The consequences of a recurrence seizure vary with age. In a young child who is generally well-supervised, the consequence of recurrence may be small because it is unlikely that the child will be seriously injured if another seizure occurs. But an older, more independent individual who is farther from home on a bicycle or driving a car may be at a greater risk.

Treatment of Childhood Epilepsy

The most common forms of childhood epilepsy respond best to medication treatment and are also most likely to be outgrown:

- Familial neonatal epilepsy (seizures in newborns)

- Febrile seizures

- Absence seizures

- Benign focal epilepsy.

These disorders are sometimes called "benign epilepsies of childhood," and they occur in children between the ages of two and thirteen. Children with these benign epileptic syndromes respond well to a single AED and are able to live an active, normal childhood. They are often able to discontinue the

160

medicine after they have been seizure-free for two years. At that time, physicians may recommend a slow tapering off and an eventual withdrawal of the medication.

About sixty-five to eighty percent of children with this type of epilepsy will continue to do well and will have no further seizures after stopping the AEDs. If seizures return, medication is resumed. Usually, it is as successful in controlling seizures as it was before.

The Objective of Treatment

The objective in the treatment is a complete control of seizures, or at least a reduction in their frequency so that they no longer interfere with physical and social well-being. It is not uncommon for a single AED to be all that is needed to achieve satisfactory seizure control.

In some cases, complete seizure control may not be possible. An occasional seizure is more appropriate than using multiple AEDs for prolonged periods that tend to cause cognitive and behavioral side effects. If the risks of therapy outweigh the possible benefits, you and your child's doctor should understand that it may be better to stop medication therapy when the seizures are infrequent or not likely to happen again.

Factors in Drug Choice

Prescribing medication for epilepsy is as much an art as a science. For either medical or social reasons, some individuals may prefer or be better suited by one medication over another. If the physician and you decide to use an AED to control the seizures, you must choose the appropriate one. Various factors including seizure type, age of the patient, neurological function, and social circumstances are part of the decision-making process. The individual and his/her family may have limited access to medical care or limited funds, and there may be a problem in administering medications multiple times a day. In that situation, an AED that is inexpensive and can be taken once a day may be the first choice.

A medication is the right one if seizures are controlled, and the individual continues to feel well and perform at his maximum ability. If there are adverse changes in function, then it is probably the wrong medication. In spite of the cost and ease of administration, the medication should be changed.

Each individual medication has the potential for causing different side effects. The choice of an AED should be based on the seizure type balanced with the risk of acceptable side effects. For example, Dilantin is an excellent AED for a variety of seizure types. Because of its potential for cosmetic side effects such as gum hypertrophy (enlargement) and excessive hair growth, you and the physician may reconsider its use by adolescents and teenagers if another suitable medication is available.

General Guidelines to AED Therapy

The best procedure is to begin treatment with one AED. If the AED does not control seizures, it is discontinued gradually while a second AED is instituted and its dosage is increased. Doctors should change drug dosage gradually, usually not more frequently than once every five-to-seven days, until the seizures are under control or until clinical toxicity appears.

On occasion, a person will not respond to an AED commonly used for his seizure type. When this occurs, the physician should determine if the type of seizure has been misclassified. If there has been an error, the physician can make the appropriate changes in the medication.

Once seizures are in control, the patient should take the medication for a prolonged period of time. If your child has infrequent seizures, the medication can be increased gradually until the blood level of the AED reaches the lower end of its therapeutic range. The dose should subsequently be increased only if there is another seizure.

Checking anticonvulsant blood levels is necessary in all cases. Monitoring blood levels serves as a guideline to indicate sub-therapeutic levels and possible problems with compliance. Blood levels also discover impending toxicity. In more complex situations (e.g., multiple therapies), blood levels may help determine which medication is more likely to be responsible for toxicity.

When psychotherapeutic medications are under consideration, the physician should carefully assess the interactions between psychotherapeutic medications and AEDs. There is the possibility of an alteration in seizure threshold, which can induce seizure activities even in individuals with a previously well-controlled disorder.

When you notice adverse changes in your child's cognitive and emotional functioning while on AEDs, inform his doctor. If there are no other explanations for the neuro-behavioral effects, the doctor should reduce the dose or change the medication if the former approach does not produce significant improvement.

Antiepileptic Drugs (AED)—Anticonvulsants

Anticonvulsants vary in their ability to affect different types of seizures. Nonetheless, anticonvulsants may act through two mechanisms at the molecular level to achieve their effect:

1. Direct modification of neuronal membrane function The anticonvulsants decrease the spread of excitation across neurons through change of the ionic concentration across cell membranes, and

2. Change of neurotransmission (i.e., change of synaptic transmitters)

All AEDs seem to share a common action that involves reducing ionic fluxes across the neuronal membrane. Such action decreases the excitability of nerve cells, which in turn decreases the frequency of seizure attacks.

Researchers study AEDs for their effectiveness against specific types of seizures, and occasionally for their effectiveness against specific epilepsy syndromes. Doctors place patients with seizure disorders on AEDs to control their seizures. In some cases, an inappropriate anti-epileptic medication may actually worsen the condition. This is why an accurate characterization of seizures and a correct diagnosis of epilepsy itself are absolutely vital.

While AEDs can significantly decrease these individuals' seizure frequency and intensity, AEDs can also impair their memory functioning, mental functioning, motor speed (e.g., becoming overactive), and mood. Before a decision is made to place your child on AEDs, you and the doctor should carefully evaluate the possibility of life-long AED therapy, the possibility of multiple AEDs, and the potential dangers of AED therapy.

Commonly Used AEDs

See Appendix F.

When to Stop Taking AEDs

If seizures have been well under control for two years, and the EEG shows a normal result, the doctor should consider tapering off the seizure medication. Epidemiological studies have found that 70-75% of individuals who have had seizures successfully controlled can be weaned from seizure medication without recurrence.

Concerns with AED Treatment in Patients with ASD

The most common problem with AED treatment is a toxic anticonvulsant level. In one study, 16% of patients receiving TEGRETOL and 28% of those receiving DILANTIN had toxic levels. Even at therapeutic levels, AEDs may contribute to cognitive, behavioral, and emotional symptoms. The negative cognitive and behavioral effects of AEDs may be devastating, and many physicians without adequate training in managing developmental disorders are insufficiently attentive to this aspect of AED pharmacotherapy. Because of inadequate training, it is not uncommon for these physicians to prescribe a medication to control behavioral reactions to AEDs when a change in the AED regime would be more appropriate. Nor is it uncommon for an individual with ASD being placed on multiple AEDs for prolonged periods when single medication therapy would be sufficient.

On the one hand, the consequences of uncontrolled epilepsy may be catastrophic. On the other hand, considering the possible toxic effects of AEDs, the occurrence of an occasional seizure without AED treatment may be an acceptable price to pay to maintain the quality of an individual's day-to-day life. Perfect seizure control is not necessarily worth the price of severe cognitive blunting, especially in a person who already has impaired cognitive functioning. Be vigilant to the problem and work with a competent physician to make a careful decision on AED treatment for your child. Should you and your child decide to go for AED therapy, you should closely monitor the effectiveness and side effects of the medications.

Alternatives to Medication Treatment

There are several options available for the person who continues to have seizures despite treatment with various medications.

Experimental AED—FDA currently does not approve these medications for marketing, but they may be available at certain epilepsy research centers. However, your child must first qualify as a suitable candidate under specific criteria defined by the study's objectives. He may be excluded from the study if his seizures are of a different type from those being investigated. Once enrolled in a study, there are often strict protocols that are part of the research, such as having frequent blood tests and filling out questionnaires.

Ketogenic Diet—This is a special diet that consists primarily of foods rich in fat and low in carbohydrates and proteins. In the body, these fats are metabolized and form a product called ketones. For reasons not completely understood, the presence of ketones seems to protect against seizure activity. However, this diet is very difficult to administer due to unpalatable taste. It also requires meticulous measuring and weighing of foods, as well as urine testing to ensure appropriate ketone levels.

Vagus Nerve Stimulator—The FDA recently approved this device for the treatment of epilepsy. The vagus nerve is the longest nerve in the brain. It is a major communication channel from the brain stem to the neck, throat, chest, and abdomen. Similar to a pacemaker, the vagus nerve stimulator is implanted under the skin and sends small electrical impulses to the vagus nerve. For reasons currently under investigation, this repeated stimulation appears to reduce the frequency of seizures in some individuals who received such a treatment.

Epilepsy Surgery—Two criteria are generally required for epilepsy surgery. The first is that a person's seizures all arise from the same part of the brain. The second is that this area of the brain is not involved in an important function such as speech, movement, or recognizing sensations. The goal of epilepsy surgery is to remove the epileptic focus (the part of the brain causing the seizures) while preserving normal function. An epileptologist conducts a complex, extensive, pre-surgical investigation, including video-EEG monitoring and recording of several seizures, to pinpoint the part of the brain in question. After this evaluation, if all the person's seizures are found to arise from a single focus, surgery is a potential option.

Additional Therapies

Parents of children with epilepsy could develop abnormal attachment to them. These parents may also have stressful lives and have higher rates of anxiety and depression. If your relatives and friends show or express their concerns to you, you should pay attention and seek professional help. You should keep in mind that your physical and mental health is one of the key factors in the successful treatment of your child's seizure disorders.

On the other hand, if you notice that your child develops emotional or behavioral symptoms that seem to be caused by chronic seizure disorder, you should seek professional help, particularly cognitive-behavioral therapy and individual and group therapies for your child to restore his mental well-being.

Appendix A

Basic Pharmacology

If a physician is considering using psychoactive drugs (psychopharmacotherapy) for your child, he or she may give you preprinted materials about the prescribed medications. You can also look into pharmacology textbooks or consumer-oriented books to learn more about the medications. This appendix helps you understand the technical terms commonly used in the preprinted information on drugs or in medical books. It also briefly describes some basic principles that apply to all medications. Understanding a medication's effect (pharmacodynamics) and the way it is absorbed, metabolized, and eliminated by the body (pharmacokinetics) can enhance safety and effectiveness.

This appendix and the next cover the general principles of pharmacology—the characteristics or properties and effectiveness of drugs. Pharmacology requires some knowledge of biology and chemistry. Some medications in this appendix are described in more detail in Chapters 8 and 11 and Appendices H and I.

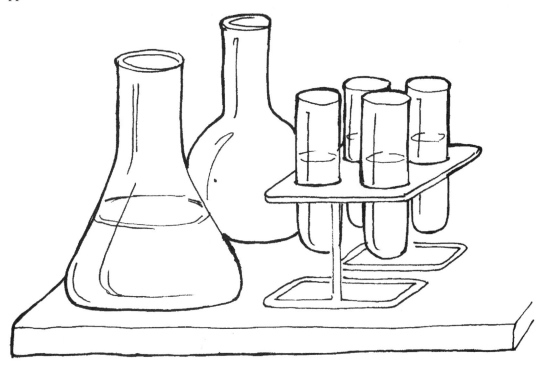

Basic Principles of Pharmacology

The goal of pharmacology is to get the appropriate medication into the target tissues (where the receptors are present) at the appropriate concentration for the right length of time. If concentrations in the target tissues are too low, therapy will be ineffective; if concentrations are too high, toxicity may result. There are two components of pharmacology that are essential for an effective medication treatment: "pharmacokinetics" and "pharmacodynamics."

Pharmacokinetics

Pharmacokinetics describes the rate at which medication is absorbed, distributed, metabolized, and eliminated from the body. This determines the minimal requirement for a medication's action. To produce the desired effects, a medication must be present in appropriate concentrations at its sites of action. Although related to the mount of medication administered, the concentrations attained also depend upon the extent and rate of its absorption, distribution, binding or localization in tissues, biotransformation, and excretion. Attaining the critical concentration may or may not occur at the same time as the clinical onset of action. Many psychotherapeutic medications take time before the desired effect is seen. For example, an antidepressant usually takes two-to-three weeks to show its effects.

Pharmacokinetics also determines how long a medication's action will continue and how frequently a patient must take the medication to maintain the desired effect. A knowledgeable physician will choose a medication based in part on how well its pharmacokinetics meets the needs for which it is prescribed. To provide an immediate but short-lived effect, the ideal medication would be rapidly absorbed and distributed to the brain, and then rapidly redistributed to other body parts for eventual excretion. The pharmacokinetic process varies between individuals and within an individual, depending on genetic differences, physiological and psychological state, diet, and other medications.

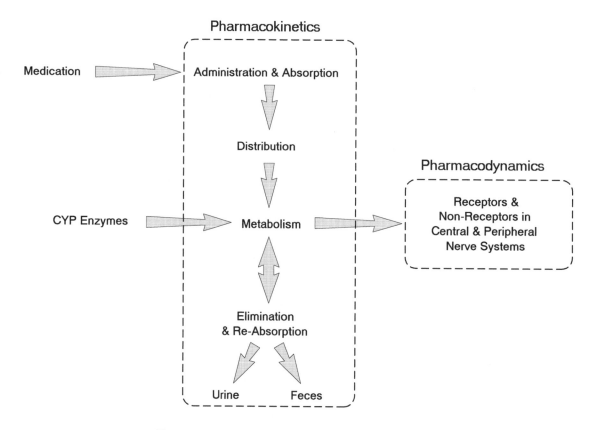

Figure A-1 Basic Psychopharmacology

Four Primary Phases of Pharmacokinetics

The four primary phases of pharmacokinetics are:

1. Administration and absorption

2. Distribution

3. Metabolism

4. Elimination

Administration and Absorption

Different routes of administration can affect the rate of absorption, as well as the ratio of a parent compound to its various metabolites. Metabolites are chemicals that result from the breakdown of a parent compound by the body. Knowing how a medication would be absorbed most effectively usually determines how that medication is administered. However, before discussing routes of administration, two important terms need a brief explanation.

- **First-Pass Elimination or Metabolism Effect**—After being absorbed from the stomach or the intestines, an orally administered medication is carried by the blood to the liver. During this first circuit through the liver, cytochrome P450 (CYP) enzymes in both the bowel wall and the liver cells can metabolize a fraction of the medication (i.e., extraction and deactivation) before it reaches the body's general circulation. Diseases or some medications can broadly alter the extent of this effect. Variations in the absorption process and extraction and deactivation by the liver after oral administration are major contributing factors to the wide range of response to a standard dose. After passage through the liver, the medication enters the general circulation for distribution to the body sites of action (e.g., the brain).

  With limited exceptions, drugs administered by any injection (parenteral) route, excluding the intra-arterial route, are subject to first-pass elimination in the lungs prior to distribution to the rest of the body. This is because all the blood in the veins has to go through the lungs to release carbon dioxide and get more oxygen before it goes into arteries. The lungs may metabolize, and thus deactivate, a number of medications that are carried through venous blood.

- **Bioavailability**—The percentage of medication that ultimately reaches the site of action is called its bioavailability. For example, a medication that is absorbed from the stomach and intestine must first pass through the liver before it reaches the systemic (general) circulation. If the medication is metabolized in the liver or excreted in the bile, some of the active medication will be deactivated or diverted before it reaches the its sites of action. If the metabolic or excretory capacity of the liver for the particular medication is great, bioavailability will be substantially decreased. On the other hand, the bioavailability of medications may be greatly increased during liver disease, resulting in an unexpected overdose. This increase or decrease in availability is a function of where in the body absorption takes place. Other anatomical, physiological, and pathological factors can also influence bioavailability. The choice of the route of medication administration must be based on understanding these conditions.

Route of Administration

Oral Administration

The most common route of medication administration is through the mouth (*per os* or *p.o.*, Latin for "by mouth") so that it is absorbed in various parts of the gastrointestinal (GI) tract. Oral administration is generally the safest, most economical, and most convenient method. However, several factors can influence absorption of medications from the GI tract, which can greatly alter the rate of medication accumulation, its concentration, and its duration, including

- Blood acidity

- Surface area for absorption

- Rate of movement of the contents through the GI tract

- Dosage form (i.e., tablet or capsule)

- Concentration of the medication

- Blood flow of the GI tract

- Digestive secretions

- Other contents of the GI tract (i.e., food).

While the oral route is the safest way to administer medications, it also has several disadvantages, including

- Medications taken orally are absorbed slower than medications taken by most other routes. It takes about 30-to-90 minutes to achieve the maximum concentration in the bloodstream, so the oral route is usually not good in an emergency.

- Patients must be conscious; otherwise, they might choke to death if the medication is given orally.

- Absorption of medication is much more variable and unpredictable due to the constantly changing conditions, including changes in stomach acidity, the presence of food or other medications, changes in the rate of stomach emptying or intestinal action due to other medications, diarrhea, or gastroenteritis.

- Some medications irritate the GI tract and may produce nausea and vomiting unless they are given with food.

- Medications in the GI tract may be metabolized before they gain access to the general circulation.

Sublingual or Buccal Administration

Blood from the mouth flows through the heart to the systematic (general) circulation without going through the liver. Thus medication administered under the tongue (sublingually) is protected from rapid first-pass metabolism by the liver, and only a small amount of medication with rapid dissolution is needed. For example, nitroglycerin (a medication for a heart attack) is effective when retained sublingually because it has high lipid solubility. Therefore, it is absorbed very rapidly. Nitroglycerin is also very potent; relatively few molecules need to be absorbed to produce the therapeutic effect. If the conventional tablet is swallowed (instead of dissolved under the tongue), the medication is destroyed in the stomach or intestines before having any therapeutic effect.

Rectal Administration

Rectal administration may serve as an alternate route for medications that tend to be destroyed in the stomach or small intestine. This route also is useful when oral ingestion is precluded by frequent vomiting or when the individual is unconscious. Approximately fifty percent of the medication that is absorbed into the blood supply from the rectum will bypass the liver, and the potential for first-pass metabolism is lower than that for an oral dose. However, rectal absorption often is irregular and incomplete, and many medications irritate the rectal mucous membrane.

Parenteral Administration

The major routes of parenteral administration are intravenous, subcutaneous, and intramuscular. Rarely used routes include intra-arterial, intra-thecal, intra-cerebroventricular, intra-peritoneal, and intra-bone marrow injections. The parenteral injection of medications has certain distinct advantages over oral administration. Availability of medication is usually more rapid and more predictable. Therefore, the physician can more accurately select the effective dose. In emergencies, parenteral administration is particularly desirable. If an individual is unconscious, uncooperative, or unable to retain anything given by mouth, parenteral therapy may be a necessity. The injection of medications also has disadvantages, including risk of infection, pain, and expense. Also, if self-medication is necessary, as in the case of diabetes, some individuals might find it difficult to inject themselves.

Intravenous Injection—The most efficient route for medication is intravenous (IV) injection, which ensures the entire dose is available for distribution by the bloodstream to its site of action. Intravenous administration results in very rapid and relatively intense effects. For example, the time it takes a medication to circulate between the vein of the forearm and the brain is less than fifteen seconds, and approximately one minute for a complete circulation of the body. Electronically controlled infusion pumps may also be used to guarantee a constant supply of medication over a long period of time, as is required for some kinds of pain relief. Certain irritating medications can only be given intravenously because the blood vessel walls are relatively insensitive and the medication, if injected slowly, is greatly diluted by the blood. Intravenous injection usually must be performed slowly, with constant monitoring of the patient's response.

The plasma and tissue may attain high concentrations of drugs very rapidly. If an overdose occurs, little can be done about it unless there is a readily available, specific antagonist for the drug. An antagonist acts against and blocks a drug's action.

Repeated injections can lead to clot formation, blood vessel irritation, or vessel collapse. There is a high incidence of allergic reaction, pronounced cardiovascular action, and side effects with intravenous administration.

Intramuscular Injection—Because of the relatively good blood supply surrounding muscles, intramuscular (IM) injection generally results in a more rapid absorption than does oral administration. Substances too irritating to be injected subcutaneously may sometimes be given intramuscularly.

Absorption from IM injection sites occurs by simple diffusion to plasma. Generally, the rate of absorption from the deltoid muscles is faster than when the injection is made into the gluteus maximus (buttock). The rate is particularly slower for females after injection into the gluteus maximus. Very obese or emaciated individuals may exhibit unusual patterns of absorption following IM injection. Medications dissolved in water are more rapidly absorbed through the IM route than when dissolved or suspended in oil. Some formulations, such as fluphenazine decanoate (used in schizophrenia), are specially formulated to provide a slow release from IM injection sites, thus providing a greatly prolonged effect over two-to-four weeks.

The intramuscular route is usually very slow and incomplete, and often results in some precipitation of the medication at the injection site, which may irritate the tissue.

Subcutaneous Injection—This method injects a medication underneath the skin into the body fat between the skin and muscle. Because of the relatively poor blood supply in fatty tissue, this method can be used with nonirritating substances to produce fairly slow and even absorption. The rate of absorption can be controlled through the form of the medication. For instance, a aqueous solution promotes fast absorption; a suspension causes somewhat slower absorption; and a solid form, such as a pellet implanted under skin, allows very slow absorption over a period of weeks or months. Such a slow absorption route solves problems for patients who have difficulty remembering to take medications.

Intra-Arterial Administration—A medication is injected directly into an artery to localize its effect in a particular tissue or organ. This practice usually has dubious therapeutic value. The medications do not go through the liver and lungs, and first-pass and cleansing effects of the liver and lungs are therefore not available. The drug is highly concentrated and can become hazardous.

Intra-Thecal Injection—The blood-brain barrier and the blood-cerebrospinal fluid barrier often preclude or slow the entrance of medications into the central nervous system (CNS). Therefore, when local and rapid effects of medications are desired, as in spinal anesthesia or acute CNS infections, medications are sometimes injected directly into the spine.

Intra-Cerebroventricular Injection—Injection of medication directly into the ventricular spaces of the brain may be used to bypass the blood-brain barrier.

Bone Marrow Injection—This route is used, for example, in an infant, or when the veins are collapsed.

Intraperitoneal Injection—The abdominal (peritoneal) cavity offers a large absorbing surface from which medications rapidly enter the circulation. Absorption by this route is faster and more uniform than with oral administration. Enzymes in the stomach or intestines do not affect the medication. This route, however, is rarely used because the dangers of producing infection and adhesions are too great.

Respiratory Tract Administration

Because the lining of the inside of the lungs provides a large surface area in close proximity to many blood vessels, medication inhalation leads to fairly rapid onset of drug action and intense effects. Gaseous and volatile drugs may be inhaled and absorbed through the pulmonary epithelium and mucous membranes of the respiratory tract. Advantages of pulmonary administration are the almost instantaneous absorption of a medication into the blood, avoidance of hepatic (liver) first-pass loss, and, in the case of pulmonary disease, local application of the drug at the desired site. For example, inhaled medications can treat bronchial asthma.

The main disadvantages are poor ability to regulate the dose, cumbersome methods of administration, and the fact that many gaseous and volatile medications produce irritation of the pulmonary epithelium, which can cause pneumonia.

Topical Application

Mucous Membrane—Doctors apply medications to the mucous membranes of the conjunctiva, nasopharynx, oropharynx, vagina, etc. for their local effects. Occasionally, this route is used to achieve rapid systematic goal (e.g., the application of an anti-diuretic hormone such as DDAVP to the nasal mucosa). Absorption through mucous membranes occurs readily. In fact, sometimes local anesthetics applied for local effect are absorbed so rapidly that they become toxic.

Skin—Adhesive skin patches can administer some medications. However, these transdermal preparations are only suitable with small doses and usually employ a rate-controlling membrane that allows a small amount of medication onto the skin. They are useful for medications with a short elimination half-life or that are destroyed in the gut and liver.

For example, a patch containing scopolamine, placed behind the ear where body temperature and blood flow enhance absorption, releases sufficient medication to protect the wearer from motion sickness. Patches containing clonidine (e.g., Catapres-TTS-1) have been used to treat hypertension and ADHD.

Eye—Topically applied ophthalmic drugs are used primarily for local effects. Local effects usually require absorption of the drug through the cornea. Corneal infection or trauma may result in more rapid absorption. Ophthalmic delivery systems that provide prolonged duration of action (e.g., suspensions and ointment) are useful additions to ophthalmic therapy. Ocular inserts, developed more recently, provide continuous delivery of a low amount of medication.

Absorption

Unless medications are injected directly into the bloodstream or applied locally, they must first pass through several lipid membranes in order to be absorbed by the circulatory system. In addition, medications taken orally or injected into the peritoneal (abdominal) cavity initially pass through the liver, where they may be structurally altered (i.e., metabolized) prior to entering the bloodstream. Once in the bloodstream, the free, unbound drug molecules (those not bound to plasma proteins) will be distributed to various organs, including the brain, liver, kidney, and adipose tissue, and then redistributed to other organs and tissues by the blood. At some point, the concentration of medication in tissue and blood is maintained at a constant level (steady state).

Metabolism of medications may occur in many tissues, but most metabolisms occur in the liver. From the liver, medications or their metabolites may then reenter the bloodstream or may be absorbed into the bile, which eventually ends up in the intestinal tract. From the intestinal tract, medications or their metabolites may be eliminated in feces or reabsorbed into the circulatory system. Water-soluble medications or their metabolites enter the kidneys and are excreted in urine. Lipid-soluble medications and metabolites will be reabsorbed into the circulatory system. A negligible amount of medications may be eliminated via lungs, sweat, tears, saliva, or mother's milk.

The most important factor in a medication's ability to pass through biological membranes is its *lipid solubility*. A lipid-soluble medication is one that dissolves in fat (lipid material). Although very small water-soluble molecules and ions can diffuse through small aqueous channels located in membranes, most drug molecules are too large to cross membranes in this manner and must diffuse through the substance of the membrane. Because most membranes are lipid, medications must be lipid-soluble to cross these membranes.

In order to dissolve in plasma and be effectively transported by the bloodstream, medications must also be somewhat soluble in water. For these reasons, most effective psychotherapeutic medications are soluble to some extent in both oil and water. Moreover, the relative solubility in each medium is a major factor in a medication's ability to get into the brain.

Transfer of Medications Across Membranes

The passage of medication usually occurs through cells, rather than between cells. In keeping with their roles of bringing essential supplies like oxygen and glucose and taking away breakdown products, most blood capillaries are relatively porous, allowing rapid interchange of drug molecules between the blood and surrounding cells. These intercellular gaps are sufficiently large that diffusion across most capillaries is affected by blood flow and not by the lipid solubility of medications.

When a medication permeates a cell, it must traverse the cellular plasma membrane. Membranes from all types of cells are remarkably similar, consisting of a bi-layer of phospholipids (lipids containing phosphorous). Membrane proteins embedded in the bi-layer serve as receptors to elicit electrical or chemical signaling pathways and provide selective targets for medication actions.

Passive Diffusion—There are several mechanisms by which molecules can cross cell membranes. Of these, passive diffusion is by far the most important for medications. Lipid-soluble medications easily dissolve in the lipid bi-layer and move down the concentration gradient into the cell (or out again). Such a transfer is directly proportional to the magnitude of the medication concentration across the cell membrane; the higher the concentration of medication is in the membrane, the faster it diffuses through that membrane.

Carrier-Mediated Membrane Transport—Active transport for a wide variety of molecules that are vital to the cell (ions, sugars, amino acids, etc.) occurs in specialized membranes like the nervous system, gut, kidney, and liver. This is necessary for the transport of compounds whose rate of movement across cell membranes by passive diffusion is too slow. This carrier-mediated transport requires energy, which is supplied by the cell, and has the ability to move molecules against their concentration gradient. However, active transport of medications appears to be limited to agents that are structurally similar to endogenous (existing within the body) molecules. For example, the dopamine precursor, dihydroxyphenylalanine (DOPA), is transported into the brain by an amino acid active-transport system.

Passage Through Voltage-Gated Ion Channels—Voltage-gated ion channels are proteins that contain a water-filled pore that allows the passage of specific ions [e.g., K^+ (potassium), Na^+ (sodium), Ca^{++} (calcium)] across a membrane. Greater than a million ions per second can pass through an ion channel. Changes in the electrical field across a membrane produce changes in the channel's molecular structure, resulting in the opening or closing of the channels. These changes in molecular structure are responsible for the electrical excitability of nerve cells and their processes.

Hydrogen ion concentration, called "pH," measures acidity and alkalinity. A fluid with pH of 7 is neutral (neither acid nor alkaline), fluids with pH less than 7 are acidic, and fluids with pH higher than 7 are alkaline. As pH decreases, fluid becomes more acidic; as pH increases, fluid becomes more alkaline. This is important because blood, gastrointestinal, and kidney systems have variable pH, which can significantly affect the absorption of medications.

The pH of the aqueous environment greatly influences the electrical charge (called "ionization") of weak electrolytes, including medications. Non-ionized molecules are more lipid-soluble. If a medication is in an acid environment, more of the medication will be non-ionized, and more lipid-soluble, which favors transfer across any cell membrane. In contrast, as the pH falls, the environment becomes more alkaline and more of medication molecules will be ionized. Ionized molecules are less lipid-soluble and less able to cross a biological membrane.

Rate of Absorption.

If a medication is absorbed very rapidly (e.g., a dose given rapidly through intravenous route) and has a small central volume (e.g., the portion of blood stream that carries the medication), the concentration of medication initially will be high. It will then fall as the medication is distributed to its final and larger volume, such as in the whole brain. If the same medication is absorbed more slowly, it will be distributed while it is being given, and peak concentrations will be lower and occur later. A given medication may act to produce both desirable and undesirable effects at several sites in the body, and the rates of distribution of medication to these sites may not be the same. For example, when a neuroleptic (tranquilizing) drug such as Haldol is given intramuscularly, it quickly calms an individual's mania, but the side effects of acute dystonia usually show up a few hours or few days later in abnormal involuntary movements and prolonged muscle contraction.

Availability is potentially erratic and incomplete for medications that are poorly soluble, slowly absorbed, unstable, or extensively metabolized by the liver, stomach, or intestines.

The amount of time required for an orally administered medication to exit the stomach and enter the small intestine will also affect absorption. The stomach is lined by a thick, mucus-covered membrane with a small surface area and high electrical resistance. The primary function of the stomach is digestion, rather than absorption. In contrast, the small intestine has the primary function of facilitating the absorption of nutrients. The lining ("epithelium") of the intestines has an extremely large surface area, it is thin, and has low electrical resistance; all of which aid absorption. Thus, any factor that accelerates emptying the stomach will likely increase the rate of drug absorption because it allows the medication to reach the intestines more quickly. Any factor that delays stomach emptying will probably have the opposite effect, regardless of the characteristics of the medication.

In general, the non-ionized form of a medication will be absorbed more rapidly than the ionized form in either the stomach or the intestines. However, the rate of absorption of a medication from the intestines will be greater than that from the stomach even if the medication is predominantly ionized in the intestines and largely non-ionized in the stomach.

Medications that are destroyed by gastric juice or that cause gastric irritation are sometimes administered in dosage forms with a coating that prevents dissolution in the gastric acid. However, some of these enteric-coated medications may also resist dissolution in the intestines, and very little of the medication may be absorbed.

Controlled-Release Preparations—The rate of absorption of a medication administered as a tablet or other solid oral-dosage form partly depends on its rate of dissolution in the gastrointestinal fluids. This factor is the basis for the so-called controlled-release, extended-release, sustained-release, or prolonged-action pharmaceutical preparations that are designed to produce slow, uniform absorption of the medication for eight hours or longer. Potential advantages of such preparations are reduction in the frequency of administration, maintenance of a therapeutic effect overnight, and decreased incidence and intensity of undesired effects.

Other Factors That Affect Absorption

In addition to the physicochemical factors described above, many variables influence the absorption of medications. Each of the following factors separately or in conjunction with one another may have profound effects on the clinical efficacy and toxicity of a medication.

- **Drug Solubility**—Absorption, regardless of the site, is depends on drug solubility. Drugs given in aqueous solution are more rapidly absorbed than those given in oily solution, suspension, or solid form.

- **Drug Concentration**—Highly concentrated medications are absorbed more rapidly than less concentrated medications.

- **Dosage Form**—Dosage form (i.e., tablet or capsule), and formulation factors such as degree of tablet compaction, size of medication particles, and crystal and salt form of the medication can affect the rate of absorption. Medication release may be very rapid, but it can also be very slow in the case of special pharmaceutical formulations, such as sustained-release preparations (e.g., Ritalin SR).

- **Blood Flow**—Blood circulation also affects drug absorption. Increased blood flow, brought about by massage or local application of heat, enhances the rate of medication absorption. Decreased blood flow, produced by vasoconstrictor agents, shock, or other disease factors, can slow absorption.

- **Absorbing Area**—The area of the absorbing surface is one of the more important determinants of the rate of drug absorption. Medications are absorbed very rapidly from large surface areas such as the lungs, the intestinal mucous membrane, or, in a few cases, the skin.

- **GI Tract Contents**—Food in the GI tract can bind to the medication or dilute it so that it is slowly absorbed.

- **Rate of Movement Through the GI Tract**—The effect of the contents moving through the GI tract depends on where the medication is best absorbed. For example, rapid emptying of the stomach decreases the rate of absorption of weak acids, such as aspirin. Rapid movement through the intestines decreases the amount of medication absorbed because of a shorter duration of contact. Slow movement through the intestines generally increases medication absorption.

- **Local pH**—The pH of the local area determines the ratio of ionized to non-ionized medication in that area. Since the non-ionized form is more readily absorbed than the ionized form, the pH affects the rate of absorption. For example, weak acids like aspirin are less ionized in an acid medium and are therefore more lipid-soluble and well-absorbed in the stomach, which has a pH of less than three. On the other hand, alkaloids like heroin, morphine, and cocaine are highly ionized and poorly absorbed from the stomach.

- **Gender**—Females tend to have lower acidic environment in the GI tract and may have increased absorption of weak bases of medications (e.g., tricyclic antidepressants and some antipsychotics). In females, a slower transit time in the small intestine delays drug absorption and peak levels and causes lower peak blood concentration.

Distribution

After a medication is absorbed into the bloodstream, it is subjected to the multiple processes of distribution governed by its lipid solubility, the pH of body fluids, the extent of protein and tissue binding, and differences in regional blood flow. It passes through various body compartments and is distributed into interstitial and cellular fluids throughout the body.

An initial phase of medication distribution reflects blood flow. Heart, liver, kidney, brain, and other organs receive most of the medication during the first few minutes after absorption. With a lesser blood supply, delivery of medication to muscle, most viscera, skin, and fat is slower, and these tissues may require several minutes or hours before attaining steady state.

A second phase of drug distribution involves a far larger fraction of the body mass than does the first phase. Diffusion into the interstitial compartment occurs rapidly because of the highly permeable nature of capillary endothelial membranes (except in the brain). Lipid-insoluble medications that poorly permeate membranes are restricted in their distribution. A medication that is extensively and strongly bound has limited access to cellular sites of action, and it may be metabolized and eliminated slowly.

The distribution of medications to the CNS from the bloodstream is unique, primarily because entry of medications into the cerebrospinal fluid and extracellular space of the CNS is restricted due to the protective network of blood vessels and cells that filter blood flowing to the brain. This is called the blood-brain barrier. (See details of drug distribution in the brain in Appendix B.)

A third phase of drug distribution involves medication accumulation in various tissues. With administration of successive doses of a medication, accumulation of the medication takes place in fat and other tissues that can store large amounts of the compound. These can become *reservoirs* for the maintenance of the plasma and brain concentrations at or above the threshold required for the treatment effect. If stored medication is in equilibrium with that in plasma and is released as the plasma concentration declines, pharmacological effects of the medication are prolonged. However, medications may accumulate in these tissues in higher concentrations than would be expected. These tissues (e.g., liver and kidney) are often where the medication causes toxicity.

Medication Reservoirs

Fat Reservoirs

Many lipid-soluble drugs are stored in adipose tissue (fat), which makes up approximately ten-to-twenty percent of the body. In obese persons, the fat content of the body may be as high as fifty percent, and even in starvation it constitutes ten percent of body weight. Fat is a rather stable reservoir because it has a relatively low blood flow. Most psychotherapeutic medications are particularly prone to accumulating in adipose tissue because of their relatively high lipid solubility. Most medications stored in human fat cause no overt symptoms unless the subject undergoes a rapid period of fat utilization due to starvation or extreme dieting.

Some short-acting medications may have prolonged duration of action, and this can be explained on the basis of fat storage. For example, thiopental (an ultrashort-acting medication used in anesthesia) is a highly lipid-soluble medication. When injected intravenously, it rapidly enters the brain, leaving a relatively small concentration in the plasma. Thus, the onset of its effects is very rapid, occurring within approximately ten-to-fifteen seconds. After injection is concluded, concentration of the thiopental falls in the brain because there is little binding of thiopental to brain tissues as it diffuses into other tissues, such as muscle. The medication then enters fat tissue and remains there for some time. As a result, the intensity of the medication's effects is reduced fairly rapidly, but some small, residual effect of the medication may be experienced for many hours.

Protein Reservoirs

Most psychotherapeutic medications are highly protein-bound. Such bound medication often accounts for more than ninety percent of the total plasma concentration. The major plasma protein involved in drug binding is albumin, which binds both acidic and alkaline (basic) drugs. Another plasma protein that may play a major role in the plasma binding of a number of alkaline drugs is alpha 1-acid glycoprotein (alpha 1-AGP). Binding to other plasma proteins generally occurs to a much smaller extent.

The role of plasma proteins in medication distribution and elimination is variable, depending on the relative affinity of the plasma protein for the medication and the affinity of the various uptake mechanisms that medication might encounter. If the affinity between the plasma protein and medication is greater than the uptake mechanism of the eliminating organ, the plasma protein binding is expected to give some protection from elimination, and vice versa. In addition, for medications that might otherwise have solubility problems in plasma, these proteins act as very efficient carriers, aiding their absorption and transport around the body. As the large protein molecules are unable to leave the bloodstream, *it is the unbound medication that diffuses out of the circulation to interact with metabolic and transport sites or reach effector sites to produce a response.*

For medications that are extensively bound to plasma proteins, the volume of distribution will approach that of the plasma volume. The volume of distribution may vary widely depending on the pK of the medication, the degree of binding to plasma proteins, the partition coefficient of the medication in fat, the degree of binding to other tissues, and so forth. The volume of distribution for a given medication can change as a function of the individual's age, gender, disease, and body composition.

Cellular Reservoirs

Many medications accumulate in cells of muscle and other tissues in higher concentrations than in the cellular fluids. If the intracellular concentration is high and the binding is reversible, the tissues involved represent a sizable drug reservoir, particularly if the tissue is a large fraction of body mass. Accumulation in cells may be the result of active transport or, more commonly, binding.

Transcellular Reservoirs

Medications also cross epithelial cells and may accumulate in the transcellular fluids. The major transcellular reservoir is the gastrointestinal tract. When an oral medication is slowly absorbed, the gastrointestinal tract serves as a drug reservoir.

Bone Reservoirs

The tetracycline antibiotics and heavy metals may accumulate in bone by absorption. Bone can become a reservoir for the slow release of toxic agents, such as lead or radium, into the blood. Their effects can persist long after exposure has ceased. Local destruction of the innermost part of the bone may also lead to reduced blood flow and prolongation of the reservoir effect because the toxic agent becomes sealed off from the circulation. This may further enhance the direct local damage to the bone. A vicious cycle results whereby the greater the exposure to the toxic agent the slower is its rate of elimination.

Concentration

Although body tissue concentrations are typically 10-100 times greater than plasma concentrations (depending on the organ), the latter provides an indirect measurement of the former. When a single oral dose is administered, the medication reaches *peak concentration* (C_{MAX}) and then undergoes a relatively rapid decline. This initial decline is due primarily to drug distribution rather than to elimination. Therefore, the initial drug concentration drop is a function of the rate of uptake into other bodily compartments rather than elimination from the body. Generally, C_{MAX} will be inversely correlated to *time to the peak concentration* (T_{MAX}) (i.e., the shorter the time for a medication to be absorbed, the higher the peak concentration). A higher C_{MAX} and shorter T_{MAX} typically mean a more rapid appearance of clinical activity following administration.

Multiple Dosing and Steady-State Drug Concentrations

Most medications are not given in a single, isolated dose, but are administered in a repetitive fashion over a prolonged period when the aim is to have a sustained therapeutic level over several days or weeks without rising to toxic levels. If doses are administered at widely spaced intervals, or if elimination of the medication is very rapid, the body will eliminate most of the medication before the next dose is given. Therefore, a medication is generally taken with an interval short enough to allow a buildup of the medication in the body to therapeutic levels and to achieve a *"steady state."* This occurs when the rate of drug administration equals the rate of elimination, so there is no net change in the plasma concentration with time. As the drug enters the body, some is removed, but the concentration continues to rise, as does the elimination rate. In general, more than ninety percent of the *steady-state concentration* is achieved after four times the *half-life* (t 1/2). Thereafter, if administration of medication is kept constant and there is no change in elimination rate, the steady state is maintained. For example, Prozac has a half-life of two-to-three days. The steady-state concentration of Prozac is established after the patient takes the medication daily for about ten days.

Half-Life

With few exceptions, the rate at which medications are absorbed, distributed, and eliminated is directly proportional to the drug concentration present. This means that a constant fraction of the medication remaining in the body is removed per unit of time. The particular time interval in which the plasma concentration falls to half its initial value is called the *elimination half-life (t ½).* In general, about fifty percent of a drug is removed in one t ½, seventy-five percent in two, eighty-seven percent in three, and ninety-four percent in four t ½. After four t ½, less than ten percent of the drug remains in the body. This is called *the total elimination time.* Although it can be a poor index of drug elimination, half-life does provide a good indication of the time required to reach steady state during repeated dosing, the time for a medication to be removed from the body, and a means to estimate the appropriate dosing interval.

Therapeutic Index

During continued oral administration, a true steady-state concentration is not achieved, but rather a series of peaks and troughs within a dosing interval. The magnitude of the difference between peak and trough concentration is determined by:

- Frequency of dosing

- Absorption rate

- Elimination half-life

Thus, a medication that is slowly absorbed will not have as exaggerated a peak and trough difference as would the identical dose given in a formulation that was rapidly absorbed in the bloodstream. The acceptable magnitude of the peak and trough differences is primarily defined by a medication's *therapeutic index,* i.e., the ratio between the therapeutic and toxic levels. If a drug has a very large therapeutic index (e.g., most neuroleptics), it may be administered infrequently in large doses, where high and low concentrations are acceptable for therapeutic effect without producing serious toxic side effects. In contrast, if a drug has a narrow therapeutic index, or where high concentrations are associated with serious toxicity (e.g., lithium, antidepressants), it must be given in smaller doses on a more frequent basis in order to maintain therapeutic levels without producing concentrations that cause toxic side effects.

Maintaining a Relatively Constant Concentration

In clinical practice, the choice of dosage interval usually represents a compromise between the desire to minimize dose variations and the inconvenience of frequent dosing. Some of the problems of frequent dosing and having to take medication during the night may be overcome by the use of *controlled-release* dosage, which is available for some drugs with a shorter half-life (i.e., less than four hours). The purpose of such preparations is to reduce the dosing frequency to make therapy more convenient and thus promote better patient compliance. In addition, by maintaining a relatively constant concentration of the medication in plasma, excessive peaks of concentration are avoided, and side effects that may be associated with peak concentrations might be reduced. The controlled-release dosage forms are sometimes developed for medications with long half-lives (greater than twelve hours). However, these usually more expensive products should not be prescribed unless specific advantages have been demonstrated. Furthermore, there is a greater risk of toxicity with the controlled-release medications when the "slow-release form" fails. They may cause "dose dumping" because the total medication ingested at one time may be several times the amount contained in the conventional preparation.

Redistribution

Termination of medication effect is usually by biotransformation and excretion, but it may also result from redistribution of the medication from its site of action into other tissues or sites. Redistribution is primarily a factor in terminating medication effect when a highly lipid-soluble medication that acts on the brain or cardiovascular system is administered rapidly by intravenous injection or by inhalation. The acute effects of a single dose of most psychotherapeutic medications are terminated by redistribution.

Factors Affect Medication Distribution

- **Gender**—Because men and women generally differ in the proportion and distribution of their muscle and fat, the intensity and duration of drug action may differ between the sexes.

- **Age**—Drug distribution in the body is influenced by a number of age-dependent factors, such as the size of body water and fat compartments and the quantity and binding capacity of plasma and tissue proteins. Generally, children have less fat proportionately than adults and thus have smaller volumes of distribution for fat-soluble medications. Many other factors, such as the amount and type of protein present, the number of binding sites, the presence and amounts of endogenous compounds (e.g., free fatty acids and bilirubin), and the blood and tissue pH, may affect the binding of medications to plasma and tissue proteins and do change during the various stages of childhood. However, there is little information on the clinical significance of these binding changes.

There are several factors that can alter the distribution phases in the elderly and make them more prone to the effect of psychotherapeutic medications. The factors include a decrease in intracellular water, a decrease in protein binding, a decrease in tissue mass, and an increase in total body fat. These changes act together to increase the effect of most psychotherapeutic medications in the elderly. The end result is that medications tend to persist longer.

Metabolism (Biotransformation)

Once a medication is introduced into the body, it generally undergoes several metabolic changes before it is eliminated. The term metabolism (also known as biotransformation) refers to any process that causes a chemical change in the medication in the body. This chemical change may result in the drug molecule becoming more active, less active, or unchanged in terms of its activity at its binding sites.

Major Metabolic Processes

- **Phase I Metabolism**—*Cleavage reactions*, the splitting of the molecule into two or more simpler molecules, and *oxidation*, combining the molecule with oxygen or increasing the electropositive charge of the molecule through the loss of hydrogen or one or more electrons

- **Phase II Metabolism**—*Conjugation*, the combining of the molecule with glucuronic or sulfuric acid, and *reduction*, the opposite of oxidation, where the molecule becomes more negatively charged by gaining one or more electrons

Nearly all tissues are capable of carrying out some type of medication metabolic activity. The most active tissues are generally those involved in the excretion of medications, particularly the liver, kidneys, and intestines. Within the cells of these tissues, the different sub-cellular parts carry out different metabolic activities.

Psychotherapeutic medications are generally lipid-soluble. Before there is any significant elimination of them from the body, the medications must become more water-soluble because the excretion of medications and their metabolites by way of the kidneys into the urine is, by far, the most important in terms of volume.

First-Pass Metabolism

Oral medications must initially pass through portions of the GI tract where various enzymes may metabolize them. After the drug molecules cross the membranes of the cells in the GI tract, they move into a blood circulation system that goes directly to the liver before getting into the blood that supplies the body and brain. The molecules can be further metabolized in the liver, a phenomenon known as *first-pass metabolism*. This is why plasma or brain concentrations of medications administered in this fashion are generally lower than those of medications administered through other routes.

Drug-Metabolizing Enzymes

The organ most responsible for metabolizing medications is the liver. Within the membranes of the primary liver cells exists a large complex of enzymes. Enzymes are proteins secreted by cells that act as a catalyst to induce chemical changes in other substances, but they themselves are unchanged in the process. To differentiate between these enzymes and a multitude of others in the body, they are called *drug-metabolizing enzymes*.

As blood passes through the liver, medications diffuse into the liver cells and are acted on by drug-metabolizing enzymes. The metabolites (or, in some cases, the unchanged medications) then diffuse back into the plasma or are secreted into the bile. Those metabolites that are in the plasma and are sufficiently water-soluble are excreted primarily in the urine. If they are not sufficiently water-soluble, they may undergo further metabolization in the liver. Metabolites in the bile are delivered into the intestines. If they are water-soluble, they are excreted in the feces. However, if they are still lipid-soluble, they may be reabsorbed from the intestines to undergo further metabolization.

Metabolization Rate

In most cases, the rate of medication metabolization is proportional to the concentration of the medication. The rate is also dependent upon the number of drug-metabolizing enzymes in the liver. This enzyme level can be elevated several times with continuous exposure to certain medications, although the process generally takes several days or weeks.

In fact, most medications that depress brain functions (such as sedatives) tend to induce higher levels of the drug-metabolizing enzymes. Such effects are not restricted to sedative-type medications. Tobacco smoking, for example, can enhance the clearance rate of Haldol by over forty percent because of its ability to enhance the hepatic microsomal enzyme system.

Biotransformation

The enzyme systems involved in the biotransformation of medications are localized in the liver, although every tissue has some metabolic activity. Other organs with significant metabolic capacity include the kidneys, gastrointestinal tract, skin, and lungs. Following oral or local administration of a medication, a significant portion of the dose may be metabolically inactivated in either the liver or intestines before it reaches the systemic blood circulation.

Cytochrome P450 Monooxygenase System—The cytochrome P450 (CYP) enzyme family is the major catalyst of drug biotransformation reactions. More than twelve cytochrome P450 gene families have been identified in human beings, and a number of distinct CYP enzymes often exist within a single cell. Three families (CYP1, CYP2, and CYP3) encode the enzymes involved in the majority of all drug biotransformations.

Classification (nosology) of CYP enzymes—CYP enzymes are grouped into families and subfamilies according to structural similarity. All CYP enzymes in the same family have at least a 40% structural similarity, and those in the same subfamily have at least a 60% structural similarity. CYP enzymes are designated as follows:

- The family by the first Arabic number (**2**D6)

- The subfamily by an alphabetic letter (2**D**6)

- The gene that codes for a specific CYP enzyme by the second Arabic number (2D**6**)

Drug-CYP Enzyme Interaction

Researchers are focusing on identifying which CYP enzymes are involved in the biotransformation of specific medications and also determining whether specific medications can induce or inhibit specific CYP enzymes.

CYP Enzyme Induction—Certain medications, such as nicotine, anticonvulsants, alcohol, and environmental pollutants, can increase the synthesis of CYP enzymes. This increase leads to an increased rate of biotransformation and corresponding decreases in the availability of the parent medication. For example, adding Tegretol to control mood swings in a patient on an antipsychotic medication may increase psychotic symptoms because Tegretol induces synthesis of CYP enzymes, causing plasma levels of antipsychotic medications to fall.

CYP Enzyme Inhibition—Competition between two or more medications for the active site of the same enzyme may lead to a decrease in the metabolism of one of these agents, depending on the relative concentrations of each medication and their affinities for the enzyme. For example, Prozac and Paxil can inhibit CYP2D6 enzyme. This effect can result in a quadrupling of a tricyclic antidepressant (TCA) plasma concentration and cause serious toxicity unless the TCA dose is reduced.

Inhibition of drug-biotransformation-enzymes results in elevated levels of the parent medication, prolonged pharmacological effects, and an increased incidence of drug-induced toxicity.

Factors Affecting Drug Biotransformation

Individuals may show a wide variation in their response to the same dose of a medication. Much of this inter-individual variability in medication response can be explained by differences in absorption, distribution, excretion, and, in particular, biotransformation.

Genetic, environmental, and physiological factors are involved in the regulation of drug biotransformation reactions. These factors have been thought to be responsible for decreased efficacy, prolonged pharmacological effects, and increased toxicity.

- **Genetic Effect**—Hereditary differences in the amount or structure of key metabolizing enzymes may result in significant variations in the rate of drug biotransformation. Genetic differences in the ability of individuals to metabolize a medication are an important contributor to the large inter-individual differences in biotransformation. Hereditary differences determine individuals as *extensive (rapid)* or *poor (slow) metabolizers*. Slow metabolizers tend to have an increased risk of getting adverse effects. Large-scale studies indicate that five to ten percent of Caucasians and one percent of Asians are slow metabolizers.

   The importance of all this is to emphasize the possibility of genetically influenced individual variations in drug response and the need to take family histories.

- **Nutrition and Disease**—In the initial stages of starvation, drug metabolization may be enhanced while in later stages, it will be reduced.

   Impairment of liver function in individuals with hepatitis, alcoholic liver disease, fatty liver disease, biliary cirrhosis, and hepatocarcinomas potentially can lead to changes in hepatic drug biotransformation.

   Decreases in hepatic blood flow resulting from cardiac insufficiency can affect the rate of hepatic biotransformation. The metabolism of medications with a high hepatic extraction ratio is limited by liver blood flow. For such medications, a decreased hepatic blood flow results in a decrease in the rate of biotransformation and clearance of the parent drug, and therefore a prolonged effect. Inderal and Elavil are examples of medication with high extraction ratio whose elimination is likely to be altered by changes in liver blood flow.

- **Age**—Drug biotransformation varies with age especially among the very young and the very old. In the developing fetus and in newborn infants, medications are metabolized mainly in the liver. The activity and concentration of many metabolizing enzymes in newborns is less than in adults. Therefore, newborns have prolonged and exaggerated medication effects.

  Children do not have a full complement of drug-metabolism enzymes until they are one or two years-of-age. During infancy, the metabolic rates are markedly elevated for the most part and then gradually decline with age until puberty. This decrease in metabolism rates may parallel increases in steroid hormone production as the child matures. The various renal functions also develop at different rates until adult function is achieved at about one year. After the first year of life, *children will inactivate and eliminate medications somewhat faster than adults and adolescents, and in general require a greater dose (proportional to body weight) than adults to achieve the same response.*

  In the elderly there may be a diminished dose requirement for many medications because of age-related decreases in liver mass, hepatic enzyme activity, and hepatic blood flow.

- **Gender**—Although very little work has been done on human sex differences in metabolizing medications, recent studies have indicated that there may be large differences in the ways in which men and women metabolize medications. In general, drug concentration is greater in young women than in men; protein binding is lower in women than in men; estradiol and progesterone used in oral contraceptives inhibit specific CYP enzyme activity and increase blood levels of antipsychotics such as clozapine.

- **Metabolic Drug Interactions**—Concurrent use of two or more medications often changes the clearance of one of the drugs. Medications that are metabolized by the same enzyme will competitively interact with each other for a binding site on the enzyme, thereby decreasing the rate of metabolism of the lower affinity drug. If the affected pathway represents the major route of elimination, then increased plasma levels of the parent drug and prolonged or exaggerated pharmacological effects are possible. For example, erythromycin can inhibit the metabolism of Tegretol (the parent drug) by CYP3A4, causing toxic levels of Tegretol.

  Drug-drug interactions also can occur when one drug induces the metabolism of a second drug. In this case, the clearance of the second drug will be increased and the pharmacological effect diminished. Barbiturates are recognized as inducers of the metabolism of a number of drugs, including Thorazine and Dilantin.

- **Medications and Chemicals**—A number of medications and chemicals, including alcohol, can affect the rate of drug biotransformation. Chronic alcoholism is a major cause of liver disease leading to abnormal and deficient drug biotransformation. Alcohol itself (independently of liver disease), however, influences the biotransformation of medications in adolescents. Acute exposure to alcohol generally depresses the rate of biotransformation. For example, acute alcohol intake increases plasma concentrations of many benzodiazepines, including Valium and chlordiazepoxide.

- **Inhibitors**—Some drugs inhibit biotransformation of other drugs and may result in exaggerated and prolonged drug responses, with an increased risk of toxicity. Cimetidine, widely used in the treatment of peptic ulcers, is a potent inhibitor of the biotransformation of many medications that are oxidized by the hepatic monooxygenase system. These include theophylline, nifedipine, Dilantin, Tegretol, Depakote, and many benzodiazepines.

- **Smoking**—Researchers have extensively studied the influence of smoking on drug biotransformation. Most studies indicate that heavy smoking causes a selective induction of certain hepatic drug-metabolizing enzymes. Increased metabolism of Tofranil, nicotine, pentazocine, and theophylline has been reported.

- **Diet**—Diet is an important source of inter- and intra-individual variability in drug biotransformation. Cabbage and Brussels sprouts, charcoal-broiled beef, and high-protein diets stimulate the metabolism of some medications, such as theophylline and phenacetin, whereas a high-carbohydrate diet tended to decrease the rate of biotransformation. The effect of diet on psychotherapeutic medications is unclear at this time.

Elimination

The last step in a medication's clearance from the body is elimination, which depends mainly on two processes: biotransformation by the liver and excretion by the kidney. Biotransformation by the liver was described earlier. The following sections describe how the body eliminates medications.

Clearance

The efficiency of elimination is measured by clearance. Clearance is expressed as a volume per unit of time (e.g., ml/min or liters/hr). Clearance usually is further defined as blood clearance, plasma clearance, or clearance based on the concentration of unbound or free drugs. Elimination of medication occurs as a result of processes that occur in the kidney, liver, and other organs and metabolism at other sites. Adding the separate clearances will equal total systemic clearance:

$$CL_{RENAL} + CL_{HEPATIC} + CL_{OTHER} = CL_{SYSTEMIC}$$

There are other factors that may affect the clearance of medication from the body including

- **Hepatic (Liver) Blood Flow**—The clearance of a medication is mainly limited by hepatic blood flow. The rate of elimination of a medication that is cleared efficiently by the liver (e.g., Thorazine, Tofranil, lidocaine, morphine, and Inderal) is not determined by the processes within the liver, but by the rate at which the medication can be transported in the blood to hepatic sites of elimination.

- **Metabolic Capacity**—The clearance of a medication for which the liver has limited metabolic capacity is sensitive to changes in enzyme activity but is insensitive to changes in hepatic blood flow. In this case, the clearance also depends on the extent to which the medication is protein-bound because only free drug is available for uptake by the liver when the liver has a low capacity to metabolize a medication.

Excretion

This is the process that removes medications from the body to the external environment. At this point, most medications have been converted into metabolites that are more water-soluble and less lipid-soluble than the parent compound. Excretory organs (except the lungs) eliminate water-soluble metabolites more efficiently than substances with high lipid solubility.

The kidneys are the most important organs for elimination of medications and their metabolites, but there are other potential excretory pathways. These include the bile tract, respiratory tract, sweat glands, tear ducts, saliva, vaginal secretions, and breast milk.

Renal Excretion

Renal excretion of medications and metabolites in the urine involves three processes: glomerular filtration, active tubular secretion, and passive tubular reabsorption.

Glomerular filtration—All plasma elements, except macromolecules like proteins, are filtered to urine in the glomerulus by the simple action of blood pressure. Glomerulus are clusters of capillaries in the nephrons of the kidney that act as blood filters. The rate of filtration of a medication depends on the volume of fluid that is filtered in the glomerulus and the unbound concentration of medication in plasma. Medication bound to protein is not filtered.

Tubular secretion—After passing through the capillaries (the smallest blood vessels), the unfiltered fraction of plasma and blood cells passes into the vessels surrounding the proximal convoluted tubules of the kidneys. These possess two highly active transport systems, one for acidic medications and one for basic ones. Transport may occur in either direction. For example, penicillin is almost exclusively secreted, while bile acids are almost exclusively reabsorbed. Medications and their metabolites must be in their ionized form for secretion by these mechanisms. In this regard, the pH of the urine is important for some medications, as it determines whether they are present in the ionized (water-soluble) or non-ionized (fat-soluble) form. When the tubular urine is made more alkaline, weak acids are excreted more rapidly, primarily because they are more ionized and passive reabsorption is decreased. When the tubular urine is made more acidic, the excretion of weak acids is reduced. Alkalinization and acidification of the urine have the opposite effects on the excretion of weak bases.

Tubular Re-Absorption—Re-absorption into the blood of all medications that cross cell membranes takes place in the proximal tubule, loop of Henle, and distal tubule of the kidney. Tubular re-absorption is by passive diffusion and depends on drug concentration and the urinary flow rate.

Biliary and Fecal Excretion

After secretion in the bile, medications and their metabolites are concentrated in the gallbladder, which, upon contraction, releases its content into the intestinal tract. Thereafter, medications are metabolized by the normal bacterial flora in the gut. They are then re-absorbed back into the portal bloodstream and carried to the kidney for excretion in urine. This is known as the *enterohepatic circulation*. Highly water-soluble drug metabolites, however, are not re-absorbed. The are removed from the body by way of the feces without going through enterohepatic circulation.

<u>Excretion by Other Routes</u>

Pulmonary excretion is important mainly for the elimination of anesthetic gases and vapors. Occasionally, this route excretes small quantities of other medications or their metabolites.

Excretion of medications into sweat, saliva, and tears is quantitatively unimportant. The concentration of some medications in saliva parallels that in plasma. Saliva may be useful in determining drug concentrations when it is difficult or inconvenient to obtain a blood sample. For example, the level of lithium can now be measured through saliva.

Non-electrolytes, such as ethanol and urea, readily enter breast milk and reach the same concentration as in plasma. Although excretion into hair and skin is also quantitatively unimportant, sensitive methods of detection of toxic metals in these tissues have forensic significance.

Factors Affecting Drug Elimination

- **Kidney Diseases**—In all diseases that affect the nephron, the glomerular filtration rate (GFR) is decreased when the number of functioning glomeruli is decreased, or when renal blood flow is severely reduced. Reduced GFR will result in a reduced elimination of those medications (e.g., lithium) that are largely excreted in the urine unchanged. In dehydration, kidney disease, or shock, low rates of urine flow will enhance concentration and consequently increase passive re-absorption of fat-soluble drug molecules from urine into plasma. Conversely, increased urinary flow decreases tubular absorption and thus enhances excretion.

- **Other Diseases**—Diseases such as cirrhosis, viral infections, collagen vascular diseases, and cardiac disease can directly or indirectly affect liver function and affect the drug elimination from the body.

- **Urine pH**—An increase in the urinary pH (i.e., a decrease in acidity) enhances the excretion of a weak organic acid like aspirin, but reduces the rate of excretion of a weak base like morphine. Therefore, the rate of excretion of certain acidic medications can be enhanced by alkalinization of the urine with bicarbonate of soda (Alka Seltzer®), while the excretion of alkaline medications can be enhanced by acidification with vitamin C. Urine is usually acid, although it may not be if a person's drinking water is highly alkaline.

- **Drugs**—Drugs can indirectly affect the clearance of other drugs through an effect on hepatic arterial blood flow. The rate of drug conversion depends on the rate of delivery to the liver, which is determined by arterial flow.

- **Age**—The ability to excrete medications varies considerably with age. Excretion through urine increases to maximal levels in humans between the ages of five and ten. Renal functioning then declines somewhat, tends to stabilize between the ages of ten and forty, and then begins to decline thereafter. Older people frequently clear medications much more slowly than younger people, making the elderly more susceptible to dose-dependent, adverse effects.

- **Gender**—It takes longer for women to eliminate drugs from their bloodstream than it takes for men. This means that women are prone to accumulate higher, and potentially more dangerous, levels of the medication with repeated administrations.

Appendix B

Basic Neuropharmacology

All thoughts, emotions, and behaviors occur because of biochemical and physiological (electrochemical) processes that take place in specialized cells in the nervous system called neurons. Medications affect these variables by interacting with molecular components of the nervous system.

This appendix briefly describes the biochemical and electrochemical processes that activate the nervous system and how psychotherapeutic medications affect these processes. This discussion of medication therapy is limited to those drugs specifically intended for the nervous system, and some of the information is theoretical rather than factual. Functions of the central nervous system (CNS) cannot be directly studied, and neuroscience is still quite limited in understanding the CNS. Nevertheless, knowing medication action at cellular levels is important because some day we will fully understand how psychotherapeutic medications cause changes in mood, emotion, and cognitive functioning.

Medication Absorption and Distribution in the Brain

For medications to interact with the CNS in the brain, they first have to enter the brain through the bloodstream. The distribution of medications to the CNS from the bloodstream is unique because entry of medications into the cerebrospinal fluid (CSF) and extra-cellular space of the CNS is restricted. The brain comprises only about two percent of the body's entire mass, but it receives approximately twenty percent of the blood flow from the heart. Based on the volume of blood flow, one would expect a relatively large amount of a medication to enter the brain. The brain, however, prevents most nonnutritive substances from entering it and affecting the nervous tissue. This is called the *blood-brain barrier (BBB)*, and it is a vital source of stability, as well as a defense.

The BBB is actually a feature of the physical structure of the smallest blood vessels (capillaries) supplying blood to brain tissue. The brain capillaries are made up of endothelial cells that are packed tightly together and are surrounded with a protective sheath of glial cells that make it difficult for drug molecules to pass through. Endothelial cells selectively transport nutrients or drugs into the brain while acting as a barrier to others. In order for a medication to get to the CNS nerve cells (neurons), the molecules must be: (a) very small, (b) lipid soluble, or (c) compatible with one of the several carrier-mediated or active transport systems developed in the capillaries and glial cells.

Active-transport systems are systems in which ions or molecules are able to attach themselves to proteins embedded in the cell membrane. The proteins then transport the ions or molecules across the membrane. Apparently, these active transport systems have evolved in such a way that nutrients, such as glucose, vitamins, and minerals, can get into the brain.

Other factors limiting medication penetration in the CNS involve protein binding and degree of ionization. Medications that are highly bound to plasma proteins are less likely to penetrate the BBB, because only free drug molecules can pass through. Medications that are weak acids are less likely to enter the CNS because their lipid solubility is low.

The BBB excludes medications and other foreign agents, thus protecting the CNS against severely toxic effects. However, the barrier is neither absolute nor invariable. Inflammation of the brain or of the membranes that envelop the brain (meninges) increases permeability.

Almost all psychotherapeutic medications seem to primarily act on the synapses of neurons. To understand how medication enters and interacts with neurons, we must know the basic structure and function of neurons.

Neuronal Conduction and Neurotransmission

The neurons of the CNS are packed tightly together and mixed in with numerous nonneuronal cellular elements called *glia*. Their functions are so interrelated that it is extremely difficult to say precisely what happens in the CNS. Therefore, much of the speculation about the activities of these cells is based on what has been demonstrated in neurons of the peripheral nervous system (PNS). These are all the neurons outside the brain and spinal cord and are much easier to isolate and manipulate. Nevertheless, most evidence suggests that the neurons and the interactions among them in the two systems (CNS and PNS) are very similar, so in most cases information we learn from one system should provide us with a reasonably good idea of what goes on in the other.

The human nervous system contains between ten billion and one thousand billion neurons, with perhaps one hundred trillion connections among them. Neurons comprise a communication network in which the information is analogous to codes made up of *on* and *off* signals. Various neurons perform different functions. For example, some communicate between the senses and the nervous system, some communicate between neurons within the nervous system, and some communicate between the nervous system and the organs of the body like the heart, blood vessels, and muscles. However, they all appear to work in basically the same fashion.

There are two basic processes in the communication network.

- **Conduction** refers to changes within a neuron that allow the information to be transmitted from one part of the neuron to another part.

- **Neurotransmission** refers to the changes that take place within one neuron because of the release of biologically active chemicals from adjacent neurons.

Psychotherapeutic medications are simply chemicals that alter the normal processes of conduction, neurotransmission, or both. One must identify the primary parts of the neuron before learning more about conduction and neurotransmission.

Structure and Function of the Neuron

The main body of the neuron is called the *soma*. It integrates information received from other neurons. Extensions from the soma are termed *dendrites* and *axons*. Normally, there are many dendrites extending from the soma; they receive information from other neurons. But there is only one axon, which serves as the pathway over which signals pass from the soma to other neurons. Dendrites tend to be relatively short, but axons can be quite long. For example, a spinal motor neuron may have an axon several meters long.

The enlarged region where the axon emerges from the soma is called the *axon hillock*. Many axons have a coating called the *myelin sheath*. Gaps in the myelin sheath, where the axon comes into direct contact with the extra-cellular fluid, are called the *nodes of Ranvier*. The presence of these gaps allows a more rapid conduction of information down the axon. Conduction in non-myelinated axons tends to be rather slow. Near the end of the axon are the axon branches, and at the tip of each branch is an enlargement called the *axon terminal*. Chemicals found within the axon terminal can be released into an exceedingly small gap between the neurons, called a *synaptic cleft*, allowing the neuron to affect the excitability of adjacent neurons. The region itself is called a *synapse*, and it consists of the presynaptic membrane of the axon terminal, the cleft, and the postsynaptic membrane of the "target" neuron.

Each neuron releases a specific type (or types) of neurotransmitter(s). Neurons are generally referred to by the neurotransmitter that is released. This is commonly done by adding the suffix "ergic" to a prefix designating the neurotransmitter. For example, "adrenergic" neurons are those that release adrenaline, "noradrenergic" neurons release noradrenaline, "dopaminergic" neurons release dopamine, "cholinergic" neurons release acetylcholine, and so forth.

Neurons and Conduction

As with all body cells, neurons consist of a cell membrane filled with fluid, within which are subcellular structures that sustain the cell and help carry out its particular function. There is also fluid surrounding neurons (i.e., extra-cellular fluid), from which the cells take up oxygen, various nutrients, and, if present, medications. Waste products and medication metabolites are discharged into this fluid. In the intra- and extra-cellular fluids are different concentrations of negatively and positively charged ions. The four primary ions important for conduction are the positively charged sodium atom (Na+), the positively charged potassium atom (K+), the negatively charged chloride atom (Cl-), and large, negatively charged, protein molecules (A-), so-called because the general term for a negatively charged particle is "anion." A fifth ion Ca++ (a calcium ion with two positive charges) is also involved.

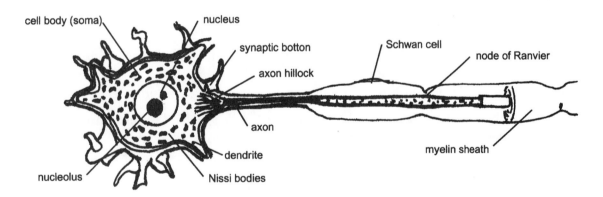

Figure B-1 The Neuron

Neurons can be in one of two states. One is called the *resting state*. In this state, there is a much higher concentration of negatively charged ions on the inside of the cell membrane than on the outside. In the resting state, we say the cell is *polarized*. In the other state, there is a rapid exchange of ions across the neuron membrane, and we say the neuron is *depolarized*. This latter process results in an activity called *action potential*, which begins the process of conduction.

The axon hillock (where the axon emerges from the cell body) integrates all the inputs (some of which are inhibitory and some of which are excitatory) from other neurons. The integration of these inputs leads to depolarization of adjacent regions (the nodes of Ranvier in myelinated axons). This results in *propagation of the impulse* down the axon, eventually reaching the axon terminals. The rate of propagation depends directly on the size of the axon and the thickness of the myelin sheath—the larger the fiber and the thicker the sheath, the faster the propagation (See Figure B-1).

Effect of Medication on Neuronal Conduction

Conduction is the ability of nerve cells (neurons) to transmit signals that control all bodily functions. Some medications have important effects on conduction and thus affect the transmission of nerve signals. There are three ways medication can affect conduction:

1. Medications can affect the properties of the membrane itself. For example, DILANTIN (an anticonvulsant) has a variety of neuronal membrane-stabilizing properties. These properties lead to a reduction of the cell's excitability. In addition, DILANTIN decreases the depolarization-linked release of several types of neurotransmitters. These effects of DILANTIN modify the pattern of seizure activities; that is, DILANTIN can abolish all types of partial and tonic-clonic seizures.

2. Medications can alter the structure or function of sodium channels located in the axonal membranes. For example, cocaine can occupy sodium channels and prevent the influx of Na+. This prevents any sensory information from reaching the CNS. This mechanism is useful as a local anesthetic.

3. Medications can alter the balance of ions on the two sides of the membrane. For example, lithium is a small, positively charged ion (Li+). When Na+ and K+ are deficient outside neurons, Li+ can substitute for K+ and is pumped inside. When Na+ and K+ are deficient inside the cell, Li+ can substitute for Na+ and is pumped outside the cell. The ramifications of these actions are still not understood, but they may have something to do with the ability of lithium salts to stabilize mood.

Neurons and Neurotransmission

Information gets across the vast majority of neurons and synapses through a chemical process called *neurotransmission*. Although medications do affect conduction, most psychotherapeutic medications appear to induce their effects by altering the neurotransmission process.

On one side of the synaptic cleft is the axon terminal, which contains enzymes that synthesize the active neurotransmitter from precursor molecules, the neurotransmitters, and small granular spheres called vesicles, which store and release the neurotransmitters. The membrane of the axon terminal at the synaptic cleft is the *presynaptic membrane*.

On the other side of the cleft is the *postsynaptic membrane*. This membrane may be part of a dendrite, soma, or axon terminal of another neuron, or it may be part of a non-nervous system cell under neuronal control, such as a muscle cell. In most instances, synaptic transmission is the passage of chemicals called *neurotransmitters* from the endings of one neuron to an adjacent neuron.

Pre-Synaptic Transmission

Neurotransmitter Synthesis

Before neurotransmission can take place, the synthesis of the active neurotransmitters must occur. In many cases, this requires a series of enzymatically induced changes in chemicals obtained in the food we eat. Because these chemicals come before the neurotransmitter, they are known as *precursors*. Precursor molecules (amino acids) are transported across the BBB and then taken up from the extra-cellular fluid. Neurotransmitter synthesis generally takes place in various parts of the neuron. If synthesized in a part of the neuron other than the axon terminal, the neurotransmitter travels down the axon until it reaches the terminal. Neurotransmitter synthesis takes place continuously, and the rate of synthesis is influenced by dynamic processes taking place inside and outside the cell, as well as by the amount of synthesis enzymes and precursor molecules. The speed with which a neurotransmitter is used and replenished is the *turnover rate*.

Release of Neurotransmitters

Neurotransmitters are found in heavy concentrations in the axon terminals. The heaviest concentrations are in the synaptic vesicles. Only those vesicles close to the membrane fuse with it, while other vesicles seem to be held in reserve some distance away. The contents of the fused vesicles, including the neurotransmitters, enzymes, and other proteins, are then discharged into the synaptic cleft. Once released into the cleft, the neurotransmitters passively diffuse to the postsynaptic membrane. They briefly bind to postsynaptic receptors and alter the cellular functions of the receiving cell.

Some neurotransmitters never reach the postsynaptic receptors. They are inactivated rapidly by diffusion into the extra-cellular fluid by enzymatic degradation or by reuptake. In the case of reuptake, the neurotransmitters are actively taken back through *autoreceptors* (presynaptic receptors) into the neurons that released them. Neurotransmitters that have undergone reuptake by the neuron may rebind to vesicles for use at a later time.

Neurons may simultaneously release more than one type of chemical that can serve as a neurotransmitter. They all play a modulating role in the activity of postsynaptic cells.

Reuptake of Neurotransmitters by Autoreceptors

There are receptors called *presynaptic receptors or autoreceptors*. These receptors appear to be located in regions of the neuron outside of synapses. They are most likely activated under conditions where there is a relatively high concentration of extra-cellular neurotransmitter. They appear to perform an "inhibitory feedback" function; that is, they decrease the neuron's synthesis or release of its neurotransmitters, which then reduces the influence of the neuron on its target cells' activity. Some neurons have autoreceptors located on their cell bodies or dendrites. These appear to play a role in the modulation of the physiological activity of the neurons, such as their rate of firing. Autoreceptors may also be localized on the axon terminals of some neurons. These appear to modulate the rate of both neurotransmitter biosynthesis and neurotransmitter release.

Stimulation of autoreceptors reduces the overall influence of the neuron on its target post-synaptic cells, while blockade of autoreceptors enhances the neuron's influence on the post-synaptic cells. Several medications alter neurotransmission because of their high affinity for these autoreceptors. For example, CATAPRES works by activating specific autoreceptors for noradrenaline and reduces the amount of noradrenaline released into the synapse. Other medications, such as PROZAC and PAXIL, block the autoreceptors and enhance the function of post-synaptic neurons.

Factors Affecting Release of Neurotransmitters

The process of releasing neurotransmitters from the axon terminal appears to be graded; that is, the amount of neurotransmitter released is dependent on the degree of polarization existing at the axon terminal when the action potential arrives. The greater degree of polarization, the more neurotransmitters are released. The degree of polarization may be affected because of activation of the neuron's autoreceptors, or because receptors on the terminal have been activated by neurotransmitters released from another axon terminal.

A neuron's activity may also be modulated by collateral feedback mechanisms via other neurons. In such cases, the activity of one neuron on another is modulated via collateral axons, which form a kind of negative feedback loop.

Specific Neurotransmitters

There are only a few neurotransmitters that have been identified with respect to drug action, although even in these cases there is a great deal of speculation. Some of these neurotransmitters are briefly described here in terms of some of their properties.

Acetylcholine (Ach) is found in various parts of the PNS and numerous areas of the CNS. It has excitatory properties in the PNS, whereas in the CNS it can have either excitatory or inhibitory influences on neurons. Ach undergoes inactivation in the synaptic cleft by an enzyme (acetylcholinesterase). Reuptake then occurs with one of the metabolites (choline).

Medications that block Ach in the brain are called *anticholinergics*. They can profoundly reduce the ability to form new memories. On the other hand, medications that enhance Ach activity may be useful in improving some types of memory dysfunction. Ach is probably involved in certain forms of aggression and grand mal seizures. Excessive Ach activity, when coupled with low norepinephrine activity, may also be a factor in certain kinds of depression.

Cholinergic mechanisms play an important role in the initiation and maintenance of rapid eye movement (REM) sleep. Abnormalities in REM sleep are found in clinical disorders like major depression, narcolepsy, obsessive-compulsive disorder, and some forms of schizophrenia, so it is possible that abnormal activation of central cholinergic mechanisms may be involved in these disorders.

Ach is released from the nerve endings of the preganglionic nerves of both parasympathetic and sympathetic nervous systems, the postganglionic nerve of the parasympathetic nervous system, and nerve ending at neuromuscular synapses. The reduction of Ach activity at some of these synapses causes many of the peripheral side effects of medications used for mental illnesses.

Ach has two primary types of receptors: muscarinic and nicotinic. The former receptor is easily activated by the drug muscarine and the latter by nicotine. In addition to nicotine and muscarine, some other drugs known to alter cholinergic functioning are curare, which blocks Ach at neuromuscular synapses; atropine, which blocks Ach at muscarinic receptors; and physostigmine, which enhances cholinergic activity at both nicotinic and muscarinic sites by inhibiting acetylcholinesterase.

Norepinephrine (NE, also known as noradrenaline) has a major influence on both the PNS and CNS. On PNS neurons, it is excitatory. In the CNS, it appears to be predominantly inhibitory with respect to its target neurons. While the brain content of NE is quite small relative to other neurotransmitters, it appears to play an important role in arousal and mood. Decreased NE activity is associated with low arousal and depression; high levels are associated with mania and increased motor activity.

NE also has two primary types of receptors, alpha and beta, with at least two subtypes for each. Stimulation of alpha receptors, which are postsynaptic receptors, generally produces an excitatory effect on the target organ, whereas stimulation of beta receptors depresses ongoing functions (except at the heart).

Epinephrine (Epi, also known as adrenaline) is closely related to NE, which is an immediate precursor to Epi in both structure and function in the PNS. Because Epi is found in very small amounts in the brain, our understanding of Epi's role in CNS functions is very limited. It may be a factor in the control of neuroendocrine function and blood pressure.

Dopamine (DA) is closely related to NE and Epi. It is one of the neurotransmitters whose primary role appears to be inhibitory on its target neurons in the CNS. It is the immediate precursor to NE in those neurons where NE is the neurotransmitter. Most DA undergoes reuptake and some undergoes COMT transformation. COMT (catechol-O-methyltransferase) is an enzyme that degrades dopamine, helping to inactivate it. Intraneuronal metabolization by way of MAO may also occur with DA.

At least four subtypes of DA receptors have been identified. The D1 receptor appears to be primarily responsible for the antipsychotic activity of many medications, as well as the motor disturbances induced by them. Both DA synthesis and DA release in CNS neurons may be regulated via DA autoreceptors, and both processes are independent of each other.

Like NE, DA comprises a relatively small proportion of neurotransmitters in the brain, but it appears to exert profound influence on many emotional, mental, and motor functions, as well as drug-induced effects. Brain DA systems are believed to mediate the euphoric effects of drugs like cocaine. An overactive DA system due to overly sensitive receptors, too many DA receptors, too much DA being released, or too little DA being re-taken-up might be the cause of many symptoms of most cases of schizophrenia. The destruction of a small subset of DA-containing neurons in the brain is responsible for Parkinson's disease. DA neurons may also be involved in tic and movement disorders, such as Huntington's chorea and Tourette syndrome, affective disorders, sexual activity and drive, hyperactivity in children and adults, and long-lasting motor disturbances associated with prolonged use of antipsychotics.

Because NE, Epi, and DA molecules have two common parts, a "catechol" nucleus and an amine group, they are often referred to as catecholamines.

Serotonin (5-hydroxytryptamine or 5-HT) is structured somewhat along the lines of the catecholamines. It also comprises one amine group. 5HT and the catecholamines are often referred to as monoamines. Termination of 5-HT action appears to be entirely through reuptake. At least thirteen distinct subtypes of 5-HT receptors have been identified. Although 5-HT has some PNS activity (e.g., it regulates contractions of various blood vessels), it plays a profound role in many CNS activities as an inhibitory neurotransmitter.

Decreased 5-HT activity has been associated with compulsive sexual activity, some forms of depression, heightened pain sensitivity, aggression, insomnia, and some psychotic symptoms. Several depression-relieving medications, such as ELAVIL, as well as hallucination-inducing drugs (e.g., LSD and mescaline) appear to act by altering serotonergic functioning.

Some amino acids, including glutamic acid and aspartic acid, are excitatory neurotransmitters; others, including γ-aminobutyric acid (GABA) and glycine, are inhibitory neurotransmitters. GABA-ergic neurons are perhaps the most widespread inhibitory neurons in the CNS. Enhancing the activity of GABA at its receptor appears to be a major common pathway for a diversity of medications with sedative and sleep-inducing properties (e.g., alcohol, VALIUM, and barbiturates).

Histamine is generally found in non-CNS cells made up of connective tissue (mast cells). It is also found in the brain. Blocking its action with antihistamines produces substantial CNS actions like drowsiness and hunger. The role of histamine in brain function is still very speculative. There are at least three histamine receptors.

Endorphins (a contraction of "endogenous morphine-like") are a type of peptides that have neuroactive properties. Endorphins may be involved in a wide variety of processes and activities, including pain perception, attention, primary reward, crying, laughing, thrills from music, stress reactions, depression, compulsive gambling, aerobics, masochism, massage, labor and delivery, appetite, and immunity.

Post-Synaptic Transmission

What happens after the neurotransmitters bind to the post-synaptic receptors is still not clear. In some cases, receptors are directly responsible for opening ion channels, whereas in other cases, receptor-transmitter binding appears to activate specific enzymes in the target cell membrane that convert energy-carrier molecules into small molecules called *nucleotides* inside the target cell. The nucleotides then trigger the internal biochemical machinery leading to a momentary opening up of channels in the neuronal membrane. In either case, receptor activation allows for negatively or positively charged ions on the two sides of the membrane to pass through the membrane.

Receptors

Receptors are fairly large molecules (usually protein) that comprise the sites where biologically active chemicals of the body such as ligands (neurotransmitters, hormones such as insulin, testosterone, estrogen, and adrenaline) or medications induce their effects.

- When a chemical (ligand or medication) occupies a receptor, it is referred to as being "bound" to it. In most cases, binding is temporary or reversible.

- If the receptor then starts some biological activity, it is said to be *activated*.

- When the chemical leaves the receptor, it is said to "dissociate" from the receptor.

- "Affinity" refers to the capacity of a compound to maintain contact with or be bound to a receptor.

- Intrinsic activity is the relative capability of a compound to activate the receptor after being bound to it.

- Chemicals, including medications with both an affinity for and capable of activating a receptor are called *agonists*.

- Chemical agents that are only partly as effective as agonists are called *partial agonists*.

- Other chemicals exert their effects by blocking the action of agonists. They are called *antagonists*.

- Ligands and some medications can be agonists or antagonists.

- In some cases, medications do not combine directly with a receptor, but instead enhance the amount of the endogenous ligands available for the receptor. These medications are *indirect agonists*.

A critical number of receptors of some specific type have to be occupied by an agonist before a biological response can occur. An agonist with high intrinsic activity causes a maximal response by activating proportionately fewer receptors. An agonist with low intrinsic activity may fail to elicit a maximal response.

Receptor Subtypes

As the diversity and selectivity of medications have increased, it has become clear that multiple subtypes of receptors exist within many previously defined classes. Moreover, molecular cloning frequently has revealed the presence of several closely related subtypes of receptors where only a single receptor was thought to exist, and some receptor subtypes have shown differential expression during development. As mentioned earlier, at least four dopaminergic receptors, at least three histaminergic receptors, and at least thirteen serotonergic receptors have been identified.

Although the mechanisms of action of some receptor subtypes may be very similar, other receptor subtypes display fundamental differences in their biochemical and cellular regulatory activities. Knowledge of receptor subtypes is of interest to the researcher and the clinician because, regardless of their mechanistic implications (or lack thereof), schemes of receptor classification have facilitated the development of a number of therapeutic medications that have selectivity for specific types or subtypes of receptors. Such drug development has provided the clinician with medications having higher ratios of therapeutic effects to toxic or unwanted effects.

Receptor Number and Distribution

The number and distribution of receptors are important in determining the magnitude of the medication's effect. In many cases, however, a full agonist does not have to occupy all receptors to produce a maximal effect. This is because there are "spare" receptors (receptor reserve). For example, if a medication needs to occupy twenty receptors to produce a maximal effect, and tissue M has thirty receptors, the medication will act like a full agonist on this tissue and produce a maximal effect. However, if tissue N has only ten receptors, the same medication will act like a partial agonist on this tissue and produces a submaximal effect. This is why changes in receptor number (up- or down-regulation) have important implications for medication action.

Chronic administration of medications can influence receptor numbers in two ways.

1. Chronic use of an antagonist produces an increase in receptors (e.g., chronic use of neuroleptics can increase dopamine receptors).

2. Chronic exposure to agonists produces a decrease in receptor numbers (e.g., chronic use of VALIUM produces a decrease in GABA receptors).

Interaction between Medications and Receptors

Many medications work by binding to specific receptors for endogenous ligands. They then either function as an agonist and mimic the action of the natural ligand, or act as an antagonist and prevent (block) the ligand from acting. Receptors have the dual ability of recognizing (binding) a medication with both sensitivity and specificity (selectivity), and then converting the process of recognition into a signal to produce a medication effect.

The interaction between a medication and a receptor can be described as affinity or efficacy.

- Affinity is a measure of the attraction of the medication to a receptor. If a medication has a high affinity for a receptor, a low concentration of medication can bind, whereas with low affinity, a high concentration of medication is required to bind.

- Efficacy is the ability of a drug-receptor combination to produce an effect.

A full agonist produces maximum effect and usually has both high affinity for the receptor and high efficacy. A partial agonist can have high affinity for a receptor but less than maximal efficacy. An antagonist produces no biological effect.

Structures, Subsystems, and Function of Nervous System

Moods, thoughts, and behaviors are not produced by the activity of single neurons. Medications also do not act at single neurons. Neurons make up a number of structures and subsystems of the nervous system. Some of these structures and subsystems are briefly described here.

Peripheral Nervous System Structures and Functions

The peripheral nervous system (PNS) composes all nervous tissue outside of the spinal cord and the brain. The PNS has nerves serving sensory functions (allowing light, sound, and chemicals from the environment to impact on the CNS) and motor functions (allowing the CNS to induce changes in bodily functions). Motor nerves are further differentiated into the somatic nervous system, which controls skeletal muscles; and the autonomic nervous system, which controls smooth and cardiac muscle activity and several glands, including the adrenal glands, salivary glands, and sweat glands.

Virtually all of these organs are connected to nerves of two opposing systems within the autonomic nervous system. One is called the *parasympathetic nervous system*, which is responsible for controlling vegetative, restorative, and energy-saving processes. It is particularly active in calm situations. The other is called the *sympathetic nervous system*, which is responsible for preparing the body for dealing with situations requiring fighting or fleeing, or times when the organism is frightened (the fight-flight-fright system). It is particularly active during times of acute stress and excitement.

The axons from both the parasympathetic and sympathetic systems that originate from neurons in the spinal cord and brain are referred to as preganglionic fibers. The target neurons for these fibers are clustered together in groups of cell bodies called *ganglia* (a ganglion is a grouping of neuron cell bodies outside the CNS). The axons that originate from these ganglionic cells and connect with the organs are referred to as postganglionic fibers. Postganglionic axons of the sympathetic system release norepinephrine (NE), which activates three different types of receptors (alpha1, alpha2, and beta2) in the membranes of target neurons. Postganglionic axons of the parasympathetic system release acetylcholine, which activates muscarinic receptors in the target neurons.

Much of what is thought to go on in the synapses in the CNS is based on studies conducted on the PNS, on the assumption that the two operate in basically the same fashion.

Central Nervous System: Structures and Functions

The brain and spinal cord comprise the central nervous system. The top portion of the brain actually comprises two semi-symmetrical halves called the *cerebral hemispheres*. The outer surface of these is called the *cerebral cortex*, and it has several densely packed layers of neuron cell bodies. Certain parts of the cortex are called sensory projection areas because these are areas of the cortex where the information from the senses is processed.

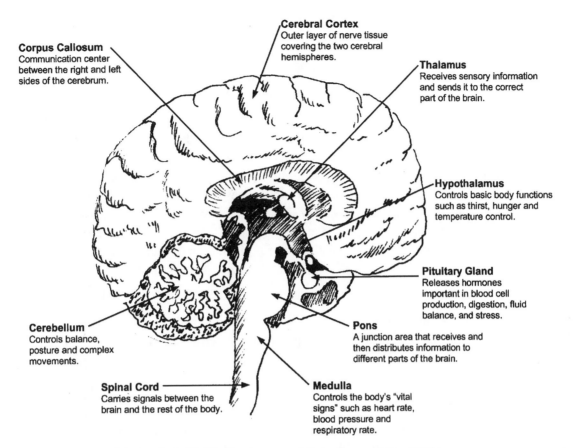

Corpus Callosum
Communication center between the right and left sides of the cerebrum.

Cerebral Cortex
Outer layer of nerve tissue covering the two cerebral hemispheres.

Thalamus
Receives sensory information and sends it to the correct part of the brain.

Hypothalamus
Controls basic body functions such as thirst, hunger and temperature control.

Pituitary Gland
Releases hormones important in blood cell production, digestion, fluid balance, and stress.

Pons
A junction area that receives and then distributes information to different parts of the brain.

Cerebellum
Controls balance, posture and complex movements.

Spinal Cord
Carries signals between the brain and the rest of the body.

Medulla
Controls the body's "vital signs" such as heart rate, blood pressure and respiratory rate.

Figure B-2 Major Regions and Functions of the Brain

- The *temporal lobes* contain the primary receiving area for auditory information and visual recognition.

- The *parietal lobes* are the primary receiving area for bodily sensations and are involved in spatial perception.

- The *occipital lobes* are the primary receiving area for visual information.

- The cortex in the *frontal lobes* allows us to ascribe meaning to the incoming stimuli initially processed in the sensory projection areas. It is essential for higher-order, thought processing, such as synthetic reasoning and abstract thought. It allows us to organize events from independent places and times and to make plans.

The two cerebral hemispheres are connected by some 200 million nerve axons collectively referred to as the *corpus callosum*, which allows them to communicate with one another.

The thalamus relays incoming sensory information to the appropriate areas of the cortex, as well as relaying information from higher regions of the brain to lower ones. It also appears to play a part in regulating the overall level of excitability of cortical neurons.

The *limbic system* is a conglomeration of diverse structures in the cerebral hemispheres where a large number of circuits relating to different functions come together. Researchers think it plays a key role in the cognitive arousal of emotion and the formation of memory. The primary reward and punishment centers are believed to exist in this diffuse system. Limbic structures may also be involved in many mood and thought disorders. Key parts of the limbic system are the hippocampus and amygdala (believed to be concerned with emotional reactions and memory storage), the cingulate gyrus, the mammillary bodies (also may play a role in emotion and memory), and the fornix (which connects the hippocampus and mammillary bodies). Relatively heavy concentrations of catecholamines (primarily norepinephrine) and enkephalins have been found in the limbic system.

The *hypothalamus* regulates the expression of basic drive states, such as hunger, thirst, sex, aggression, and body temperature, and exerts major control over the autonomic nervous system. It is also the nervous system's way of mediating control over the endocrine system because it has numerous neuronal connections and hormones that can influence the activity of the pituitary gland, whose hormones control numerous functions of the other endocrine glands of the body. The hypothalamus has heavy concentrations of catecholamines and enkephalins that regulate its function. Medications that alter activity at catecholamine receptors (such as cocaine, amphetamine, and chlorpromazine) or enkephalin receptors (such as morphine and heroin) profoundly influence mood, emotion, emotional reaction, and primary drive because they indirectly affect hypothalamus function.

The *medulla* controls vital reflex functions such as respiration, heartbeat, and blood pressure.

The *pons* connects higher brain centers with the cerebellum and, along with the medulla, contains most of the cell bodies of the reticular activating system. These regions of the brain contain relatively high concentrations of catecholamines, serotonin, and enkephalins.

The *cerebellum* controls automatic skeletal motor activities and coordinates balance and the body's movements.

The *midbrain* contains primitive centers for auditory and visual processing. It is also important for the perception of pain. The midbrain has a high concentration of enkephalins. The midbrain also contains dopaminergic neurons, whose axons project into areas in the frontal cortex and the basal ganglia.

The reticular activating system (RAS) comprises a diffuse network of neurons whose cell bodies originate in the pons and medulla. The RAS sends axons (ascending and descending) to most regions of the brain and spinal cord. The RAS participates in a wide variety of psychological processes ranging from perception to mood to our ability to associate events. It may set "brain tone" by regulating mood and the responsiveness of incoming stimulation from the senses or internally produced stimuli (mental activity). The ascending RAS regulates the level of alertness and screen information by filtering out unimportant sensory information and allowing important information to reach higher brain centers for further processing.

These functions also suggest that thought and perceptual disturbances may be the result of malfunctions in the reticular activating system. Although several types of neurons play roles in this system, serotonergic and noradrenergic neurons appear to be particularly important. Their influence is primarily inhibitory with respect to their target neurons if the organism is in a vegetative state or there is little environmental stimulation. With sudden changes in environmental stimulation, the activity of the target neurons may actually be enhanced with RAS noradrenergic input. During certain stages of sleep, these serotonergic and noradrenergic neurons cease firing almost completely.

Along with the descending RAS, numerous brain structures, including the motor cortex and cerebellum, are involved in regulating the activity of motor neurons that control the skeletal muscles. One group of these brain structures comprises the basal ganglia that are just above and to the side of the thalamus. Basal ganglia serves in the regulation of slow, voluntary, smooth movement of different speeds, which can be modified by sensory feedback while the movement is occurring.

Loss of dopaminergic input to the basal ganglia leads to progressive deterioration of walking, standing, and many other postures and movements involving the body as a whole. Excessive dopaminergic input may result in repetitive or stereotypic movements. The symptoms of Parkinson's disease and several side effects of medications used to treat schizophrenia arise from disturbances in the basal ganglia.

Appendix C

Sample Medical Forms

Sample 1—Medication Consent Form

Patient's Name: _____

Registration Number: _____

Medication: _____

1. I understand that this medication is being prescribed for my child/ward for treatment of symptoms of a mental or emotional disorder. It is the clinician's opinion that use of this medication at this time may benefit the conditions for which my child seeks treatment. I understand that there is no guarantee that this medication will be beneficial. _____ (Prescribing Physician) has discussed alternative treatment options with me (including no treatment).

2. I understand that arrangements have been made to monitor my child's response to this medication to assess its effectiveness, and it will be discontinued if it is no longer found to be necessary or effective. It will be prescribed in the lowest dose that is thought to be effective.

3. I understand that all medication may produce side effects, and some side effects may be serious or permanent. I have received oral and written instructions regarding this medication, including a list of the common and serious side effects of this medication. I understand the importance of reporting side effects or unusual reactions to my child's physician. I have read and understood the written material provided to me explaining the medication my child will be taking. I have had the opportunity to ask any questions and have received full and complete answers.

4. I have told the physician about my child's medical conditions, current medications, and history of reactions to medication.

5. I understand the importance of taking this medication in the manner prescribed by the physician.

6. I understand that it will be necessary to monitor my child's condition with blood studies, cardiograms, height and weight measurements, and blood pressure measurements, and that I will be consulted prior to other studies. I agree to follow these recommendations.

7. I consent voluntarily to the prescription of this medication for my child and understand that I may withdraw this consent at any time without prejudice to further treatment.

Parent/Guardian Signature _____

Date_____ Time _____ Print Name: _____

Prescribing Physician's Signature _____

Date_____ Time _____ Print Name: _____

Sample 2—Medication Consent Form[1]

My [My child's _____ (Name)] treatment with _____ (Name of drug) has been personally explained to me by Dr._____. The following points of information, among others, have been specifically discussed and made clear, and I have had the opportunity to ask any questions concerning this information.

1. _____ (Patient's Name) understands [I _____ (Name of the parent/guardian) understand] that _____ (Name of drug) is used to treat certain types of _____ (e.g., seizures) and my (my child's) physician has told me that I have (my child has) this type(s) of _____ (e.g., seizures)

2. I understand that _____ (name of the drug) is being used since my (my child's) _____ (e.g., seizures) have not been satisfactorily treated with other drugs

3. I understand there is a serious risk that I (my child) could develop _____ (e.g., aplastic anemia and/or liver failure, both of which are potentially fatal), by using _____ (Name of drug)

4. I understand that there are no laboratory tests which will predict if I am (my child is) at an increased risk for one of the potentially fatal conditions

5. I understand that I (my child) should have the recommended blood work before my (my child's) treatment with _____ (Name of drug) is begun or continued and then every _____ (e.g., 1-2) weeks while taking _____ (Name of drug). I understand that although this blood work may help detect if I (my child) develop(s) one of these conditions, it may do so only after significant, irreversible, and potentially fatal damage has already occurred

6. If I am (my child is) currently taking other drugs, I understand that the manufacturer of _____ (Name of the drug) recommends that the dosage of these other drugs be decreased by a certain amount when _____ (Name of the drug) is started; if my (my child's) physician determines that this should not be done in my (my child's) case, he/she has explained the reason(s) for this decision

7. I understand that I must immediately report any unusual symptoms to Dr._____ and be especially aware of any _____ (e.g., rashes, easy bruising, bleeding, sore throats, fever, and/or dark urine).

I now authorize Dr._____ to begin my (my child's) treatment with _____ (Name of the drug); or, if my (my child's) treatment has already begun with _____ (Name of the drug), to continue such treatment.

Patient Signature _____

Parent/Guardian Signature _____

Date _____ Time _____

Address _____

_____

[1] A signed copy of the informed consent should be given to you for your child's home record, and an additional copy should be retained in your child's medical record.

Physician Statement Regarding Medication

I have fully explained to the patient _____ (Name) [or patient's parent/guardian _____ (Name)] the nature and purpose of the treatment with _____ (Name of the drug) and the potential risks associated with that treatment. I have asked the patient (or patient's parent/guardian) if he/she has any questions regarding this treatment or the risks and have answered those questions to the best of my ability. I also acknowledge that I have read and understand the prescribing information listed above.

Physician Signature _____

Date _____ Time _____

Appendix D

Diagnostic Tools

Diagnostic Interview Instruments

Overall Psychopathology

Schedule for Affective Disorder and Schizophrenia (SADS)—The SADS is a semi-structured, diagnostic interview designed to ascertain and record past and current episodes of psychopathology in adults. There is a children and adolescents' version of the schedule (Kiddie-SADS or K-SADS). There are also epidemiological versions: SADS-E and K-SADS-E. The epidemiological version includes all the major mental disorder categories. Only individuals trained in diagnostic assessment should use the schedule, and the interviewer should be thoroughly familiar with the structure of the interview and the DSM-IV criteria.

Other structured and semi-structured interviews include the Diagnostic Interview Schedule for Children (DISC) modeled on the adult DIS used in the U.S. National Institute of Mental Health's Epidemiological Catchment Area (ECA) Study, the Diagnostic Interview for Children (DICA); and the Interview Schedule for Children (ISC).

Depression

Children's Depression Rating Scale-Revised (CDRS-R)—The CDRS-R is a clinically derived scale for practitioners to screen and assess severity of depression in children aged 6-to-12 years by integrating information from all available sources. It has 17 items (scored 1-7)—14 based on verbal responses and 3 on behavior (e.g., hyperactivity). The scoring of all behavioral items is described to minimize subjectivity. The scale takes 20-to-30 minutes to complete.

Bellevue Index of Depression (BID)—The BID consists of 40 items that are scored on a severity scale (0-3) and duration ("less than one month" to "always"). It takes 15 to 30 minutes to work through all 40 questions, although a shortened version of the BID also exists. In order to be scored as a symptom of depression, a given item must be present for longer than a month but not more than two years. This is a unique feature of the BID and clearly ties it to depression as a disorder that usually lasts from a few weeks to two years.

Diagnostic Interview for Depression in Children and Adolescents (DIDCA)—The DIDCA is a semi-structured interview to diagnose and assess Major Depressive Episode in youngsters. It covers ten key symptoms (e.g., sad/dysphoric mood, appetite disturbances) and each is further broken down with several specific examples. There is one version for interviews with the child (DIDCA-C) and one with the primary caregiver (DIDCA-P). Items are rated for presence over the last four weeks. In addition, there are follow-up questions to determine whether the symptom ever occurred in the child's lifetime.

Other Interview Schedules—Other interview systems for assessing depression in children and adolescents include all the structured diagnostic interviews discussed earlier (DISC, DICA, ISC, and the K-SADS) and the School Age Depression Listed Inventory (SADLI). The SADLI is the only one of these interview schedules that was devised solely as an assessment instrument for depression.

Mania

Mania is ordinarily diagnosed by using a DSM-IV or ICD-10 oriented interview such as DICA, K-SADS, or more often, an unstructured clinical interview.

Anxiety Disorder

The anxiety disorders portions of structured interviews discussed above (such as the DICA, K-SADS, or ISC) can be used for diagnosis of anxiety disorders. There is also a specialized Anxiety Disorders Interview Schedule (ADIS), developed to permit differential diagnoses among the anxiety disorders in children 6-to-18 years of age.

Schizophrenia

For diagnosis, a DSM IV- or ICD-10-oriented interview is needed, where possible, using one of the recommended semi-structured interviews, either child (e.g., K-SADS, DICA, ISC), or for older adolescents, adult types (SADS, DIS, etc.) If these are thought too cumbersome, a symptom checklist like the Stony Brook may be used instead. The K-SADS, in particular, and a derivative covering the psychosis section, the Interview for Childhood Disorders and Schizophrenia (ICDS), have shown promising reliability for child schizophrenia.

Preschooler

The Behavioural Screening Questionnaire (BSQ)—This is a brief interview comprising 12 items of problem behavior scored 0-2 to provide a Behavior Score. A score of 10 or above is regarded as clinically significant.

Rating Scales for Assessing Behavioral Profiles in a Variety of Diagnostic Groups

General Considerations

Rating scales have a number of features that make them attractive for assessing psychopathologies:

- Rating scales are generally economical, as they can typically be completed in a few minutes, usually by caregivers

- Rating scales enable raters to aggregate behaviors across a wide range of settings and over time, unlike certain indices (such as direct observations of behavior). Therefore, raters can detect and record infrequent behaviors and problems.

- Behavior rating scales usually comprise behavioral items of importance to caregivers, and hence tend to be clinically relevant and consumer-oriented

- Most good rating scales have norms, which assist clinicians in determining how "abnormal" the problem is.

Although rating scales are an extremely efficient and inexpensive way of assessing treatment effects, they also have some limitations:

- There is the problem of rater subjectivity in determining whether a given behavior constitutes a problem and, if so, how serious. As a way of minimizing this, whenever possible the same rater (e.g., parent, teacher) should always repeat the ratings on a given child. In this way, changes occurring across time and treatments can be attributed largely to changes in the individual's behavior rather than changes in standards across raters

- There is the problem of "halo effects," which may be described as the tendency of some raters to score the child in terms of the rater's overall impression of the child, regardless of the content of various items and their contribution to different domains or subscales. The appearance of consistently high scores, irrespective of behavioral domain, may cause the clinician to question a rater's judgment and seek a replacement. To alleviate this problem, employ more than one rater whenever possible

- Another important issue relates to the type of problem being assessed. Generally, caregivers are fairly reliable in reporting acting-out problems and disorders (e.g., hyperactivity, fighting, conduct disorders) but seem less so with internalizing or emotional problems (e.g., anxiety, dysphoria, depression) that create discomfort for the child but little disruption for society. This differential sensitivity is the reason for the prominence of self-rating scales for internalizing disorders.

General-Purpose Rating Scales

Not all practices will be able to use the array of instruments for particular disorders/problems discussed in this appendix. Therefore, general instruments suitable for most individuals (particularly children and adolescents) seen in most practices are described below.

Child Behavior Checklist and Its Analogues

Child Behavior Checklist (CBCL)—This is a parent-rating instrument for assessing children aged 4-to-16 years. Items are rated on a three-point scale. It comprises two main sections.

1. Social Competence has 20 items on amount and quality of the child's involvement in sports, hobbies, organizations, jobs, friendships, etc., scored on three-point scales from "below average" to "above average."

2. A Behavior Problem scale comprises 112 specified items plus one for the parent to write in additional difficulties.

Although different item pools were formerly used depending on age and sex group, the CBCL now has the same eight-factor, analytically derived subscales, regardless of the child's age or gender:

1. Aggressive behavior

2. Depressed

3. Attention problems

4. Delinquent behavior

5. Social problems

6. Somatic complaints

7. Thought problems

8. Withdrawal

This new, uniform factor structure can now be used to follow the same child over time without the former complications that otherwise occurred when the child reached a given age or when boys and girls were to be compared. Although some of the factor labels are similar to those used in diagnostic systems like the DSM-IV, they are not intended to imply that such a diagnosis would be appropriate for a child who scores high on the dimension. There are two broadband factors: Internalizing and Externalizing, based on second-order factor analysis.

Child Behavior Checklist for Preschoolers—The CBCL, discussed in detail above, has norms for children as young as 4 years-of-age. More recently, the CBCL/2-3 was introduced for children aged 2-to-3 years. Half of its 100 items were taken from the CBCL and other items from scales such as the Behavioural Screening Questionnaire and the Preschool Behavior Questionnaire. There are six analytically derived factor subscales, of which Sleep and Destructive are unique to this age group, the others being also found in the CBCL:

1. Social Withdrawal (14 items)

2. Depressed (15 items)

3. Sleep Problems (8 items)

4. Somatic Problems (12 items)

5. Aggressive (32 items)

6. Destructive (14 items)

Child Behavior Checklist Teacher Report Form (CBCL-TRF)—The TRF requests information about the child's background, academic performance, and adaptive functioning. It contains behavior problem items, most of which are the same or analogous to those in the CBCL. The TRF is scored in a similar fashion to the CBCL, and it results in a similar set of subscales. The major differences are that the TRF was designed for children aged 6-to-16 years (instead of 4-to-16), and certain behaviors not readily observed in the classroom have been replaced with unrelated items that may be salient in school.

Youth Self-Report (YSR)—This is one of the rare adolescent scales that allows youngsters aged 11-to-18 years to rate themselves. The behavior problem items are generally the same as those in the CBCL except that they have been worded in the first person. The YSR may prove to be especially helpful in assessing internalizing disorders, where the level of agreement between the child and significant adults is often very poor and where personal discomfort is often the principal target of treatment.

Revised Behavior Problem Checklist (RBPC)—The RBPC is an 89-item revised version of the extensively investigated and used 51-item Behavior Problem Checklist. It comprises six subscales, as follows:

1. Conduct Disorder (22 items)

2. Socialized Aggression (17 items)

3. Attention Problem-Immaturity (16 items)

4. Anxiety-Withdrawal (11 items)

5. Psychotic Behavior (6 items)

6. Motor Excess (5 items)

Any adult having a good knowledge of the youngster can fill in the RBPC; it is a well-established instrument and a good "general-purpose" rating scale.

The Preschool Behavior Questionnaire (PBQ)—This is a screening instrument for problems in preschoolers, with most of the 30 items taken from the Children's Behaviour Questionnaire plus 10 additional items. There are three subscales and a total score as well:

1. Hostile-Aggressive

2. Anxious-Fearful

3. Hyperactive-Distractible

The Symptom Checklist for Preschoolers—This Symptom Checklist is derived by factor analysis of behavior ratings of children in preschool, kindergarten, or day-care centers. This is for teachers or assistant teachers to complete. It has 49 items on an Apathy-Withdrawal or an Anger-Defiance subscale, and a three-point scale is used for each item.

The Behaviour Check List for Preschoolers—This is a parent rating form that closely parallels the BSQ. The scales are worded in a way that is highly relevant to the behavior of preschool children, but they provide only a global severity score and do not convey information about different symptom areas.

Symptom- or Disorder-Specific Rating Scales

Hyperactivity (ADHD)

Teacher Rating Scales

ADHD-Only Instruments

Childhood Attention Problems (CAP) Scale—Derived from the CBCL-TRF by extracting items that consistently loaded heavily on the Hyperactivity factor of the TRF *and* that were consistent with DSM-III-R criteria for ADHD. There are two factor subscales obtained by adding item scores: Inattention and Hyperactivity. There are no age differences for norms.

Conners Abbreviated Symptom Questionnaire (CASQ) —Uses ten key items describing inattention and disruptive behaviors common to both Conners Teacher Rating Scale and Conners Parent Rating Scale. The CASQ has also been called the Hyperactivity Index, the Hyperkinesis Index, the Abbreviated Parent-Teacher Questionnaire, Conners Abbreviated Teacher Rating Scale, the Abbreviated Conners Teacher Rating Scale (ACTRS), and the Abbreviated Teacher-Parent Rating Scale (ATRS), which only tends to cause confusion. The latter two acronyms (ACTRS and ATRS) are especially troublesome because they are so readily confused with the ACTeR, which is also used with hyperactive children (discussed below).

The ADHD Rating Scale—A 14-item instrument based on the symptoms specified in the DSM-III-R. Separate factor analyses of teacher and parent ratings gave nearly identical factor structures, each with an Inattention-Hyperactivity subscale and an Impulsivity-Hyperactivity subscale.

Scales for ADHD plus Other Symptoms

Conners Teacher Rating Scale (TRS), also called Conners Teacher Questionnaire (CTQ)—The TRS/CTQ has been the most popular teacher scale in ADHD. There are 53 items and four subscales:

1. Hyperactivity (17 items)

2. Conduct Problem (13 items)

3. Emotional Overindulgent (8 items)

4. Anxious/Passive (6 items)

5. Asocial (5 items)

6. Daydreams/Attendance Problem (4 items)

The IOWA Conners Teacher's Rating Scale—This is a scale that measures aggression and hyperactivity by using items (five of each) that are correlated only on Hyperactivity and Conduct Problem (Aggression) factors in TRS. The IOWA Conners has the advantages of being brief and soundly derived, but the small number of items and the fact that it was derived solely with teacher ratings may limit its application.

The ADD-H: Comprehensive Teacher Rating Scale (ACTeRS)—is a more recent scale, empirically derived and specifically designed for clinical management and research with ADHD children. Its 24 items score onto four subscales:

1. Attention

2. Hyperactivity

3. Social Skills

4. Oppositional

Parent Rating Scales

ADHD-Only Instruments

Parents and Teachers can use both the CASQ and the ADHD Rating Scale discussed earlier under teacher instruments.

Scales for ADHD Plus Other Symptoms

Conners Parent Rating Scale (CPRS) also called Parent Symptom Questionnaire (PSQ)—There are two versions of this well-known scale, namely the original, cumbersome, 93-item scale and a revised 48-item scale. In completing the CPRS, parents rate the presence and severity of symptoms in the child as currently functioning.

The longer scale has eight subscales, partly empirically, and partly intuitively, derived:

1. Conduct Disorder

2. Anxious-Shy

3. Restless/Disorganized

4. Learning Problem

5. Psychosomatic

6. Obsessive Compulsive

7. Antisocial

8. Hyperactive-Immature

The shorter 48-item scale has five subscales:

1. Conduct Problems

2. Learning Problems

3. Psychosomatic

4. Impulsive-Hyperactive

5. Anxiety

The Yale Children's Inventory (YCI)—This newer instrument assesses attention deficits and learning disabilities in children. The YCI has 62 items and takes about 10 minutes to complete. Parents are asked to rate the child on each item using a four-point scale that ranges from *never* to *often*. These would be key areas to monitor during medication trials in ADHD. There are eight factor-analytically derived subscales:

1. Attention (7 items)

2. Hyperactivity (5 items)

3. Impulsivity (5 items)

4. Tractability (6 items)

5. Habituation (4 items)

6. Conduct Disorder-Socialized (5 items)

7. Conduct Disorder-Aggressive (5 items)

8. Negative Affect (6 items)

Self-Rating Hyperactivity Scales

ADD-H Adolescent Self-Report Scale, has 52 items with seven subscales as follows: (1) Problems with concentration, (2) Problems of restlessness, (3) Problems of self-control, (4) Problems with anger, (5) Problems with friends, (6) Problems with confidence, and (7) Problems with learning.

Situation-Specific Scales

These scales differ from all those described above because the questions concern behavior in specific situations.

Werry-Weiss-Peters Activity Scale—Designed for use by parents and other domestic caregivers. The scale is widely used and drug-sensitive, but it correlates as much with conduct problems as with attention-overactivity problems.

Home Situations Questionnaire (HSQ) and School Situations Questionnaire (SSQ)—These are parallel instruments. There are 16 situations in the HSQ and 12 in the SSQ, each of which yields two scores: number of situations and mean severity score.

Rating Scales for Obsessive-Compulsive Disorder (OCD)

In diagnosing children and adolescents, most work has been done with the self-report Leyton Obsessional Inventory–Child version, which is an adaptation of the adult scale. There are two versions: a 44-item (for diagnosis) and a short 20-item scale (for surveys). Items are scored for resistance, interference, and presence versus absence.

Rating Scales for Tic and Tourette syndromes

The Tourette Syndrome Severity Scale (5-10 minutes) and the Tourette Syndrome Global Scale are the most popular, are easy to use, and seem reliable. A more recent effort, aimed at greater clarity of items, better reliability, and greater construct purity, is the Yale Global Tic Severity Scale. It is psychometrically robust but takes 15-to-20 minutes to administer.

Rating Scales for Measuring Oppositional, Conduct, and Aggressive Problems

Aggression is a complex behavior and may be (a) physical or verbal, (b) adult-directed or peer-directed, (c) reactive and retaliatory, (d) planned and proactive, and (e) eruptive or antisocial/hostile. It may be covert (as in the case of stealing) or overt (as in fighting). Hence, comprehensive coverage with a single instrument is difficult. Several instruments are available that either have been used for assessing drug effects on hostility in children or have obvious potential in that regard. As with most externalizing behavior, the majority are for use by the child's caregivers.

Informant Instruments

The Conners Scales—Conners Teacher Rating Scale (TRS) and Parent Rating Scale (PRS) described above have subscales for Conduct Problems and, in the 93-item PRS, an Antisocial subscale. Hyperactivity often occurs with conduct disorder, and these scales also measure this.

The Peer Conflict Scale—assesses physical and verbal interactions between the patient and other children. It comprises ten items, rated on a four-point scale, that were derived from a behavior observation code for assessing social and aggressive behavior.

Child Behavior Checklist (CBCL) and Teacher Report Form (TRF)—The CBCL and TRF, described earlier, have two subscales relevant to assessing hostility—a Delinquent Behavior subscale and an Aggressive Behavior subscale.

The Revised Behavior Problem Checklist—The RBPC places a heavy emphasis on conduct problems, aggression, and hostility, with 39 of its 89 items scoring on either Conduct Problem or

Socialized Aggression subscales. As such, it has considerable relevance to the assessment of aggressive types of disorders.

Inpatient Rating Scales

Overt Aggression Scale, Staff Observation Aggression Scale, Social Dysfunction and Aggression Scale—These scales may be modified and used in outpatient settings if parents and caregivers can be trained to rate the behaviors. The Overt Aggression Scale calls for each episode of aggression to be rated on four categories: 1) verbal aggression, 2) physical aggression against objects, 3) physical aggression against self, and 4) physical aggression against other people.

The Staff Observation Aggression Scale (SOAS) requires that incidents be reported in five categories: 1) type of provocation, 2) means used by the patient, 3) aim of the aggression, 4) consequences for the victim, and 5) Measures taken to stop the aggression.

Categories 2 to 4 contribute to a Global Severity score. The Social Dysfunction and Aggression Scale (SDAS) includes milder forms of aggressive behavior than might be captured in the two just described. It has 11 items, 9 of outward aggression and 2 of inward aggression.

Self-Rating Scales

These are not particularly good for externalizing behavior because of underreporting due to limited communication abilities in individuals with ASD or lack of insight in individuals with Asperger Syndrome, especially those with delinquency. They may, however, give some perspective on the child's view of his own problems.

The Youth Self-Report—The YSR, described above, has a Delinquent Behavior subscale (11 items) and an Aggressive Behavior subscale (19 items). Its utility for assessing aggression in youth is unknown.

Children's Inventory of Anger—This is an instrument for measuring self-perceived anger in children. Scales of this type are worth considering in assessing children having aggressive disorders, although their rightful place is unknown.

Rating Scales for Depression

There has been a proliferation of instruments for assessment of depression in the last decade. The following are some of the more commonly used rating scales.

Self-Rating Scales

Children's Depression Inventory (CDI)—The development of the CDI was based on the Beck Depression Inventory for adults, with items added relating to school and peer functioning. The CDI comprises 27 items scored 0 to 2. The child chooses one of three sentences (normal through depressive) that describe him over the previous two weeks. Usually the examiner reads the instructions and items aloud while the youngster marks the answers. Normative data are available, and scores are affected by age (nonlinear) and gender (females score higher).

Children's Depression Scale (CDS)—The CDS comprises 66 items, 48 of which are depressive in content and 18 euthymic items. The youngster inserts each card into the appropriate box arrayed before him, identified with the words "Very wrong" through "Very right." Higher scores on the depressive items indicate greater severity of depression. The CDS has eight subscales:

1. Affective response

2. Social problems

3. Self esteem

4. Preoccupation with sickness

5. Guilt

6. Miscellaneous D (Depression) items

7. Pleasure and enjoyment

8. Miscellaneous P (Positive) items

The first six are combined into a Total Depression Score and the last two into a Total Positive Score. The scale's developers support the use of the scoring boxes because of their "game-like quality," although a modified paper-and-pencil format may be more practical in an office setting.

Depressive Self-Rating Scale—This 18-item (scored 0-2) scale has the virtue of brevity.

The Reynolds Scales—There are two related instruments, the 30-item Child Depression Scale and the Reynolds Adolescent Depression Scale (RADS). The Child Scale, for ages 8 to 13 years, comprises 29 symptoms of depression scored on a four-point scale, and one consisting of five faces ranging from sad to happy. The RADS comprises 30 items rated on a four-point scale reflecting DSM-III symptomatology for major and minor depression. There are obvious similarities between the two Reynolds scales, which may be a strength, as they presumably could be used as parallel tools for assessing children and adolescents. Unlike most instruments for assessing affective symptomatology, the Child Depression Scale and the RADS use DSM-III-R symptoms, which makes its concept of "depression" clear. Also, it uses a refined four-point scoring format that should be sensitive to modest and/or subtle treatment effects. However, many items were selected for relevance to a school setting, which may reduce its applicability in clinical practice.

Informant (Parent and Teacher) Scales

Children's Depression Inventory (CDI)—Several authors have developed informant versions of the CDI by rewording the items in the third person.

Children's Depression Scale (CDS)—The CDS contains both a self-rating and an informant version. The adult version is purely a paper-and-pencil instrument.

Bellevue Index of Depression (BID)—The BID has been described above and it also can be used as a paper-and-pencil (informant) instrument.

Emotional Disorders Rating Scale (EDRS)—The EDRS has 59 items and eight component subscales: Anxiety, Hostility/Anger, Psychomotor Retardation, Depressed Mood Verbal, Depressed Mood Nonverbal, Somatic Vegetative, Sleep Disturbance, Irritability, and Elated/Manic Mood. Each item is rated for frequency and severity. It also has the advantage of simultaneously assessing anxiety, which often occurs with depression.

Rating Scales for Bipolar Mood Disorder

Among scales for children and adolescents, the EDRS is discussed above.

Rating Scales for Anxiety Disorders

Self-Rating Scales

There is a general lack of data concerning the validity of child versus adult informant ratings of children's anxiety (which have low agreement with each other). With this in mind, it is wise to use both the child's appraisal of his own internal state as well as that of significant others when assessing anxiety. Self-rating scales are only useful in higher functioning older individuals with ASD.

Fear Survey Schedule for Children (FSSC-R)—This is adapted from the adult Fear Survey Schedule 80 items with three-point scale. Factor analysis yielded five factors:

1. Fear of failure and criticism

2. Fear of the unknown

3. Fear of injury and small animals

4. Fear of danger and death

5. Medical fears

Revised Children's Manifest Anxiety Scale (RCMAS)—The original Children's Manifest Anxiety Scale and the revised version were adaptations of a popular adult scale. The RCMAS comprises 37 statements to which the child is asked to respond "true" or "false." There are 9 lie-scale items, and the remainder load on one of three empirically derived subscales:

1. Physiological

2. Worry and oversensitivity

3. Concentrational

Childhood Anxiety Sensitivity Index (CASI) and Child Anxiety Frequency Checklist (CAFC)—The CASI is an 18-item modification of the adult instruments and assesses sensitivity to anxiety (i.e., perceptiveness to anxiety) by asking children to rate how aversively they view 18 anxiety symptoms on a three-point scale. The CAFC, adapted from the adult AFC, evaluates the frequency of eight anxiety symptoms, such as rapid heartbeat, shakiness, and trouble catching one's breath.

State-Trait Anxiety Scale for Children—The STAIC is a self-report inventory that can be administered singly or in groups. It was developed for children of elementary school age and is in two parts: Anxiety-State and Anxiety-Trait scales, both of which are 20 items long and take about 7 to 10 minutes to complete. The Anxiety-State scale asks the child to respond as he feels *right now,* and the Anxiety-Trait scale how he *usually feels.* Both use a three-point scale for items. Norms are available only for fourth- to sixth-grade children.

Behavior Rating Scales for Anxiety

These are intended for completion by significant caregivers.

Louisville Behavior Check List—In the revised version, there is an 18-item Fear subscale containing items referring to specific fears such as fear of the dark and death. Some reflect difficulty in coping alone, and others have worrying behaviors that are general and repetitious. There is also a

15-item (17 for girls) Sensitivity subscale relating to internal and external cues and inappropriate reactions to stress (e.g., cries easily, feels more pain than normal).

Louisville Fear Survey for Children—This clinically derived scale has 81 items (each scored 1-3) covering many fears in children aged 4 to 18 years, which can be completed by children or adult informants. There are three factor-analytically derived subscales:

1. Fear of physical injury

2. Fear of natural events

3. Fear of psychic stress (taking tests, being criticized, etc.).

Specific Anxiety Disorders

Panic Disorder—It is likely that the DIS scales developed for the International Study of Panic Disorder would serve for this age group, but for routine diagnosis, the DSM-Ill-R based interviews like DICA and K-SADS, discussed above, have limited (and inadequate) screening sections on panic disorder.

Separation Anxiety Disorder—Only ad hoc or general-purpose diagnostic or anxiety instruments already described seem to have been used in diagnosis.

Phobic Disorders—These are best diagnosed and evaluated by using the FSSC-R (see above).

Posttraumatic Stress Disorder—While ordinarily it would be diagnosed using DSM-III-R-oriented interviews or checklists, there is at least one specific technique, the PTSD Reaction Index, which evaluates 16 PTSD symptoms following a special semi-structured interview.

Behavior Rating Scales or Interviews for People with Challenging Cognitive Function

Scales already described for assessing specific symptoms and disorders in other groups of children and adolescents can often be applied to children and adolescents with challenging cognitive function, but limitations in self-expression and developmental variations may make many instruments described above unacceptable. In this section, selected instruments developed specifically for behavior rating in individuals with challenging cognitive function will be discussed briefly.

Vineland Adaptive Behavior Scales—The Vineland is a semi-structured interview that assesses capacities for self-sufficiency in various domains of functioning including Communication (receptive, expressive, and written language), Daily Living Skills (personal, domestic, and community skills), Socialization (interpersonal relationships, play and leisure time, and coping skills), and Motor Skills (gross and fine). The Scales is administered to a parent or other primary caregivers. The Vineland is available in three editions:

1. Survey form for use primarily as a diagnostic and classification to normal to low-functioning individuals

2. Expanded form for use in the development of individual education or rehabilitative planning

3. Classroom edition for use by teachers.

AAMR Adaptive Behavior Scale—Residential and Community, Second Edition (ABS-RC:2)—The revised version of the original AAMR (American Association of Mental Retardation) Adaptive Behavior Scales consists of maladaptive behavior ratings for a large number of behaviors. The items are rated as do not apply, occasionally occurring, or occurring frequently. The 14 domains include

1. Violent and destructive behavior

2. Antisocial behavior

3. Rebellious behavior

4. Untrustworthy behavior

5. Withdrawal

6. Stereotypic behavior and odd mannerism

7. Inappropriate interpersonal manners

8. Unacceptable vocal habits

9. Unacceptable or eccentric habits

10. Self-abusive behavior

11. Hyperactive tendencies

12. Sexually aberrant behavior

13. Psychological disturbances

14. Use of medications.

The Aberrant Behavior Checklist (ABC)—The ABC is a 58-item informant rating scale specifically designed to assess treatment effects. The five factor-derived subscales are:

1. Irritability/agitation/crying (15 items)

2. Lethargy/social withdrawal (16 items)

3. Stereotypic behavior (7 items)

4. Hyperactivity, noncompliance (16 items)

5. Inappropriate speech (4 items).

Each item is rated on a 4-point scale from 0 (not present) to 3 (the problem is severe). A newer version (the ABC-Community) has been normed with a community sample. The ABC was largely institutional in origin and derived with a sample of people with severe to moderate mental retardation. The newer ABC-Community was also studied with adults living in group homes.

The Reiss Screen for Maladaptive Behavior (Reiss Screen)—The Reiss Screen was developed as a screening tool to identify mental health problems in people with mild, moderate, and severe mental retardation. The scale contains 38 items. The scale is to be completed by two caregivers and the scores are averaged. Ratings are on a 3-point scale of no problem, problem, and major problem. A 26-item total score provides an index of the severity of a person's problems. This rating scale is well-designed and easy to use.

The Reiss Scale for Children's Dual Diagnosis—This scale is similar to the Reiss Screen in that two caregivers are asked to rate items on a 3-point scale. Ten scales were derived from factor analysis, all with 5 items each:

1. Anger/self-control

2. Anxiety disorder

3. Attention-deficit

4. Autism/pervasive

5. Conduct disorder

6. Depression

7. Poor self-esteem

8. Psychosis somatoform behavior

9. Withdrawn/isolated

The instrument also assesses significant maladaptive behaviors such as crying spells, enuresis/encopresis, hallucinations, involuntary movements, lies, obesity, pica, fire setting, sexual problem, and verbal abuse.

Developmental Behavior Checklist (DBC)—The format for this instrument was based on the Child Behavior Checklist. The Developmental Behavior Checklist has two forms, one for parents and one for teachers. A 3-point rating scale is used: not true, sometimes true, and often/very true. The original items were derived from the study of case files, and factor analysis resulted in six subscales:

1. Disruptive behavior (20 items)

2. Self-absorbed behavior (20 items)

3. Language disturbance (9 items)

4. Anxiety (12 items)

5. Autistic related (9 items)

6. Antisocial behavior (4 items)

Emotional Problems Scales: Behavior Rating Scales (BRS) and Self-Report Inventory (SRI)— These instruments offer an informant rating scale and a self rating scale companion set.

The Behavior Rating Scales (BRS) were developed for individuals with mild mental retardation or borderline intelligence. This scale takes some time to complete because of the large number of items. As with some of the other measures, the number of items in each subscale varies considerably, from 8 on Sexual Maladjustment and Verbal Aggression to 19 on Physical Aggression and Distractibility. It is recommended that raters be professionals in the field of mental retardation. The BRS has 12 subscales, for which scores are plotted over a cumulative frequency distribution of percentiles.

1. Thought/behavior disorder (15 items)

2. Verbal aggression (8 items)

3. Physical aggression (19 items)

4. Sexual maladjustment (8 items)

5. Noncompliance (15 items)

6. Hyperactivity (19 items)

7. Distractibility (19 items)

8. Anxiety (11 items)

9. Somatic concerns (12 items)

10. Withdrawal (19 items)

11. Depression (11 items)

12. Low self-esteem (15 items)

The SRI has 162 items derived from the same sample as the BRS. Six scales were developed:

1. Thought and behavior disorder (20 items)

2. Impulse control (33 items)

3. Anxiety (25 items)

4. Depression (36 items)

5. Low self-esteem (20 items)

6. Lie scale (12 items)

The lie scale is intended to assess the validity of the patient's responses. Items are read to the client and the clinician marks "yes" or "no."

The Psychopathology Inventory for Mentally Retarded Adults (PIMRA)—This instrument is available both as a 56-item informant rating scale and as a 56-item inventory self-report scale. Each is designed for individual administration either to the informant or to the client. The PIMRA, which was designed to correspond to DSM-III, has the following scales, each with seven items:

1. Schizophrenia

2. Affective disorder

3. Psychosexual disorder

4. Adjustment disorder

5. Anxiety disorder

6. Somatoform disorder

7. Personality disorder

8. Inappropriate adjustment

There is also a total score based on all 56 items. Items are judged as either being true or false. The self-report inventory is typically read aloud to the individual who rates himself. This inventory is intended for adolescents or adults with mild mental retardation, although some adults with moderate mental retardation are able to complete the inventory. Respondents are required to answer yes or no.

Emotional Disorders Rating Scale for Developmental Disabilities—This scale is a close relative of the EDRS, discussed previously.

Maladaptive Behavior Scale—This global index was discussed under general rating instruments. It is suitable for use with individuals who have developmental disability, because it can be used to assess any observable symptom or behavior and is able to be repeated.

The Diagnostic Assessment of the Severely Handicapped (DASH)—The DASH is a 96-item informant rating scale, closely tied to the DSM-III-R, for assessing adults with severe to profound mental retardation.

Neuropsychological Tests

Achievement Tests

This is a complex area and there is a long range of instruments extending from readiness and diagnostic to content-oriented tests. In the early grade levels, content of achievement tests tends to differ markedly. Some tests emphasize memory of factual material, whereas others stress higher cognitive abilities, such as analysis and interpretation. A multitude of different scores may be available including grade norms, percentiles, standard scores, and grade placement scores, and these may be interpreted differently. *You should learn to understand the interpretation of the testing results*.

Wide Range Achievement Test-Revised (WRAT-R)—WRAT-R and its predecessor, the WRAT are the most frequently used tests. It assesses performance in the areas of reading, spelling, and arithmetic, and administration time is approximately 20 to 30 minutes.

Other tests include the following:

- Gilmore Oral Reading Test

- Gray Oral Reading Test

- Gates-McKillop Reading Diagnostic Tests

- Neale Analysis of Reading

- Gates MacGinitie Reading Tests

- Iowa Tests of Basic Skills.

All of these except the Iowa Tests are primarily for the assessment of reading disorder.

Continuous Performance Task (CPT)—This is a vigilance task in which the child is required to make a response whenever a target stimulus appears. Two versions are often used. In the simpler, the child presses a switch whenever the target (an *X)* appears; in the more difficult, the child responds to the letter X but only when preceded by the letter A. Errors of omission (failures to detect the X), errors of commission (false detections), and response time are recorded. There are numerous versions of the CPT available, both visual and auditory versions, in which letters or numbers are recorded onto cassette tape. The latter might easily be integrated into clinical practice, but now there are computerized versions available as well as a commercial version. Hyperactive (ADHD) children make substantially more errors than control subjects.

Cancellation Tasks—This test involves marking a specified form or letter on a sheet usually interspersed with non-targets as distracters. Only limited time is allowed so that the child cannot complete the task. The number of target stimuli correctly marked, the number missed, incorrect cancellations, and the total numbers cancelled are scored.

Matching Familiar Figures (MFF) Task Discrimination—In its most common format, the MFF task comes as a booklet with plastic binding. The child's task is to identify which of six test stimuli is identical to one on an adjacent page. The original MFF contains 12 sets of stimuli, whereas a more recent version contains 20 sets. Measures include time required for the child to make a response and the number of errors before the match is identified.

Analogue Classroom Tests—These involve several sheets containing problems in arithmetic, spelling, and reading, all within the child's demonstrated ability range. Usually, the child is given a standard amount of time to solve the problems, and the measures obtained may include the number of problems attempted and the number completed correctly.

Paired Associate Learning (PAL)—In this paradigm, the subject is required to learn pairs of objects not naturally associated in any way, such as pictures of common objects or words. The first part of the pair (the stimulus) is presented and the child is asked to name the other member before it is re-presented. Testing continues until some criterion (such as one or two perfect trials) is reached or until the completion of a predetermined number of trials. Dependent measures can include errors to criterion and trials to criterion, although the former is more sensitive. PAL appears to be largely a measure of short-term and medium-term memory, and unlike many of the tasks previously described, PAL measures *effortful* performance.

Delay Task—The Delay Task was devised to measure impulsivity in ADHD children using the differential reinforcement of low (DRL) rate behavior, in which the child responds by pressing a button on a portable monitor. The Delay Task is part of the commercially available Gordon Diagnostic System and is a companion to the CPT mentioned above. The child is told that if he waits long enough between responses, a point will be forthcoming each time on a counter. The actual delay required is six seconds, although the child is not told this. The Delay Task lasts eight minutes and has been shown to discriminate between hyperactive and control groups of children

Short Term Recognition Memory Task—The Short Term Memory (STM) task was originally developed to assess memory in children with challenging cognitive function and involves the presentation of arrays of cartoon figures followed by a single figure. The child indicates whether the test figure is a member of the previous array by pressing a "same" or "different" response key.

Computer Tests

Gordon Diagnostic System—This system was developed for assessing children with ADHD and comprises a continuous performance test (CPT), a delay test, and a distractibility test. The Gordon Diagnostic System is a compact, self-contained test.

Serial Recall—This is a norm-referenced test of linguistic and nonlinguistic sequential recall evaluating short-term memory and is the first of four planned programs collectively referred to as the *Michigan Memory Series Software*. The test involves the presentation of strings of characters (e.g., numbers), which are then automatically adjusted to the child's ability, and the youngster must indicate the position that a test character held within the string. Summary data include accuracy and response time, a breakdown by serial position, and an analysis that compares the child's results to age-related norms.

Test of Variables of Attention (TOVA)—This program controls a continuous performance task of the A-X type (but using squares instead) that lasts 23 minutes and yields six dependent variables. Dependent measures include (1) errors of omission, (2) errors of commission, (3) mean response time, (4) variability of response time, (5) anticipatory responses, and (6) response time following commission errors. There are norms, comparison data on ADHD versus control subjects, and findings for premedication versus postmedication, but many details are lacking, so these data are difficult to judge.

Mechanical Device Measures

Automated Measures of Activity Level—The wrist actometer is a self-winding wristwatch that has been modified to indicate the total amount of movement (rather than time). Another device is a special simple-to-construct stabilimetric seat that the person being tested uses in conjunction with performance tests. Another method may use pressure-sensitive mats to measure activity of children. The most sophisticated is a solid-state unit fastened to the trunk, which can measure free-range activity over 24 hours.

Appendix E

University of Michigan Medical Center
Department of Psychiatry
Child and Adolescent Psychiatry Division
Developmental Disorders Clinic

Parent Global Impression Scale

Child name _____ ___ Father ____ Mother

Date _____/_____/_____ ____ Other (Specify _____)

Baseline Overall Severity

How do you rate your child's overall problem severity at this time? (check one)

1 =__ Normal   5 = __ Marked

2 =__ Borderline   6 = __ Severe

3 =__ Mild   7 = __ Among the most extremely ill patients

4 =__ Moderate

Baseline Severity of Symptom Cluster _____ (e.g., hyperactivity)

Baseline Severity of Symptom Cluster _____

1 =   __   Normal   5 = __ Marked

2 =   __   Borderline   6 = __ Severe

3 =   __   Mild   7 = __ Among the most extremely ill patients

4 =   __   Moderate

Baseline Severity of Symptom Cluster _____

1 =   __   Normal   5 = __ Marked

2 =   __   Borderline   6 = __ Severe

3 =   __   Mild   7 = __ Among the most extremely ill patients

4 =   __   Moderate

Baseline Severity of Symptom Cluster _____

1 =   __   Normal   5 = __ Marked

2 =   __   Borderline   6 = __ Severe

3 =   __   Mild   7 = __ Among the most extremely ill patients

4 =   __   Moderate

Baseline Severity of Symptom Cluster _____

1 = __ Normal	5 = __ Marked
2 = __ Borderline	6 = __ Severe
3 = __ Mild	7 = __ Among the most extremely ill patients
4 = __ Moderate	

Baseline Severity of Symptom Cluster _____

1 = __ Normal	5 = __ Marked
2 = __ Borderline	6 = __ Severe
3 = __ Mild	7 = __ Among the most extremely ill patients
4 = __ Moderate	

Baseline Severity of Symptom Cluster _____

1 = __ Normal	5 = __ Marked
2 = __ Borderline	6 = __ Severe
3 = __ Mild	7 = __ Among the most extremely ill patients
4 = __ Moderate	

Baseline Severity of Symptom Cluster _____

1 = __ Normal	5 = __ Marked
2 = __ Borderline	6 = __ Severe
3 = __ Mild	7 = __ Among the most extremely ill patients
4 = __ Moderate	

Baseline Severity of Symptom Cluster _____

1 = __ Normal	5 = __ Marked
2 = __ Borderline	6 = __ Severe
3 = __ Mild	7 = __ Among the most extremely ill patients
4 = __ Moderate	

Baseline Severity of Symptom Cluster _____

1 = __ Normal	5 = __ Marked
2 = __ Borderline	6 = __ Severe
3 = __ Mild	7 = __ Among the most extremely ill patients
4 = __ Moderate	

* Add additional symptom cluster ratings if necessary

Appendix F

University of Michigan Medical Center
Department of Psychiatry
Child and Adolescent Psychiatry Division
Developmental Disorders Clinic

Parent Global Impression Scale

Child name _____ ___ Father ____ Mother

Date _____/_____/_____ ____ Other (Specify _____)

Overall Severity at Follow-Up

How do you rate your child's overall problem severity at this time? (check one)

1 = __ Normal   5 = __ Marked

2 = __ Borderline   6 = __ Severe

3 = __ Mild   7 = __ Among the most extremely ill patients

4 = __ Moderate

Overall Improvement at Follow-Up

In your opinion, how much has your child changed since s/he began to receive treatment from the Developmental Disorders Clinic (not since last visit)?

1 = __ Very Much Improved   4 = __ No Change

2 = __ Much Improved   5 = __ Worsened

3 = __ Minimally Improved

Improvement of Symptom Cluster (_____)

In your opinion, how much has your child changed since (____/____/____) s/he began to receive medication treatment (_____) from the Developmental Disorders Clinic (not since last visit)?

1 = __ Very Much Improved   4 = __ No Change

2 = __ Much Improved   5 = __ Worsened

3 = __ Minimally Improved

Improvement of Symptom Cluster (_____)

In your opinion, how much has your child changed since (____/____/____) s/he began to receive medication treatment (_____) from the Developmental Disorders Clinic (not since last visit)?

1 = __ Very Much Improved   4 = __ No Change

2 = __ Much Improved   5 = __ Worsened

3 = __ Minimally Improved

Improvement of Symptom Cluster (_____)

In your opinion, how much has your child changed since (____/____/____) s/he began to receive medication treatment (_____) from the Developmental Disorders Clinic (not since last visit)?

1 = __ Very Much Improved   4 = __ No Change

2 = __ Much Improved   5 = __ Worsened

3 = __ Minimally Improved

Improvement of Symptom Cluster (_____)

In your opinion, how much has your child changed since (____/____/____) s/he began to receive medication treatment (_____) from the Developmental Disorders Clinic (not since last visit)?

1 = __ Very Much Improved   4 = __ No Change

2 = __ Much Improved   5 = __ Worsened

3 = __ Minimally Improved

Improvement of Symptom Cluster (_____)

In your opinion, how much has your child changed since (____/____/____) s/he began to receive medication treatment (_____) from the Developmental Disorders Clinic (not since last visit)?

1 = __ Very Much Improved   4 = __ No Change

2 = __ Much Improved   5 = __ Worsened

3 = __ Minimally Improved

* Add additional symptom cluster ratings if necessary

Appendix G

University of Michigan Medical Center
Department of Psychiatry
Child and Adolescent Psychiatry Division
Developmental Disorders Clinic
Medication Side-Effects Checklist

Child's Name: _____ Rater: _____ Date: ____/____/____

Medications: 1) _____ 2) _____

Based on your observation of your child during the past week including today, please rate the following side effects on a scale of **0-4**:

0 = None	1 = Minimal / Rarely	3 = Moderate / Frequently
	2 = Mild / Occasionally	4 = Severe / Always

Digestive
____ Increased appetite
____ Decreased appetite
____ Dry mouth
____ Thirst
____ Nausea
____ Vomiting
____ Diarrhea
____ Constipation

Skin & Appendages
____ Photosensitivity
____ Skin rash
____ Acne
____ Dry skin
____ Urticaria (Hives)

Urogenital
____ Urinary retention
____ Frequent urination

Cardiovascular
____ Tachycardia
____ Fainting spell
____ Nasal congestion
____ Nasal bleeding

Musculoskeletal
____ Eye blinking
____ Grimacing
____ Mouth twitching
____ Lips smacking
____ Chewing
____ Teeth grinding
____ Tongue in & out
____ Sustained tongue protruding
____ Drooling
____ Head tilting
____ Rolling eyes
____ Postural rigidity
____ Pacing
____ Hand tremor
____ Shoulder shrugging
____ Head /arm jerking
____ Clapping
____ Hopping
____ Incoordination

Body as a Whole
____ Fever
____ Edema of face/ankles
____ Weight increase
____ Weight decrease
____ Sweating/clamminess

Nervous
____ Headache
____ Insomnia
____ Nightmares
____ Drowsiness
____ Dizziness
____ Confusion
____ Slurred/difficult speech
____ Seizure

Psychiatric
____ Depression
____ Agitation
____ Nervousness
____ Excitement
____ Elevated mood
____ Talkativeness

Appendix H

Psychotherapeutic Medications

ADDERALL

(Dextro-Amphetamine Sulfate, Amphetamine Sulfate, Dextro-Amphetamine Saccharate, and Amphetamine Aspartate)

Pharmacodynamics

Amphetamines are non-catecholamine sympathomimetic amines with central nerve system (CNS) stimulant activity. They may have a direct effect on both alpha- and beta-receptor sites in the peripheral system, as well as release stores of norepinephrine in adrenergic nerve terminals. The CNS action is thought to occur in the cerebral cortex and reticular-activating system. The anorexigenic effect is probably secondary to the CNS-stimulating effect; the site of action is probably the hypothalamic-feeding center.

Pharmacokinetics

Pharmacokinetic information is not currently available.

Indications

1. Attention Deficit Disorder with Hyperactivity (ADHD)

2. Narcolepsy

3. Unlabeled use as potential augmenting agent for antidepressants

Pediatric Use—Amphetamines are not recommended for use in children under 3 years-of-age.

Contraindication

1. Advanced medical disorders including arteriosclerosis, cardiovascular disease, moderate to severe hypertension, hyperthyroidism, glaucoma

2. Agitated states

3. Individuals with a history of drug abuse

4. During or within 14 days following the administration of monoamine oxidase inhibitors

Potential Side Effects

Cardiovascular System—Palpitations, rapid heartbeat, hypertension, cardiomyopathy

Neurological System—Dyskinesia, tremor, headache, exacerbation of motor and phonic tics and Tourette syndrome

Psychiatric Disorders—Over-stimulation, restlessness, dizziness, insomnia, euphoria, dysphoria, psychotic episodes (rare)

Gastrointestinal System—Dry mouth, unpleasant taste, diarrhea, constipation, other gastrointestinal disturbances, anorexia, weight loss

Dermatological System—Urticaria

Sexual Function—Impotence, changes in libido

Potential Drug Interactions

1. Gastrointestinal acidifying agents (reserpine, ascorbic acid, fruit juices, etc.) lower absorption of amphetamines. Urinary acidifying agents (ammonium chloride, sodium acid phosphate, etc.) increase urinary excretion of amphetamines. Both groups of agents lower blood levels and efficacy of amphetamines.

2. Gastrointestinal alkalinizing agents (sodium bicarbonate, etc.) increase absorption of amphetamines. Urinary alkalinizing agents (acetazolamide, some thiazides) increase the concentration of the non-ionized species of the amphetamine molecule, thereby decreasing urinary excretion. Both groups of agents increase blood levels and therefore potentiate the actions of amphetamines.

3. Amphetamines decrease the effect of adrenergic blockers (e.g., INDERAL).

4. Amphetamines may enhance the activity of tricyclic or sympathomimetic agents and increase cardio-vascular effect.

5. NORPRAMIN and possibly other tricyclics may increase the concentration of d-amphetamine in the brain.

6. MAO inhibitors slow amphetamine metabolism. This slowing may increase the release of norepinephrine and other monoamines from adrenergic nerve endings and cause headaches and other signs of hypertensive crisis. A variety of neurological toxic effects and malignant hyperpyrexia can occur, sometimes with fatal results.

7. Amphetamines may decrease the sedative effect of antihistamines.

8. Amphetamines may decrease the hypotensive effects of antihypertensives.

9. THORAZINE and HALDOL block dopamine and norepinephrine reuptake, thus inhibiting the central stimulant effects of amphetamines, and can be used to treat amphetamine poisoning.

10. The antiobesity and stimulatory effects of amphetamines may be inhibited by lithium carbonate.

11. Amphetamines enhance the adrenergic effect of norepinephrine.

12. Amphetamines may delay intestinal absorption of Phenobarbital, DILANTIN, ZARONTIN; co-administration of Phenobarbital or DILANTIN, or ZARONTIN may produce a synergistic anticonvulsant action.

13. Amphetamines inhibit the hypotensive effect of CALAN.

Potential Laboratory Test Interactions:

Amphetamines can cause a significant elevation in plasma corticosteroid levels. This increase is greatest in the evening. Amphetamines may interfere with urinary steroid determinations.

Drug Abuse and Dependence

ADDERALL is a Schedule II controlled substance.

Amphetamines have been extensively abused. Tolerance, extreme psychological dependence, and severe social disability have occurred.

Withdrawal Symptoms

Abrupt cessation following prolonged high dosage administration results in extreme fatigue and mental depression; changes are also noted on the sleep EEG.

Laboratory Tests

Therapeutic range of blood concentration for ADDERALL has not been established.

Dosage and Administration

ADDERALL should be administered at the lowest effective dosage and dosage should be individually adjusted. Late evening doses should be avoided because of the resulting insomnia.

Treatment of ADHD—In children from 3 to 5 years-of-age, start with 2.5mg daily usually given in the morning; daily dosage may be raised in increments of 2.5mg at weekly intervals until optimal response is obtained.

In children 6 years-of-age and older, start with 5mg once or twice daily; daily dosage may be raised in increments of 5mg at weekly intervals until optimal response is obtained. Only in rare cases will it be necessary to exceed a total of 4Omg per day. Give first dose on awakening; give additional doses (1 or 2) at intervals of 4 to 6 hours.

Where possible, medication administration should be interrupted occasionally to determine if there is a recurrence of behavioral symptoms sufficient to require continued therapy.

Treatment of Narcolepsy—Usual dose is 5mg to 60mg per day in divided doses, depending on the individual patient response. Narcolepsy seldom occurs in children under 12 years-of-age; however, when it does, ADDERALL may be used. The suggested initial dose for children aged 6-12 is 6mg daily; daily dose may be raised in increments of 5mg at weekly intervals until optimal response is obtained.

In individuals 12 years-of-age and older, start with 10mg daily; daily dosage may be raised in increments of 10mg at weekly intervals until optimal response is obtained. If bothersome adverse reactions appear (e.g., insomnia or anorexia), dosage should be reduced. Give first dose on awakening; give additional doses (1 or 2) at intervals of 4 to 6 hours.

Overdosage

Toxic symptoms rarely occur with doses of less than 15mg; 30mg can produce severe reactions. Symptoms of overdosage include: restlessness, hyperactivity, irritability, tremor, hyperreflexia, rapid respiration, nausea, vomiting, diarrhea, abdominal cramps, arrhythmias, hypertension, hypotension, circulatory collapse, confusion, assaultiveness, hallucinations, panic states, hyperpyrexia and rhabdomyolysis.

ANAFRANIL

(Clomipramine)

ANAFRANIL is an antiobsessional drug that belongs to the class of pharmacologic agents known as tricyclic antidepressants.

Pharmacodynamics

ANAFRANIL is presumed to inhibit the reuptake of serotonin (5-HT) in the brain.

Pharmacokinetics

- The bioavailability of ANAFRANIL is not significantly affected by food.

- ANAFRANIL distributes into cerebrospinal fluid, the brain, and breast milk.

- The protein binding of ANAFRANIL is approximately 97%, principally to albumin.

- Maximum plasma concentrations of ANAFRANIL occur within 2-6 hours (mean, 4.7 hr).

- The half-life of ANAFRANIL ranges from 19 hours to 37 hours (mean, 32 hr).

- Steady-state levels after multiple dosing are typically reached within 7-14 days.

- ANAFRANIL and its metabolites are excreted in urine and feces following biliary elimination.

Indications

1. For the treatment of Obsessive-Compulsive Disorder (OCD)

2. May also relieve depression, panic attack, and chronic pain

Pediatric Use -The safety and effectiveness in pediatric patients below the age of 10 have not been established.

Contraindications

1. In individuals with a history of hypersensitivity to ANAFRANIL

2. Given in combination, or within 14 days before or after treatment, with an MAOI

3. During the acute recovery period after a myocardial infarction

Potential Side Effects

Body as a Whole—Malaise, flushing, chest pain, fever, allergy, pain, local edema, chills, weight decrease, otitis media, asthenia, general edema, increased susceptibility to infection, and malaise

Neurological System—Vertigo, tremor, headache, myoclonus, paresthesia, twitching, hypertonia, speech disorder, migraine, paresis, abnormal coordination, abnormal EEG, abnormal gait, apathy, ataxia, coma, convulsions, delirium, dyskinesia, dysphonia, encephalopathy, extrapyramidal disorder, hyperkinesia, hypnagogic hallucinations, hypokinesia, leg cramps, neuralgia, sensory disturbance, teeth-grinding

Psychiatric Disorders—Abnormal thinking, somnolence, dizziness, insomnia, nervousness, memory impairment, impaired concentration, anxiety, depression, sleep disorder, psychosomatic disorder, yawning, confusion, abnormal dreaming, agitation, depersonalization, irritability, emotional lability, panic reaction, aggressive reaction, delusion, euphoria, hallucinations, hostility, hypomanic or manic reaction, paranoia, phobic disorder, psychosis, somnambulism, stimulation, suicidal ideation, and suicide attempts

Cardiovascular System—Postural hypotension, palpitation, tachycardia, syncope, ECG changes, intraventricular conduction abnormalities, arrhythmia, bradycardia, cardiac arrest, extrasystoles, pallor

Gastrointestinal System—Dry mouth, tongue ulceration, tooth caries, tooth disorder, dysphagia, esophagitis, increased appetite, nausea, dyspepsia, anorexia, vomiting, diarrhea, constipation, abdominal pain, flatulence, gastrointestinal disorder, eructation, ulcerative stomatitis, abnormal hepatic function, blood in stool, colitis, duodenitis, gastric ulcer, gastritis, gastroesophageal reflux, gingivitis, glossitis, hemorrhoids, hepatitis, increased saliva, irritable bowel syndrome, peptic ulcer, rectal hemorrhage

Endocrine System—Weight increase, lactation, breast enlargement, breast pain, hypothyroidism

Hematological and Lymphatic Systems—Purpura, anemia, leukopenia, agranulocytosis, thrombocytopenia, and pancytopenia, lymphadenopathy

Metabolic System—Thirst, elevations in SGOT and SGPT, dehydration, diabetes mellitus, gout, hypercholesterolemia, hyperglycemia, hyperuricernia, hypokalemia

Muscular and Skeletal Systems—Myalgia, back pain, arthralgia, muscle weakness, arthrosis

Respiratory System—Pharyngitis, rhinitis, sinusitis, coughing, bronchospasm, epistaxis, dyspnea, laryngitis, bronchitis, hyperventilation, increased sputum, pneumonia

Dermatological System—Increased sweating, dry skin, rash, pruritus, dermatitis, acne, urticaria, abnormal skin odor, alopecia, cellulitis, cyst, eczema, erythematous rash, genital pruritus, maculo-papular rash, photosensitivity reaction, psoriasis, pustular rash, skin discoloration

Genitourinary System—Micturition disorder, urinary tract infection, micturition frequency, urinary retention, dysuria, cystitis, dysmenorrhea, menstrual disorder, vaginitis, leukorrhea, amenorrhea, endometriosis, epididymitis, hematuria, nocturia, oliguria, ovarian cyst, polyuria, prostatic disorder, renal calculus, renal pain, urethral disorder, urinary incontinence, uterine hemorrhage, vaginal hemorrhage

Sexual Function—Change of libido, ejaculation failure, impotence

Special Senses—Abnormal vision, taste perversion, tinnitus, abnormal lacrimation, mydriasis, conjunctivitis, anisocoria, blepharospasm, ocular allergy, vestibular disorder, abnormal accommodation, deafness, diplopia, earache, eye pain, foreign body sensation, hyperacusis, parosmia, photophobia, scleritis, taste loss

Withdrawal Symptoms

Abrupt discontinuation of ANAFRANIL may cause a variety of withdrawal symptoms including dizziness, nausea, vomiting, headache, malaise, sleep disturbance, hyperthermia, and irritability.

Potential Drug Interactions

1. Hyperpyretic crisis, seizures, coma, and death may occur when ANAFRANIL is given with an MAOI

2. Co-administration of HALDOL with ANAFRANIL increases plasma concentrations of ANAFRANIL

3. Co-administration of ANAFRANIL with phenobarbital increases plasma concentrations of phenobarbital

4. ANAFRANIL may block the pharmacologic effects of CATAPRES or similar agents

5. ANAFRANIL plasma level may be increased by the concomitant administration of RITALIN or CONCERTA or hepatic enzyme inhibitors (e.g., TAGAMET, PROZAC) and decreased by the concomitant administration of hepatic enzyme inducers (e.g., barbiturates, DILANTIN)

6. An individual who is stable on a given dose of ANAFRANIL may become abruptly toxic when given one of the cytochrome P450 2D6 inhibiting drugs (e.g., TAGAMET, SRIs) as concomitant therapy.

Laboratory Tests

Therapeutic range of blood concentration is 80-100 μg/mL.

Dosage and Administration

During initial titration, ANAFRANIL should be given in divided doses with meals to reduce gastrointestinal side effects. The goal of this initial titration phase is to minimize side effects by permitting tolerance to side effects to develop or allowing the individual time to adapt if tolerance does not develop.

In older adolescents and adults, ANAFRANIL should be initiated at a dosage of 25mg daily and gradually increased, as tolerated, to approximately 100mg during the first 2 weeks. Thereafter, the dosage may be increased gradually over the next several weeks up to a maximum of 250mg daily. After titration, the total daily dose may be given once daily at bedtime to minimize daytime sedation.

In children 10 years and older, the starting dose is 25mg daily and should be gradually increased (given in divided doses) during the first 2 weeks, as tolerated, up to a daily maximum of 3mg/kg or 100mg, whichever is smaller. Thereafter, the dosage may be increased gradually over the next several weeks, up to a daily maximum of 3mg/kg or 200mg, whichever is smaller. After titration, the total daily dose may be given once daily at bedtime to minimize daytime sedation.

As OCD is a chronic condition, it is reasonable to consider continuation for a responding individual. However, dosage adjustments should be made to maintain the individual on the lowest effective dosage, and these individuals should be periodically reassessed to determine the need for further treatment. During maintenance, the total daily dose may be given once daily at bedtime.

Overdosage

Critical manifestations of overdose include cardiac dysrhythmias, severe hypotension, convulsions, and CNS depression including coma. Other CNS manifestations may include drowsiness, stupor, ataxia, restlessness, agitation, delirium, severe perspiration, hyperactive reflexes, muscle rigidity, and athetoid and choreiform movements. Cardiac abnormalities may include tachycardia, signs of congestive heart failure, and in very rare cases, cardiac arrest. Respiratory depression, cyanosis, shock, vomiting, hyperpyrexia, mydriasis, and oliguria or anuria may also be present.

ARTANE

(Trihexyphenidyl)

Pharmacodynamics

ARTANE is a synthetic antispasmodic drug that exerts a direct inhibitory effect upon the parasympathetic nervous system, i.e., it blocks acetylcholine at cerebral synapses. It also has a relaxing effect on smooth musculature; exerted both directly upon the muscle tissue itself and indirectly through an inhibitory effect upon the parasympathetic nervous system.

Pharmacokinetics

- ARTANE is absorbed rapidly after oral administration and the peak plasma level is reached within 1-2 hours of ingestion.

- Peak effect is reached within 1 hour.

- Elimination half-life is 3-4 hours.

- ARTANE is eliminated primarily in urine.

Indications

1. As an adjunct treatment of all forms of Parkinsonism

2. For the control of extrapyramidal disorders caused by medications such as antipsychotic medications

Contraindications

1. Hypersensitivity to the medication or any component

2. Narrow-angle glaucoma, pyloric or duodenal obstruction, stenosing peptic ulcers, bladder neck obstructions, achalasia, or myasthenia

Potential Side Effects

Neurological System—Dizziness, headache

Psychiatric Disorders—Drowsiness, nervousness, delusions, hallucinations, confusion, agitation, disturbed behavior

Dermatological System—Dry skin, skin rashes

Gastrointestinal System—Dry mouth, suppurative parotitis, constipation, mild nausea or vomiting, dilatation of the colon, paralytic ileus

Cardiovascular System—Tachycardia

Genitourinary System—Urinary hesitancy or retention

Special Senses—Dilation of the pupils, blurring of vision, eye pain

Potential Drug Interaction

1. ARTANE may decrease effect of levodopa.

2. Co-administration with narcotic analgesics, phenothiazines, TCAs, or anticholinergics may increase the risk of ARTANE toxicity.

Dosage and Administration

The initial dose should be low and then increased gradually. Whether ARTANE may best be given before or after meals should be determined by the way the individual reacts. If ARTANE tends to dry the mouth excessively, it may be better to take it before meals, unless it causes nausea. If taken after meals, mint candies, chewing gum, or water can allay the thirst that ARTANE sometimes induces.

Treatment of Drug-Induced Parkinsonism—It is recommended to begin therapy with a single 1mg dose. If the extrapyramidal manifestations are not controlled in a few hours, the subsequent doses may be progressively increased until satisfactory control is achieved. The total daily dosage usually ranges between 5 and 15mg although, in some cases, these reactions have been satisfactorily controlled on as little as 1mg daily.

Temporarily reducing the dosage of the antipsychotics or instituting ARTANE therapy and then adjusting dosage of both drugs until the desired therapeutic effect is retained without onset of extrapyramidal reactions may sometimes achieve satisfactory control more rapidly.

The total daily intake of ARTANE is tolerated best if divided into 3 doses and taken at mealtimes. High doses (more than 10mg daily) may be divided into 4 parts with 3 doses administered at mealtimes and the fourth at bedtime.

It is sometimes possible to maintain the individual on a reduced ARTANE dosage after the reactions have remained under control for several days. ARTANE may be discontinued after the maintaining period (1-2 weeks) and restarted when the symptoms reemerge.

Overdosage

Signs and symptoms of ARTANE overdose include blurred vision, urinary retention, and tachycardia.

ATIVAN

(Lorazepam)

Pharmacodynamics

ATIVAN has a tranquilizing action on the central nervous system with no appreciable effect on the respiratory or cardiovascular systems. ATIVAN interacts with the GABA benzodiazepine receptor complex. This interaction is presumed to be responsible for ATIVAN's mechanism of action. ATIVAN exhibits relatively high and specific affinity for its recognition site but does not displace GABA. Attachment to the specific binding site enhances the affinity of GABA for its receptor site on the same receptor complex. The pharmacodynamic consequences of benzodiazepine agonist actions include antianxiety effects, sedation, and reduction of seizure activity. The intensity of action is directly related to the degree of benzodiazepine receptor occupancy.

Pharmacokinetics

- ATIVAN is readily absorbed with an absolute bioavailability of 90 percent.

- Peak concentrations in plasma occur approximately 2 hours following oral administration.

- The mean half-life of unconjugated ATIVAN in plasma is about 12 hours.

- ATIVAN is approximately 85% bound to plasma proteins.
- ATIVAN is eliminated mainly by the kidneys.

Indications

1. For the treatment of anxiety disorders or for the short-term relief of the symptoms of anxiety or anxiety associated with depressive symptoms

2. Unlabeled use in management of rages

Pediatric Use -Safety and effectiveness of ATIVAN in children of less than 12 years have not been established.

Contraindication

Individuals with known sensitivity to the benzodiazepines or with acute narrow-angle glaucoma should not take ATIVAN

Potential Side Effects

Adverse reactions, if they occur, are usually observed at the beginning of therapy and generally disappear with continued medication or upon decreasing the dose.

The most frequent adverse reaction to ATIVAN is sedation, followed by dizziness, weakness, and unsteadiness. Less frequent adverse reactions are disorientation, depression, nausea, change in appetite, headache, sleep disturbance, agitation, dermatological symptoms, and eye-function disturbance, together with various gastrointestinal symptoms and autonomic manifestations. Transient amnesia or memory impairment has been reported in association with the use of ATIVAN.

Potential Drug Interactions

1. ATIVAN may increase CNS-depressant effects of phenothiazines, narcotic analgesics, barbiturates, antidepressants, scopolamine, monoamine-oxidase inhibitors, and alcohol.

2. Concomitant use of LOXITANE (loxapine) and ATIVAN may cause significant respiratory depression, stupor, or hypotension.

3. Marked sedation, excessive salivation, or ataxia may be caused by concomitant use of CLOZARIL and ATIVAN.

4. Concomitant use of HALDOL and ATIVAN may cause apnea, coma, bradycardia, arrhythmia, and heart arrest.

5. Concurrent administration of ATIVAN with DEPAKOTE may result in decreased total clearance of ATIVAN, thus increasing ATIVAN plasma concentrations.

6. Co-administration of ATIVAN with oral contraceptive steroids may increase the total clearance of ATIVAN. Thus it may be necessary to increase the dose of ATIVAN in females who are concomitantly taking oral contraceptives.

7. Concurrent administration of ATIVAN with probenecid may result in a prolongation of ATIVAN half-life and a decrease in its total clearance. Thus ATIVAN dosage needs to be reduced when co-administered with probenecid.

Physical and Psychological Dependence

ATIVAN is a controlled substance in Schedule IV.

ATIVAN may produce psychological and physical dependence.

Withdrawal Symptoms

Convulsions, tremor, abdominal and muscle cramps, vomiting, and sweating have occurred following abrupt discontinuance of ATIVAN. The more severe withdrawal symptoms have usually been limited to those individuals who received excessive doses over an extended period of time. Generally milder withdrawal symptoms (e.g., dysphoria and insomnia) have been reported following abrupt discontinuance of benzodiazepines taken continuously at therapeutic levels for several months. Consequently, after extended therapy, abrupt discontinuation should be avoided and a gradual dosage-tapering schedule should be followed.

Laboratory Tests

Some individuals on ATIVAN have developed leukopenia, and some have had elevations of LDH. Periodic blood counts and liver function tests are recommended for individuals on long-term therapy.

Dosage and Administration

For optimal results, dose, frequency of administration, and duration of therapy should be individualized according to individual response. The dosage of ATIVAN should be increased gradually when needed to help avoid adverse effects. When higher dosage is indicated, the evening dose should be increased before the daytime doses.

In older adolescents and adults, the usual range is 2 to 6mg/day given in divided doses, the largest dose being taken before bedtime, but the daily dosage may vary from 1 to 10mg/day.

For children 6 years and older, an initial dosage of 1-to-2mg/day in divided doses is recommended, to be adjusted as needed and tolerated.

For anxiety, most individuals require an initial dose of 2-to-3mg/day given two-to-three times daily.

For insomnia due to anxiety or transient situational stress, a single daily dose of 2 to 4mg may be given, usually at bedtime.

Overdosage

Overdosage of ATIVAN is usually manifested by varying degrees of central nervous system depression ranging from drowsiness to coma. In mild cases, symptoms include drowsiness, mental confusion, and lethargy. In more serious cases, and especially when other drugs or alcohol are ingested, symptoms may include ataxia, hypotonia, hypotension, hypnotic state, coma, and very rarely, death.

BUSPAR

(Buspirone)

BUSPAR is an antianxiety agent that is not chemically or pharmacologically related to the benzodiazepines, barbiturates, or other sedative-anxiolytic medications.

Pharmacodynamics

The exact mechanism of action of buspirone is unknown. BUSPAR has a high affinity for serotonin (5-HTIA) receptors and has moderate affinity for brain D2-dopamine receptors.

Pharmacokinetics

- BUSPAR is rapidly absorbed and undergoes extensive first-pass metabolism.

- Food may decrease the extent of presystemic clearance of BUSPAR.

- Approximately 95% of BUSPAR is plasma protein bound.

- Peak plasma levels are reached 40 to 90 minutes after single oral doses of 20mg.

- The average elimination half-life of unchanged BUSPAR is about 2-to-3 hours.

- BUSPAR is metabolized by the liver and excreted by the kidneys.

Indications

1. For the management of anxiety disorders or the short-term relief of the symptoms of anxiety

2. Unlabeled uses in major depression, potential augmenting agent for antidepressants, premenstrual syndrome, management of aggression in mental retardation and secondary mental disorders

Pediatric Use -The safety and effectiveness of BUSPAR have not been determined in individuals below 18 years of age.

Contraindications

Hypersensitivity to buspirone hydrochloride

Potential Side Effects

Body as a Whole—Headache, fatigue, weakness, sweating or clamminess, weight gain, fever, roaring sensation in the head, weight loss, and malaise

Neurological System—Numbness (occurs frequently), paresthesia, incoordination, akathisia, tremor, involuntary movements, slowed reaction time, lightheadedness, and seizures

Psychiatric Disorders—Dream disturbances, dizziness, drowsiness, nervousness, insomnia, decreased concentration, excitement, anger/hostility, confusion, depression, dysphoria, noise intolerance, euphoria, dissociative reaction, depersonalization, fearfulness, loss of interest, hallucinations, suicidal ideation

Cardiovascular System—Chest pain, tachycardia, palpitations, syncope, hypotension, hypertension

Gastrointestinal System—Dry mouth, salivation, nausea, vomiting, anorexia, increased appetite, abdominal/gastric distress, diarrhea, constipation, flatulence, irritable colon, rectal bleeding

Muscular and Skeletal Systems—Musculoskeletal aches/pains, muscle cramps, muscle spasms, rigid/stiff muscles, and arthralgias

Respiratory System—Hyperventilation, shortness of breath, chest congestion

Dermatological System—Skin Rash, edema, pruritus, flushing, easy bruising, hair loss, dry skin, facial edema, blisters

Genitourinary System—Urinary frequency, urinary hesitancy, menstrual irregularity, spotting, dysuria

Sexual Function—Decreased or increased libido

Special Senses—Blurred vision, tinnitus, sore throat, nasal congestion, redness and itching of the eyes, altered taste, altered smell, conjunctivitis

Potential Drug Interactions

1. Elevated blood pressure when BUSPAR is added to a regimen including an MAOI.

2. Concomitant use of DESYREL and BUSPAR may cause 3-to-6-fold elevations on SGOT and SGPT.

3. Concomitant administration of BUSPAR and HALDOL may result in increased serum HALDOL concentrations.

Drug Abuse and Dependence

BUSPAR is not a controlled substance. There is no evidence that BUSPAR causes tolerance, or either physical or psychological dependence.

Laboratory Tests

No specific laboratory tests are recommended.

Dosage and Administration

In older adolescents and adults, initial dose of 15mg daily (7.5mg twice daily) is recommended. To achieve an optimal therapeutic response, an increment dosage of 5mg per day at intervals of 2-to-3 days up to maximum daily dosage of 60mg is recommended. BUSPAR should be taken in divided doses (two or three times daily)

Overdosage

Signs and Symptoms: nausea, vomiting, dizziness, drowsiness, miosis, and gastric distress. No deaths have been reported following overdosage with BUSPAR alone.

CALAN

(Verapamil)

Pharmacodynamics

CALAN is a calcium ion influx inhibitor that exerts its pharmacologic effects by modulating the influx of ionic calcium across the cell membrane of the arterial smooth muscle as well as in conductile and contractile myocardial cells. By decreasing the influx of calcium, CALAN prolongs the effective refractory period within the AV node and slows AV conduction in a rate-related manner. This property accounts for the ability of CALAN to slow the ventricular rate in individuals with chronic atrial flutter or atrial fibrillation. In individuals with sick sinus syndrome, CALAN may interfere with sinusnode impulse generation and may induce sinus arrest or sinoatrial block.

CALAN exerts antihypertensive effects by decreasing systemic vascular resistance. CALAN dilates the main coronary arteries and coronary arterioles and is a potent inhibitor of coronary artery spasm. This property increases myocardial oxygen delivery in individuals with coronary artery spasm and is responsible for the effectiveness of CALAN in vasospastic as well as unstable angina at rest.

CALAN regularly reduces the total peripheral resistance against which the heart works both at rest and at a given level of exercise by dilating peripheral arterioles. This unloading of the heart reduces myocardial energy consumption and oxygen requirements and probably accounts for the effectiveness of CALAN in chronic stable effort angina.

Pharmacokinetics

- More than 90% of the orally administered dose of CALAN is absorbed.

- Because of rapid biotransformation of CALAN during its first pass through the portal circulation, bioavailability ranges from 20% to 35%.

- Peak plasma concentrations are reached between 1 and 2 hours after oral administration.

- No relationship has been established between the plasma concentration of CALAN and a reduction in blood pressure.

- The mean elimination half-life in single dose ranged from 3 to 7 hours; after repetitive dosing, the half-life ranged from 4 to 12 hours.

- Approximately 90% is bound to plasma proteins.

- Orally administered CALAN undergoes extensive metabolism in the liver.

- Approximately 70% of an administered dose is excreted as metabolites in the urine and 16% or more in the feces within 5 days. About 3% to 4% is excreted in the urine as unchanged drug.

Indications

CALAN is indicated for the treatment of the following:

1. Angina at rest including vasospastic and unstable (pre-infarction) angina

2. Chronic stable angina (also known as classic, effort-associated angina)

3. In association with digitalis for the control of ventricular rate at rest and during stress in individuals with chronic atrial flutter and/or atrial fibrillation

4. Prophylaxis of repetitive paroxysmal supraventricular tachycardia

5. Management of essential hypertension

Contraindications

CALAN is contraindicated in:

1. Severe left ventricular dysfunction

2. Hypotension (systolic pressure less than 90 mm Hg) or cardiogenic shock

3. Sick sinus syndrome

4. Second- or third-degree AV block

5. Atrial flutter or atrial fibrillation and an accessory bypass tract

6. Individuals with known hypersensitivity to CALAN hydrochloride.

Potential Side Effects

Serious adverse reactions are uncommon when CALAN therapy is initiated with upward dose titration within the recommended single and total daily dose.

Body as a Whole—Fatigue, edema

Neurological System—Cerebrovascular accident, dizziness, confusion, headache equilibrium disorders, insomnia, muscle cramps, paresthesia

Psychiatric Disorders—Psychotic symptoms, shakiness, somnolence

Cardiovascular System—Angina pectoris, atrioventricular dissociation, chest pain, claudication, myocardial infarction, bradycardia, PR-interval prolongation, palpitations, heart failure, purpura (vasculitis), hypotension, pulmonary edema, flushing, syncope

Respiratory System—Dyspnea

Gastrointestinal System—Dry mouth, gingival hyperplasia, nausea, constipation, diarrhea, gastrointestinal distress, elevated liver enzymes (SGOT, SGPT, and alkaline phosphatase)

Hematologic and Lymphatic Systems—Ecchymosis or bruising

Dermatologic System—Rash, exanthema, hair loss, hyperkeratosis, macules, sweating, urticaria, Stevens-Johnson syndrome, erythema multiforme

Endocrine System—Gynecomastia, galactorrhea, hyper-prolactinemia, spotty menstruation

Genitourinary System—Increased urination

Sexual Function—Impotence

Special Senses—Blurred vision, tinnitus

Potential Drug Interactions

1. CALAN may increase blood alcohol concentrations and prolong its effects.

2. Concomitant therapy with beta-adrenergic blockers and CALAN may result in additive negative effects on heart rate, atrioventricular conduction, or cardiac contractility.

3. A decrease in metoprolol and propranolol clearance has been observed when either drug is administered concomitantly with CALAN.

4. Chronic CALAN treatment can increase serum digoxin levels by 50% to 75% during the first week of therapy, and this can result in digitalis toxicity.

5. CALAN administered concomitantly with oral antihypertensive agents (e.g., vasodilators, angiotensin-converting enzyme inhibitors, diuretics, beta-blockers) will usually have an additive effect on lowering blood pressure.

6. Lithium: Increased sensitivity to the effects of lithium (neurotoxicity) has been reported during concomitant CALAN-lithium therapy; lithium levels have been observed sometimes to increase, sometimes to decrease, and sometimes to be unchanged.

7. Verapamil therapy may increase TEGRETOL concentrations during combined therapy. This may produce TEGRETOL side effects such as diplopia, headache, ataxia, or dizziness.

8. Phenobarbital therapy may increase CALAN clearance.

9. CALAN may inhibit the clearance and increase the plasma levels of theophylline.

10. CALAN may potentiate the activity of curare-like and depolarizing neuromuscular blocking agents.

Dosage and Administration

Treatment of Angina—The usual dose is 80mg to 120mg three times a day. Upward titration should be based on therapeutic efficacy and safety evaluated approximately eight hours after dosing. Dosage may be increased at daily (e.g., patients with unstable angina) or weekly intervals until optimum clinical response is obtained.

Treatment of Arrhythmias—The dosage in digitalized patients with chronic atrial fibrillation ranges from 240 to 320mg/day three-to-four times daily.

Treatment of Essential hypertension—Dose should be individualized by titration. The usual initial mono-therapy dose is 80mg three times a day (240mg/day). Daily dosages of 360 and 480mg have been used but there is no evidence that dosages beyond 360mg provided added effect. Upward titration should be based on therapeutic efficacy, assessed at the end of the dosing interval.

The dose of CALAN must be individualized by titration. The usefulness and safety of dosages exceeding 480mg/day have not been established; therefore, this daily dosage should not be exceeded.

Overdosage

CALAN is known to decrease gastrointestinal transit time. It also may cause cardiovascular symptoms and signs as described above.

CATAPRES

(Clonidine)

Pharmacodynamics

CATAPRES is a centrally acting alpha-adrenoreceptor agonist hypotensive agent. It stimulates alpha-adrenoreceptors in the brain stem. This action results in reduced sympathetic outflow from the central nervous system and in decreases in peripheral resistance, renal vascular resistance, heart rate, and blood pressure.

CATAPRES acts relatively rapidly. The individual's blood pressure declines within 30 to 60 minutes after an oral dose, the maximum decrease occurring within 2 to 4 hours. Normal postural reflexes are intact; therefore, orthostatic symptoms are mild and infrequent.

During long-term therapy, cardiac output tends to return to control values while peripheral resistance remains decreased. Slowing of the pulse rate has been observed in most individuals given CATAPRES, but the medication does not alter normal hemodynamic response to exercise.

The exact relationship of the pharmacologic actions to the antihypertensive and psychotherapeutic effects of CATAPRES has not been fully elucidated.

Pharmacokinetics

- The peak plasma level of CATAPRES is reached in approximately 3 to 5 hours.

- The plasma half-life ranges from 12 to 16 hours.

- Following oral administration, about 40-60% of the absorbed dose is recovered in the urine as unchanged drug within 24 hours. The remainder of the absorbed dose is metabolized in the liver.

Indications

1. CATAPRES is indicated in the treatment of hypertension. CATAPRES may be employed alone or concomitantly with other anti-hypertensive agents.

2. Unlabeled use for ADHD, tic disorders, aggression and rages, and initial insomnia.

3. Perioperative Use: Administration of CATAPRES should be continued to within four hours of surgery and resumed as soon as possible thereafter. The blood pressure should be carefully monitored and appropriate measures instituted to control it as necessary. Blood pressure should be carefully monitored during surgery and additional measures to control blood pressure should be available if required.

Pediatric Use: Safety and effectiveness in pediatric patients below the age of twelve have not been established

Contraindications

CATAPRES should not be used in individuals with known hypersensitivity to CATAPRES.

Potential Side Effects

Body as a Whole—Weakness, fatigue, headache, withdrawal syndrome, pallor, a weakly positive Coombs' test, increased sensitivity to alcohol, fever

Neurological System—Sedation, drowsiness

Psychiatric Disorders—Nervousness and agitation, mental depression, insomnia, vivid dreams or nightmares, restlessness, anxiety, visual and auditory hallucinations, and delirium

Cardiovascular—Orthostatic symptoms, palpitations and tachycardia, bradycardia, syncope, Raynaud's phenomenon, congestive heart failure, and ECG abnormalities (sinus node arrest, functional bradycardia, high degree AV block and arrhythmias)

Dermatological—Rash, pruritus, hives, angioneurotic edema and urticaria, and alopecia

Gastrointestinal—Dry mouth, nausea and vomiting, anorexia and malaise, mild transient abnormalities in liver function tests, hepatitis, parotitis, constipation, pseudo-obstruction, and abdominal pain

Metabolic System—Weight gain, gynecomastia

Muscular and Skeletal Systems—Muscle or joint pain, and leg cramps

Genitourinary System—Nocturia, difficulty in micturition, urinary retention

Sexual Function—Decreased sexual activity, impotence, and loss of libido

Special Senses—Dryness of the nasal mucosa, dryness of the eyes, burning of the eyes, blurred vision

Potential Drug Interactions

1. CATAPRES may potentiate the CNS-depressive effects of alcohol, barbiturates, or other sedating drugs.

2. Co-administration of CATAPRES and tricyclic antidepressants may reduce the hypotensive effect of CATAPRES necessitating an increase in the CATAPRES dose.

3. Co-administration of CATAPRES and agents known to affect sinus node function or AV nodal conduction, e.g. digitalis, calcium channel blockers and beta-blockers may potentiate the additive effects such as bradycardia and AV block.

Withdrawal Symptoms

Sudden cessation of CATAPRES treatment has resulted in symptoms such as nervousness, agitation, headache, and tremors accompanied or followed by a rapid rise in blood pressure and elevated catecholamine concentrations in the plasma. The likelihood of such reactions to discontinuation of clonidine therapy appears to be greater after administration of higher doses or continuation of concomitant beta-blocker treatment. Rare instances of hypertensive encephalopathy, cerebrovascular accidents, and death have been reported after CATAPRES withdrawal. When discontinuing therapy with CATAPRES, the physician should reduce the dose gradually over 2 to 4 days to avoid withdrawal symptoms.

Dosage and Administration

There is no data based recommendation of dosage and administration for CATAPRES to be used to treat individuals with ADHD, tic disorders, agitation or rages, and initial insomnia. The followings are general guides to its administration based on clinical experiences.

Treatment of ADHD, Tic Disorders, Agitation or Rages

Young children: Begin with 0.025mg per day. Further increment of 0.025mg per day may be made at weekly interval if necessary until the desired response is achieved. The dose of CATAPRES must be adjusted according to the individual's blood pressure and clinical responses. At the optimal dosage with positive response, CATAPRES can then be taken two or three times daily.

Treatment of older children and adolescents may begin with 0.05mg per day and an increment of 0.05mg per day at weekly intervals.

For Treatment of Initial Insomnia

Young Children: Begin with 0.05mg given one hour before bedtime. Further increment of 0.025mg per night may be made every three to five nights until the desired response is achieved.

Older children and adolescents may begin with 0.1mg given one hour before bedtime. Further increment of 0.025mg per night may be made every three to five nights until the desired response is achieved.

Overdosage

Hypertension may develop early and may be followed by hypotension, bradycardia, respiratory depression, hypothermia, drowsiness, decreased or absent reflexes, weakness, irritability, and miosis. The frequency of CNS depression may be higher in children than adults. Large overdoses may result in reversible cardiac conduction defects or dysrhythmias, apnea, coma, and seizures. Signs and symptoms of overdose generally occur within 30 minutes to two hours after exposure. As little as 0.1mg of CATAPRES has produced signs of toxicity in children.

There is no specific antidote for CATAPRES overdose. CATAPRES overdosage may result in the rapid development of CNS depression; therefore, induction of vomiting with ipecac syrup is not recommended. Gastric lavage may be indicated following recent and/or large ingestions. Administration of activated charcoal and/or a cathartic may be beneficial. Supportive care may include atropine sulfate for bradycardia, intravenous fluids and/or vasopressor agents for hypotension, and vasodilators for hypertension. Naloxone may be a useful adjunct for the management of clonidine-induced respiratory depression, hypotension, or coma. Blood pressure should be monitored since the administration of naloxone has occasionally resulted in paradoxical hypertension.

CATAPRES-TTS

(Clonidine Transdermal Therapeutic System Patch)

CATAPRES-TTS is a transdermal patch providing continuous systemic delivery of clonidine for 7 days at an approximately constant rate. The amount of medication released is directly proportional to the area. The composition per unit area is the same for all three doses. Proceeding from the visible surface towards the surface attached to the skin, there are four consecutive layers:

1. Backing layer of pigmented polyester film

2. Drug reservoir of clonidine, mineral oil, polyisobutylene, and colloidal silicon dioxide

3. Microporous polypropylene membrane that controls the rate of delivery of clonidine from the system to the skin surface

4. Adhesive formulation of clonidine, mineral oil, polyisobutylene, and colloidal silicon dioxide. Prior to use, a protective slit release liner of polyester that covers the adhesive layer is removed.

Release Rate Concept—CATAPRES-TTS is programmed to release clonidine at an approximately constant rate of 0.1, 0.2 or 0.3mg clonidine per day for 7 days. Therapeutic plasma clonidine levels are achieved 2-to-3 days after initial application of CATAPRES-TTS. The 3.5, 7.0, and 10.5 CM2 systems/patches deliver 0.1, 0.2, and 0.3mg of clonidine per day, respectively. Application of a new system/patch to a fresh skin site at weekly intervals continuously maintains therapeutic plasma concentrations of clonidine. If the CATAPRES-TTS is removed and not replaced with a new system/patch, therapeutic plasma clonidine levels will persist for about 8 hours and then decline slowly over several days. Over this time period, blood pressure returns gradually to pretreatment levels.

Indications, Contraindications, Potential Side Effects, Potential Drug Interactions, and Withdrawal Symptoms

Similar to that described above under CATAPRES tablets.

Perioperative Use—CATAPRES-TTS therapy should not be interrupted during the surgical period. Blood pressure should be carefully monitored during surgery and additional measures to control blood pressure should be available if required.

Dosage and Administration

In daily practice, it is recommended to begin with oral CATAPRES. When the efficacy and total daily dosage of CATAPRES has been established, then switch to the CATAPRES-TTS. The oral CATAPRES should be continued for 2-3 days because the effect of CATAPRES-TTS may not commence until 2-3 days after initial application. Therefore, gradual reduction of prior drug dosage is advised.

Apply CATAPRES-TTS once every 7 days to a hairless area of intact skin on the upper outer arm or chest in individuals who tend to be compliant to the treatment. In individuals who tend to remove the system/patch from their body, apply the system/patch to the back near the spine so that it is difficult for the individual to remove it. Each new application of CATAPRES-TTS should be on a different skin site from the previous location. If the system loosens during 7-day wearing, the adhesive overlay should be applied directly over the system to ensure good adhesion. There have been rare reports of the need for patch changes prior to 7 days to maintain symptom control.

If an individual experiences isolated, mild localized skin irritation before completing 7 days of use, the system/patch may be removed and replaced with a new system applied to a fresh skin site.

If the system should begin to loosen from the skin after application, the individual should be instructed to place the adhesive overlay directly over the system to ensure adhesion during its 7-day use.

After use, CATAPRES-TTS should be folded in half with the adhesive sides together and discarded away from children's reach.

CELEXA

(Citalopram)

Pharmacodynamics

CELEXA is an orally administered selective serotonin reuptake inhibitor (SSRI) with a chemical structure unrelated to that of other SSRIs or of tricyclic, tetracyclic, or other available antidepressants.

Pharmacokinetics

- Following a single oral dose of CELEXA, peak blood levels occur at about 4 hours.

- The absorption of CELEXA is not affected by food.

- Biotransformation of CELEXA is mainly hepatic, with a mean terminal half-life of about 35 hours.

- With once-daily dosing, steady state plasma concentrations are achieved within approximately one week.

Indications

For the treatment of depression

Pediatric Use—Safety and effectiveness in pediatric patients have not been established.

Contraindications

1. Concomitant use of CELEXA and monoamine oxidase inhibitors (MAOIs) is contraindicated.

2. In individuals with a hypersensitivity to CELEXA or any of the inactive ingredients in CELEXA.

Potential Side Effects

Body as a Whole—Hot flushes, rigors, alcohol intolerance, syncope, influenza-like symptoms

Neurological System—Paresthesia, migraine, hyperkinesia, vertigo, hypertonia, extrapyramidal disorder, leg cramps, involuntary muscle contractions, hypokinesia, neuralgia, dystonia, abnormal gait, hypesthesia, ataxia, convulsion/seizure

Psychiatric Disorders—Impaired concentration, amnesia, apathy, depression, increased appetite, aggravated depression, suicide attempt, confusion, aggressive reaction, paranoia, drug dependence, depersonalization, hallucination, euphoria, activation of mania/hypomania, psychotic depression, delusion, paranoid reaction, emotional lability, panic reaction, psychosis

Cardiovascular System—Tachycardia, postural hypotension, hypotension, hypertension, bradycardia, edema (extremities), angina pectoris, extrasystoles, cardiac failure, flushing, myocardial infarction, cerebrovascular accident, myocardial ischemia

Gastrointestinal System—Increased saliva, flatulence, gastritis, gastroenteritis, stomatitis, eructation, hemorrhoids, dysphagia, teeth grinding, gingivitis, esophagitis

Hematologic and Lymphatic Systems—Purpura, anemia, epistaxis, leukocytoses, leukopenia, lymphadenopathy

Metabolic System—Decreased weight, increased weight increased hepatic enzymes, thirst, dry eyes, increased alkaline phosphatase, and abnormal glucose tolerance

Musculoskeletal System—Arthritis, muscle weakness, skeletal pain

Endocrine System—Amenorrhea, galactorrhea, breast pain, breast enlargement, vaginal hemorrhage

Respiratory System Disorders—Coughing, bronchitis, dyspnea, pneumonia

Dermatological System—Rash, pruritus, photosensitivity reaction, urticaria, acne, skin discoloration, eczema, alopecia, dermatitis, dry skin, psoriasis

Special Senses—Abnormal accommodation, taste perversion, tinnitus, conjunctivitis, eye pain

Genitourinary System—Polyuria, micturition frequency, urinary incontinence, urinary retention, dysuria

Sexual Function—Increased libido

Potential Drug Interaction

1. CELEXA in combination with a monoamine oxidase inhibitor (MAOI) may cause serious, sometimes fatal, reactions including hyperthermia, rigidity, myoclonus, autonomic instability with possible rapid fluctuations of vital signs, and mental status changes that include extreme

agitation progressing to delirium and coma. These reactions may also develop in individuals who have recently discontinued CELEXA treatment and have been started on an MAOI.

2. Because lithium may enhance the serotonergic effects of CELEXA, caution should be exercised when CELEXA and lithium are co-administered.

3. Given the enzyme-inducing properties of TEGRETOL, the possibility that TEGRETOL may increase the clearance of CELEXA should be considered if the two drugs are co-administered.

Dosage and Administration

Treatment of Depressive Disorders—In older adolescents and adults, the initial dose is 20mg once daily, taking any time of the day with or without food. If significant improvement is not observed after 2-to-3 weeks, the daily dose can be increased to 40mg. There is no data at the present to support daily dosage of more than 40mg.

In children 12 years and older, if indicated, the initial dose can be 10mg daily with a weekly increment of 5- 10mg/day up to 20-30mg/day.

Treatment of Obsessive-Compulsive Disorder—The dosage and administration are the same as those used in the treatment of Depressive Disorder.

Overdosage

Symptoms most often accompanying CELEXA overdose include drowsiness, sweating, nausea, vomiting, tremor, somnolence, and sinus tachycardia. In rare cases, symptoms may include amnesia, confusion, coma, convulsions, hyperventilation, cyanosis, rhabdomyolysis, and ECG changes.

CLOZARIL

(Clozapine)

Pharmacodynamics

CLOZARIL interferes with the binding of dopamine at D_1, D_2, D_3 and D_5 receptors, and has a high affinity for the D_4 receptor. CLOZARIL also acts as an antagonist at adrenergic, cholinergic, histaminergic, and serotonergic receptors.

Pharmacokinetics

- Food does not appear to affect the systemic bioavailability of CLOZARIL. Thus, CLOZARIL may be administered with or without food.

- Steady-state peak plasma concentration occurs at the average of 2.5 hours (range: 1-6 hours) after dosing.

- CLOZARIL is approximately 97% bound to serum proteins.

- The mean elimination half-life of CLOZARIL after a single 75mg dose was 8 hours (range: 4-12 hours), compared to a mean elimination half-life, after achieving steady state with 100mg b.i.d. dosing, of 12 hours (range: 4 to 66 hours).

- CLOZARIL is almost completely metabolized prior to excretion and only trace amounts of unchanged drug are detected in the urine and feces. Approximately 50% of the administered dose is excreted in the urine and 30% in the feces.

Indications

1. Because of the significant risk of agranulocytosis and seizure associated with its use, CLOZARIL should be used only in individuals who have failed to respond adequately to treatment with appropriate courses of standard antipsychotic medications (i.e., at least 2 trials, each with a different standard antipsychotic medication, at an adequate dose, and for an adequate duration), either because of insufficient effectiveness or the inability to achieve an effective dose due to intolerable adverse effects from those medications.

Pediatric Use—Safety and effectiveness in pediatric patients have not been established.

Contraindications

1. In individuals known to be hypersensitive to CLOZARIL or any component of this medication

2. In individuals with myeloproliferative disorders, uncontrolled epilepsy, or a history of CLOZARIL induced agranulocytosis or severe granulocytopenia

3. Severe central nervous system depression or comatose states from any cause

4. Simultaneous use with other medications having a known potential to cause agranulocytosis or otherwise suppress bone marrow function

Potential Side Effects

Body as a Whole—Chills, chills with fever, hypothermia, malaise, fatigue

Neurological Systems—Drowsiness, sedation, delirium, confusion, dizziness/vertigo, abnormal EEG (increases delta and theta activity and slows dominant alpha frequencies), increased REM sleep, insomnia, intensification of dream activity, disturbed sleep, nightmares, headache, myoclonic jerks, tremor, paresthesia, cataplexy, seizures, status epilepticus, slurred speech, loss of speech, stuttering, dysarthria, amentia, tics, poor coordination, ataxia, involuntary movement, rigidity, akathisia, amnesia/memory loss, histrionic movements, Parkinsonism, hyperkinesias, hypokinesia, akinesia, syncope

Psychiatric Disorders—Exacerbation of psychosis, delusions, hallucinations, paranoia, shakiness, irritability, agitation, depression, anxiety

Autonomic Nervous System—Numbness, polydipsia, hot flashes, dry throat, mydriasis

Cardiovascular System—Atrial or ventricular fibrillation, premature ventricular contraction, palpitations, tachycardia, bradycardia, hypotension, hypertension, periorbital edema, edema, phlebitis/thrombophlebitis, cyanosis, nose bleed, chest pain/angina

Gastrointestinal System—Salivary gland swelling, salivation, dry mouth, bitter taste, numb or sore tongue, heartburn, abdominal discomfort, dysphagia, nausea, vomiting, anorexia, increased appetite, acute pancreatitis, abdominal distention, gastroenteritis, nervous stomach, gastric ulcer, intestinal obstruction/paralytic ileus, constipation, fecal impaction, rectal bleeding, abnormal stools, diarrhea, hematemesis, eructation

Hepatobiliary System—Cholestasis, hepatitis, jaundice, liver test abnormality

Dermatologic System—Rash, photosensitivity, vasculitis, erythema multiforme, pruritus, pallor, eczema, erythema, sweating, bruise, dermatitis, petechiae, urticaria, Stevens-Johnson syndrome

Muscular and Skeletal Systems- Myasthenic syndrome, rhabdomyolysis, twitching, joint pain, pain (back, neck, legs), muscle spasm, muscle pain

Respiratory System—Nasal congestion, rhinorrhea, sneezing, throat discomfort, laryngitis, coughing, bronchitis, hyperventilation, wheezing, dyspnea, shortness of breath, aspiration, pleural effusion, pneumonia, pneumonia-like symptoms

Hematologic and Lymphatic Systems—Deep vein thrombosis, elevated hemoglobin/hematocrit, increased erythrocyte sedimentation rate (ESR), pulmonary embolism, sepsis, thrombocytosis, thrombocytopenia, anemia, leukocytosis, leukopenia, neutropenia agranulocytosis

Endocrine System—Hyperglycemia, hyperuricemia, hyponatremia, weight gain, weight loss, dysmenorrhea, breast pain/discomfort

Genitourinary System—Acute interstitial nephritis, priapism (prolonged penis erection), vaginal itch/ infection, urinary abnormalities, urinary urgency/ frequency, incontinence, urinary retention

Sexual Function—Impotence, libido increase or decrease, abnormal ejaculation

Special Sense—Ear disorder, eyelid disorder, bloodshot eyes, nystagmus, visual disturbances

Potential Drug Interactions

1. The risks of using CLOZARIL in combination with other drugs have not been systematically evaluated.

2. Although it has not been established that there is an interaction between CLOZARIL and benzodiazepines or other psychotherapeutic medications, orthostatic hypotension accompanied by cardiac or respiratory arrest has been reported.

3. Because CLOZARIL is highly bound to serum protein, the administration to an individual taking another medication that is highly bound to protein (e.g., warfarin, digitoxin) may cause an increase in plasma concentrations of these medications, potentially resulting in adverse effects. Conversely, adverse effects may result from displacement of protein-bound CLOZARIL by other highly bound medications.

4. Tagamet and erythromycin may both increase plasma levels of CLOZARIL, potentially resulting in adverse effects.

5. DILANTIN may decrease CLOZARIL plasma levels, resulting in a decrease in effectiveness of a previously effective CLOZARIL dose.

6. SRIs may increase serum levels of CLOZARIL.

7. Concomitant use of CLOZARIL with other medications metabolized by cytochrome P450 2D6 may require lower doses than usually prescribed for either CLOZARIL or the other medications such as antidepressants, phenothiazines, and TEGRETOL.

8. CLOZARIL may also potentiate the hypotensive effects of antihypertensive medications and the anticholinergic effects of atropine-type drugs.

Drug Abuse and Dependence

Physical and psychological dependence have not been reported or observed in individuals taking CLOZARIL.

Laboratory Tests

Individuals who are being treated with CLOZARIL *must* have a baseline white blood cell (WBC) and differential count before initiation of treatment and a WBC count every week for the first six months. Thereafter, if acceptable WBC counts [i.e., WBC greater or equal to 3,000/mm^3 and absolute neutrophil count (ANC) greater or equal 1,500 /mm^3] have been maintained during the first 6 months of continuous therapy, WBC counts can be monitored every other week. WBC counts *must* be monitored weekly for at least 4 weeks after the discontinuation of CLOZARIL.

Dosage and Administration

Initial Treatment—Begin with one-half of a 25mg tablet (12.5mg) once or twice daily and then continue with daily dosage increments of 25-50mg/day, if well-tolerated, to achieve a target dose of 300-450mg/day by the end of 2 weeks. Subsequent dosage increments should be made no more than once or twice-weekly, in increments not to exceed 100mg. Cautious titration and a divided dosage schedule are necessary to minimize the risks of hypotension, seizure, and sedation. While many individuals may respond adequately at doses between 300-600mg three times daily, it may be necessary to raise the dose to the 600-900mg/day range to obtain an acceptable response. However, dosing should not exceed 900mg/day. Because of the possibility of increased adverse reactions at higher doses, particularly seizures, individuals should be given adequate time to respond to a given dose level before escalation to a higher dose is contemplated.

Maintenance Treatment—Responding individuals should be continued on CLOZARIL, but at the lowest level needed to maintain remission. Because of the significant risk associated with the use of CLOZARIL, individuals should be periodically reassessed to determine the need for maintenance treatment.

Discontinuation of Treatment—Gradual reduction in dose is recommended over a 1-2 week period. If an individual's medical condition requires abrupt discontinuation (e.g., leukopenia), the individual should be carefully observed for the recurrence of psychotic symptoms.

Re-Initiation of Treatment in Individuals Previously Discontinued—When restarting individuals who have had even a brief interval off CLOZARIL, i.e., 2 days or more since the last dose, it is recommended that treatment be reinitiated with one-half of a 25mg tablet (12.5mg) once or twice daily. If that dose is well tolerated, it may be feasible to titrate these individuals back to a therapeutic dose more quickly than is recommended for initial treatment. However, any individual who has previously experienced respiratory or cardiac arrest with initial dosing, but was then able to be successfully titrated to a therapeutic dose, should be re-titrated with extreme caution after even 24 hours of discontinuation. On the other hand, individuals discontinued for WBC counts below 2000/mm^3 or an ANC below 1000/mm^3 *must* not be restarted on CLOZARIL.

Overdosage

The most commonly reported signs and symptoms associated with CLOZARIL overdose are: altered states of consciousness including drowsiness, delirium and coma; tachycardia; hypotension; respiratory depression or failure; and hypersalivation. Aspiration pneumonia and cardiac arrhythmias have also been reported. Seizures have occurred in a minority of reported cases. Fatal overdoses have been reported with CLOZARIL, generally at doses above 2500mg.

COGENTIN

(Benztropine Mesylate)

Pharmacodynamics

COGENTIN is a synthetic compound containing structural features found in atropine and diphenhydramine. COGENTIN possesses both anticholinergic and antihistaminic effects, although only the former have been established as therapeutically significant in the management of Parkinsonism.

Indications

1. For use as an adjunct in the therapy of all forms of Parkinsonism

2. In the control of extrapyramidal disorders (except tardive dyskinesia) due to neuroleptic drugs (e.g., phenothiazines)

Contraindications

1. Hypersensitivity to COGENTIN

2. Because of its atropine-like side effects, this medication is contraindicated in children less than three years-of-age, and should be used with caution in older children.

Potential Side Effects

Neurological System—Weakness, inability to move particular muscle groups, numbness of fingers, aggravation of tardive dyskinesia

Psychiatric Disorders—Mental confusion, excitement, nervousness, listlessness, visual hallucinations, disorientation, memory impairment, depression, toxic psychosis

Cardiovascular System—Tachycardia

Gastrointestinal System—Paralytic ileus, constipation, vomiting, nausea, dry mouth leading to difficulty in swallowing or speaking, nausea, loss of appetite, vomiting, weight loss

Genitourinary System—Dysuria, urinary retention

Special Senses—Blurred vision, dilated pupils

Dermatological System—Skin rash

Other Systems—Heat stroke, anhidrosis, hyperthermia, fever

Potential Drug Interactions

Paralytic ileus, hyperthermia and heat stroke, all of which have sometimes been fatal, have occurred in individuals taking anticholinergic-type antiparkinsonism drugs, including COGENTIN, in combination with phenothiazines and/or tricyclic antidepressants.

Dosage and Administration

COGENTIN tablets should be used when patients are able to take oral medication. The injection is especially useful for psychotic patients with acute dystonic reactions or other reactions that make oral medication difficult or impossible. It is recommended also when a more rapid response is desired than can be obtained with the tablets. Usually intramuscular injection is preferred. The improvement is sometimes noticeable a few minutes after injection. In emergency situations, when the condition of the individual is alarming, 0.5 to 2mg of the injection normally will provide quick relief. If the parkinsonian effect begins to return, the dose can be repeated. Because of cumulative action, therapy should be initiated with a low dose, which is increased gradually at five- or six-day intervals to the smallest amount necessary for optimal relief. Increases should be made in increments of 0.5mg, to a maximum of 6mg, or until optimal results are obtained without excessive adverse reactions.

Treatment of Drug-Induced Extrapyramidal Disorders—In treating extra-pyramidal disorders due to neuroleptic drugs, the recommended dosage is 1 to 4mg once or twice a day orally or parenterally. Dosage must be individualized according to the need of the individual. In acute dystonic reactions, 0.5 to 2mg of the injection usually relieves the condition quickly. After that, the tablets, 0.5 to 2mg twice a day, usually prevent recurrence.

When extrapyramidal disorders develop soon after initiation of treatment with neuroleptic drugs, they are likely to be transient. One to 2mg of COGENTIN tablets two or three times a day usually provides relief within one or two days. After one or two weeks, the drug should be withdrawn to determine the continued need for it. If such disorders recur, COGENTIN can be re-instituted.

Certain drug-induced extrapyramidal disorders that develop slowly may not respond to COGENTIN.

When COGENTIN is started, do not terminate therapy with other antiparkinsonian agents abruptly. If the other agents are to be reduced or discontinued, it must be done gradually.

Overdosage

Manifestations of overdosage of COGENTIN may include CNS depression, preceded or followed by stimulation, confusion, nervousness, listlessness, intensification of mental symptoms or toxic psychosis in individuals with mental illness being treated with antipsychotic medications (e.g., HALDOL), hallucinations (especially visual), dizziness, muscle weakness, ataxia, dry mouth, mydriasis, blurred vision, palpitations, tachycardia, elevated blood pressure, nausea, vomiting, dysuria, numbness of fingers, dysphagia, allergic reactions (eg., skin rash, headache, hot, dry, flushed skin, delirium, coma, shock, convulsions, respiratory arrest, anhidrosis, hyperthermia, glaucoma, constipation).

CONCERTA

(Methylphenidate Extended-Release Tablets)

CONCERTA is a central nervous system stimulant.

Pharmacodynamics

CONCERTA is thought to block the reuptake of norepinephrine and dopamine into the presynaptic neuron and increase the release of these monoamines into the extra neuronal space.

Pharmacokinetics

- CONCERTA is readily absorbed.

- Food Effects: Food does not affect the absorption of CONCERTA.

- Following oral administration of CONCERTA, plasma CONCERTA concentrations increase rapidly reaching an initial maximum at about 1-to-2 hours, then increase gradually over the next several hours. Peak plasma concentrations are achieved at about 6 to 8 hours after which a gradual decrease in plasma levels of CONCERTA begins.

- The half-life of CONCERTA is approximately 3.5 hours.

Indications

CONCERTA is used to treat individuals with ADHD.

Pediatric Use—CONCERTA should not be used in children under six years, since safety and efficacy in this age group have not been established. Long-term effects of methylphenidate in children have not been well established.

Contraindications

1. In individuals with marked anxiety, tension, and agitation, since the drug may aggravate these symptoms

2. In individuals known to be hypersensitive to methylphenidate or other components of the product

3. In individuals with glaucoma

4. In individuals with motor tics or with a family history or diagnosis of Tourette syndrome

5. During treatment with monoamine oxidase inhibitors, and also within a minimum of 14 days following discontinuation of a monoamine oxidase inhibitor (hypertensive crises may result)

Potential Side Effects

Neurological System—Headache, dizziness, tics, dyskinesia, drowsiness, seizures

Psychiatric Disorders—Insomnia, transient depressed mood, toxic psychosis

Gastrointestinal System—Abdominal pain (stomach ache), vomiting, nausea, anorexia, loss of appetite, weight loss, abnormal liver function

Cardiovascular System—Palpitations, hypertension, hypotension, tachycardia, bradycardia angina, cardiac arrhythmia, cerebral arteritis and/or occlusion

Hematological System—Leukopenia and/or anemia

Respiratory System—Upper respiratory tract infection, increased cough, pharyngitis, sinusitis

Dermatological System—Skin rash, urticaria, fever, arthralgia, exfoliative dermatitis, erythema multiforme with histopathological findings of necrotizing vasculitis, thrombocytopenic purpura, scalp hair loss

Special Senses—Visual disturbances with accommodation and blurring of vision

Potential Drug Interactions

1. Methylphenidate may inhibit the metabolism of coumarin anticoagulants, anticonvulsants (e.g., LUMINAL, DILANTIN, MYSOLINE), and some antidepressants (tricyclics and SRIs). Downward dose adjustment of these drugs may be required when given concomitantly with methylphenidate. It may be necessary to adjust the dosage and monitor plasma drug concentrations (or, in the case of coumarin, coagulation times), when initiating or discontinuing concomitant methylphenidate.

2. Serious adverse events have been reported in concomitant use with CATAPRES, although no causality for the combination has been established.

Drug Abuse and Dependence

CONCERTA is classified as a Schedule II controlled substance by federal regulation.

CONCERTA should be given cautiously to individuals with a history of drug dependence or alcoholism. Chronic abusive use can lead to marked tolerance and psychological dependence with varying degrees of abnormal behavior. Frank psychotic episodes can occur, especially with parenteral abuse.

Withdrawal Symptoms

Withdrawal following chronic therapeutic use may unmask symptoms of the underlying disorder that may require follow-up.

Laboratory Tests

Periodic CBC, differential, and platelet counts are advised during prolonged therapy.

Dosage and Administration

CONCERTA is available in two tablet strengths. Each extended-release tablet for once-a-day oral administration contains 18 or 36mg of methylphenidate and is designed to have a 12-hour duration of effect.

Due to the controlled-release design of the tablet, CONCERTA should only be used in individuals who are *able to swallow the tablet whole* with the aid of liquids. Tablets should not be chewed, divided, or crushed. The medication is contained within a nonabsorbable shell designed to release the drug at a controlled rate. The tablet shell, along with insoluble core components, is eliminated from the body.

Overdosage

Signs and symptoms of acute methylphenidate overdosage may include the following: vomiting, agitation, tremors, hyperreflexia, muscle twitching, convulsions (may be followed by coma), euphoria, confusion, hallucinations, delirium, sweating, flushing, headache, hyperpyrexia, tachycardia, palpitations, cardiac arrhythmias, hypertension, mydriasis, and dryness of mucous membranes.

CYLERT

(Pemoline)

CYLERT is a central nervous system stimulant. It is structurally dissimilar to the amphetamines and methylphenidate. It is an oxazolidine compound.

Pharmacodynamics

CYLERT has a pharmacological activity similar to that of other known central nervous system stimulants; however, it has minimal sympathomimetic effects and the exact mechanism and site of action of the medication in man is not known. There is neither specific evidence that clearly establishes the mechanism whereby CYLERT produces its mental and behavioral effects in children, nor conclusive evidence regarding how these effects relate to the condition of the central nervous system.

Pharmacokinetics

- CYLERT is rapidly absorbed from the gastrointestinal tract.

- Approximately 50% is bound to plasma proteins.

- Peak serum levels of the drug occur within 2 to 4 hours after ingestion of a single dose.

- The serum half-life is approximately 12 hours.

- Steady state is reached in approximately 2-to-3 days.

- CYLERT is metabolized by the liver and is excreted primarily by the kidneys with approximately 50% excreted unchanged and only minor fractions present as metabolites.

Indications

Attention Deficit Disorder (ADD) with hyperactivity, however, due to reports of hepatic-related fatalities involving individuals taking CYLERT, physicians have significantly decreased the prescribing of CYLERT.

Pediatric Use—Safety and effectiveness in children below the age of 6 years have not been established.

Contraindications

1. In individuals with known hypersensitivity or idiosyncrasy to the medication

2. In individuals with impaired hepatic function

Potential Side Effects

Hepatic System—Elevated liver enzymes, hepatitis, and jaundice

Neurological System—Seizures, precipitate attacks of Tourette syndrome, dyskinetic movements of the tongue, lips, face and extremities, nystagmus, oculogyric crisis, dizziness, headache, drowsiness

Psychiatric Disorders—Insomnia, exacerbate symptoms of behavior disturbance and thought disorder in psychotic children, transient psychotic symptoms (rare), increased irritability, mild depression, hallucinations

Gastrointestinal System—Anorexia, weight loss, nausea, and stomachache

Miscellaneous—Suppression of growth with long-term use, skin rashes.

Potential Drug Interactions

Decreased seizure threshold has been reported in individuals receiving CYLERT concomitantly with antiepileptic medications.

Drug Abuse and Dependence

CYLERT is subject to control under DEA schedule IV.

The pharmacologic similarity of CYLERT to other psychostimulants with known dependence liability suggests that psychological and/or physical dependence might also occur with CYLERT.

Laboratory Tests

Liver function tests should be performed prior to and periodically during therapy with CYLERT. The drug should be discontinued if abnormalities are revealed and confirmed by follow-up tests.

Dosage and Administration

CYLERT has a gradual onset of action. Using the recommended schedule of dosage titration, significant clinical benefit may not be evident until the third or fourth week of drug administration.

CYLERT is administered as a single oral dose each morning. The recommended starting dose is 37.5mg/day. This daily dose should be gradually increased by 18.75mg at weekly intervals until the desired clinical response is obtained. The effective daily dose for most children and adolescents ranges from 56.25 to 75mg. The maximum recommended daily dose CYLERT is 112.5mg.

Where possible, drug administration should be interrupted occasionally to determine if there is a recurrence of behavioral symptoms sufficient to require continued therapy.

Overdosage

Signs and symptoms of acute overdosage may include the following: vomiting, agitation, tremors, hyperreflexia, muscle twitching, convulsions (may be followed by coma), euphoria, confusion, hallucinations, delirium, sweating, flushing, headache, hyperpyrexia, tachycardia, hypertension and mydriasis.

DDAVP

(Desmopressin Acetate Nasal Spray, Rhinal Tube, and Tablets)

Pharmacodynamics

DDAVP is a synthetic analogue of the natural pituitary hormone 8-arginine vasopressin (ADH), an antidiuretic hormone affecting renal water conservation. DDAVP enhances reabsorption of water in the kidneys by increasing cellular permeability of the collecting ducts; possibly causes smooth muscle constriction with resultant vasoconstriction.

Intranasal DDAVP provides a prompt onset of antidiuretic action with a long duration after each administration.

The use of DDAVP Tablets in individuals with an established diagnosis will result in a reduction in urinary output with an accompanying increase in urine osmolality. These effects usually will decrease urinary frequency and nocturia.

Pharmacokinetics

After intranasal administration

- Onset of ADH effect is within 1 hour.

- Peak effect is reached within 1-5 hours.

- Duration of the effect is 5-21 hours.

Indications

1. Alone or adjunctive to behavioral conditioning or other non-pharmacological intervention

2. As antidiuretic replacement therapy in the management of central cranial diabetes insipidus

3. For management of the temporary polyuria and polydipsia following head trauma or surgery in the pituitary region

Pediatric Use—DDAVP Nasal Spray and DDAVP Rhinal Tube have been used in childhood nocturnal enuresis. Short-term (4-8 weeks) DDAVP intranasal administration has been shown to be safe and modestly effective in children aged 6 years or older with severe childhood nocturnal enuresis. Adequately controlled studies with intranasal DDAVP in primary nocturnal enuresis have not been conducted beyond 4-8 weeks. The dose should be individually adjusted to achieve the best results.

DDAVP Tablets have been used safely in children, age 4 years and older, with diabetes insipidus for periods up to 44 months. In younger children, the dose must be individually adjusted in order to prevent an excessive decrease in plasma osmolality leading to hyponatremia and possible convulsions.

Contraindication

DDAVP Nasal Spray, DDAVP Rhinal Tube, and DDAVP Tablet are contraindicated in individuals with known hypersensitivity to desmopressin acetate or to any of the components of DDAVP Nasal Spray, DDAVP Rhinal Tube, or DDAVP Tablet.

Potential Side Effects

Body as a whole—Abdominal cramp or pain, asthenia, chills, sore throat

Nervous System—Headache, depression, dizziness, seizure

Respiratory System—Epistaxis, nostril pain, rhinitis, cough, respiratory infection

Cardiovascular System—Vasodilation, flushing, slight hypertension

Gastrointestinal System—Gastrointestinal disorder, nausea, transient elevated liver enzyme SGOT

Dermatological System—Leg rash

Special Senses—Conjunctivitis, edema eyes, lacrimation disorder

Laboratory Tests

In some cases plasma osmolality measurements may be required. For the healthy individuals with primary nocturnal enuresis, serum electrolytes should be checked at least once if therapy is continued beyond 7 days.

Dosage and Administration

DDAVP Nasal Spray and DDAVP Rhinal Tube are each provided as an aqueous solution for intranasal use only. DDAVP is also available as a solution for injection or a tablet for oral intake when the intranasal route may be compromised. These situations include nasal congestion and blockage, nasal discharge, atrophy of nasal mucosa, and severe atrophic rhinitis. Intranasal delivery may also be inappropriate where there is an impaired level of consciousness.

In Primary Nocturnal Enuresis, dosage should be adjusted according to the individual. The recommended initial dose for those 6 year of age and older is 20 mcg or 0.2 mL solution intra-nasally at bedtime. Adjustment up to 40 mcg is suggested if the child does not respond. Some children may respond to 10 mcg and adjustment to that lower dose may be done if the child has shown a response to 20 mcg. It is recommended that one-half of the dose be administered per nostril. Since the spray cannot deliver less than 0.1 mL (10 mcg), smaller doses should be administered using the rhinal tube delivery system. Do not use the nasal spray in children requiring less than 0.1 mL (10 mcg) per dose.

The DDAVP Nasal Spray bottle accurately delivers 50 doses of 10 mcg each. Any solution remaining after 50 doses should be discarded since the amount delivered thereafter may be substantially less than 10 mcg of the drug. No attempt should be made to transfer remaining solution to another bottle.

When the DDAVP tablet is used, the dosage must be determined for each individual child and adjusted according to the response. In general, dosing should start at 0.05mg (1/2 of the 0.1mg tablet) given at bedtime.

There are reports of an occasional change in response with time, usually greater than 6 months. Some individuals may show a decreased responsiveness, others a shortened duration of effect.

Overdosage

Signs and symptoms include drowsiness, headache, confusion, anuria, and water intoxication.

DESYREL

(Trazodone)

Pharmacodynamics

DESYREL is an antidepressant chemically unrelated to tricyclic, tetracyclic, or other known antidepressant agents. The mechanism of DESYREL's antidepressant action in man is not fully understood. DESYREL may selectively inhibit serotonin uptake by brain synaptosomes and potentate the behavioral changes induced by the serotonin precursor, 5-hydroxytryptophan.

Pharmacokinetics

- DESYREL is well absorbed after oral administration without selective localization in any tissue.

- When DESYREL is taken shortly after ingestion of food, there may be an increase in the amount of drug absorbed, a decrease in maximum concentration, and a lengthening in the time to maximum concentration.

- Peak plasma levels occur approximately one hour after dosing when DESYREL is taken on an empty stomach or two hours after dosing when taken with food.

- Elimination of DESYREL is biphasic, consisting of an initial phase (half-life 3-6 hours) followed by a slower phase (half-life 5-9 hours), and is unaffected by the presence or absence of food.

Indications

1. For the treatment of depression

2. Unlabeled use in the treatment of Sleep Disorders

3. Unlabeled use in the control of aggressions

Pediatric Use—Safety and effectiveness in children below the age of 18 have not been established.

Contraindications

1. DESYREL is contraindicated in individuals hypersensitive to DESYREL.

2. DESYREL is not recommended for use during the initial recovery phase of myocardial infarction.

Potential Side Effects

Body as a Whole—Malaise, weakness, head full or heavy, chest pain, chills

Neurological System—Dizziness, vertigo, lightheadedness, headache, ataxia, incoordination, impaired speech, extrapyramidal symptoms, akathisia, paresthesia, tremors, muscle twitches, numbness, and aphasia, tardive dyskinesia, grand mal seizures, stupor

Psychiatric Disorders—Anger, hostility, confusion, decreased concentration, disorientation, drowsiness, excitement, fatigue, insomnia, nightmares, vivid dreams, impaired memory, nervousness, hallucinations/delusions, psychosis, paranoid reaction, hypomania, abnormal dreams, agitation, and anxiety

Cardiovascular System—Conduction block, orthostatic hypotension, syncope, palpitations, bradycardia, atrial fibrillation, congestive heart failure, myocardial infarction, cardiac arrest, arrhythmia, ventricular ectopic activity including ventricular tachycardia, hypertension, hypotension, shortness of breath, tachycardia, palpitations, cerebrovascular accident, vasodilation

Respiratory System—Nasal/sinus congestion, apnea

Hematological and Lymphatic Systems—Leukocytosis, anemia, hemolytic anemia, and methemoglobinemia (abnormal hemoglobin).

Gastrointestinal System—Dry mouth, increased salivation, abdominal/gastric disorder, bad taste in mouth, increased appetite, decreased appetite, nausea, vomiting, constipation, and diarrhea

Hepatic System—Jaundice, cholestasis, hyperbilirubinemia, liver enzyme alterations

Endocrine System—Weight gain, weight loss, early menses, hirsutism, lactation, breast enlargement or engorgement, inappropriate ADH syndrome

Muscular and Skeletal Systems—Musculoskeletal aches/pains

Dermatological System—Sweating, clamminess, pruritus, psoriasis, urticaria, rash, allergic reaction, alopecia

Genitourinary System—Increased urinary frequency, urinary incontinence, urinary retention, delayed urine flow, hematuria, priapism (prolonged penile erection)

Sexual Function—Decreased libido, increased libido, impotence, missed periods, retrograde ejaculation

Special Senses—Eyes red, tired, or Itching, blurred vision, tinnitus, diplopia

Potential Drug Interactions

1. Increased serum digoxin or DILANTIN in individuals who receive DESYREL concurrently with either of the two drugs

2. Increased and decreased prothrombin time may occur in warfarinized patients who take DESYREL.

3. Concomitant administration of antihypertensive therapy with DESYREL may require a reduction in the dose of the antihypertensive drug.

4. DESYREL may enhance the response to alcohol, barbiturates, and other CNS depressants.

Laboratory Tests

Occasional low white blood cell and neutrophil counts have been noted in individuals receiving DESYREL. The medication should be discontinued in any individual whose white blood cell count or absolute neutrophil count falls below normal levels. White blood cell and differential counts are recommended for patients who develop fever and sore throat (or other signs of infection) during therapy.

Dosage and Administration

DESYREL should be given shortly after a meal or light snack because the total drug absorption may be up to 20% higher when the drug is taken with food. The risk of dizziness/lightheadedness may increase under fasting conditions.

The dosage should be initiated at a low level and increased gradually, noting the clinical response and any evidence of intolerance. Occurrence of drowsiness may require the administration of a major portion of the daily dose at bedtime or a reduction of dosage.

Response to DESYREL may be seen as early as by the end of the first week of treatment, but generally a significant therapeutic effect is seen by the end of the second week. In some individuals, it may take 2-4 weeks for a significant therapeutic response.

For the treatment of depression or frequent rages with aggressions—In adults, begin with 150mg/day in divided doses. The dose may be increased by 50mg/day every three-to-four days. The maximum dose for outpatients usually should not exceed 400mg/day in divided doses. In more severely depressed individuals, the dose may be given up to but not in excess of 600mg/day in divided doses.

In adolescents, the initial dose may be 25-50mg/day with weekly increment dose of 25-50mg/day up to 100-150mg/day in divided doses. In children 6-12 years, the initial dose may be 1.5-2mg/kg/day in divided doses. The dose may be increased 25-50mg/day every 3-5 days up to 6mg/kg/day in 3 divided doses.

For the treatment of sleep difficulties and insomnia—In adults, the initial dose of 75-100mg may be taken at bedtime with increment of 25mg/night every 3 nights up to 300-400mg/night.

In older children and adolescents, the initial dose of 50-75mg may be given at bedtime with increment of 25mg/night every 3 nights up to 200-300mg/night. In children under 6 years-of-age, if indicated, the initial dose of 25-50mg may be given at bedtime with increment of 12.5-25mg every 3 nights up to 100-150mg/night.

Maintenance—Dosage during prolonged maintenance therapy should be kept at the lowest effective level. Once an adequate response has been achieved, dosage may be gradually reduced, with subsequent adjustment depending on therapeutic response. It is generally recommended that a course of DESYREL treatment should be continued for several months for the treatment of depression. For the treatment of sleep difficulties, DESYREL should be continued for 1-2 months if satisfactory results are achieved. Then it should be discontinued and the sleep difficulties should be re-evaluated.

Overdosage

The most severe reactions reported to have occurred with overdose of DESYREL alone have been priapism, respiratory arrest, seizures, and EKG changes. The reactions reported most frequently have been drowsiness and vomiting.

DETROL

(Tolterodine)

Pharmacodynamics

DETROL is a competitive muscarinic receptor antagonist. Both urinary bladder contraction and salivation are mediated via cholinergic muscarinic receptors.

Pharmacokinetics

- After oral administration, DETROL is rapidly absorbed from the GI tract.

- Peak serum concentrations typically occur within 1-to-2 hours after dose administration.

- Food intake increases the bioavailability of DETROL (average increase 53%) This change is not expected to be a safety concern and adjustment of dose is not needed.

- DETROL is highly bound to plasma proteins.

- DETROL is extensively metabolized by the liver following oral dosing.

- Elimination half-life is about 2 to 4 hours.

- About 77% of DETROL is excreted in urine and 17% in feces.

Indications

Overactive bladder with symptoms of urinary frequency, urgency, or urge incontinence

Pediatric Use—The safety and effectiveness of DETROL in children have not been established, but clinicians have used it for the treatment of enuresis in children.

Contraindications

In individuals with the following conditions:

1. Clinically significant bladder outflow obstruction because of the risk of urinary retention

2. Gastrointestinal obstructive disorders, such as pyloric stenosis, which may lead to gastric retention

3. History of or currently uncontrolled narrow-angle glaucoma

4. History of hypersensitivity to the drug or its ingredients

Potential Side Effects

Body as a whole—General back pain, chest pain, fatigue, headache, influenza-like symptoms, falling

Neurological System—Vertigo, dizziness, paresthesia

Psychiatric Disorders—Nervousness, somnolence, dizziness

Gastrointestinal System—Dry mouth, nausea, dyspepsia, vomiting, abdominal pain, constipation, and diarrhea

Respiratory System—Coughing, rhinitis, sinusitis, pharyngitis, bronchitis, upper respiratory infection

Genitourinary System—Dysuria, micturition frequency, urinary retention, urinary tract infection

Dermatologic System—Pruritus, rash, erythema, dry skin, fungal infection

Muscular and Skeletal Systems—Arthralgia

Metabolic System—Weight gain

Cardiovascular System—Hypertension

Special Sense—Abnormal vision (accommodation abnormalities), xerophthalmia

Potential Drug Interactions

1. Individuals receiving cytochrome P450 3A4 inhibitors such as macrolide antibiotics (erythromycin and clarithromycin) or antifungal agents (ketoconazole, itraconazole, and miconazole) should not receive doses of DETROL greater than 1mg twice daily.

2. Although PROZAC significantly inhibited the metabolism of DETROL, no dose adjustment is required when DETROL and PROZAC are co-administered.

Dosage and Administration

The initial recommended dose is 2mg twice daily. The dose may be lowered to 1mg twice daily based on individual response and tolerance.

Overdosage

Symptoms of DETROL overdose include dry mouth.

DITROPAN

(Oxybutynin)

Pharmacodynamics

DITROPAN exerts direct antispasmodic effect on smooth muscle and inhibits the muscarinic action of acetylcholine on smooth muscle. DITROPAN increases bladder (vesical) capacity, diminishes the frequency of uninhibited contractions of the detrusor muscle, and delays the initial desire to void. DITROPAN thus decreases urgency and the frequency of both incontinent episodes and voluntary urination.

Pharmacokinetics

Pharmacokinetic information is not currently available.

Indications

DITROPAN is used to treat symptoms of bladder instability associated with voiding in individuals with uninhibited neurogenic or reflex neurogenic bladder (i.e., urgency, frequency, urinary leakage, urge incontinence, dysuria).

Pediatric Use—The safety and efficacy of DITROPAN have been demonstrated for children 5 years-of-age and older. Some clinicians use DITROPAN to treat enuresis in some children. However, as there is insufficient clinical data for children under age 5, DITROPAN is not recommended for this age group.

Contraindications

1. Untreated angle closure glaucoma

2. Partial or complete obstruction of the gastrointestinal tract, paralytic ileus, megacolon, toxic megacolon complicating ulcerative colitis, severe colitis, and myasthenia gravis

3. Obstructive uropathy

4. Unstable cardiovascular status in acute hemorrhage

5. Demonstrated hypersensitivity to the medication

Potential Side Effects

Nervous System—Asthenia, dizziness, drowsiness, hallucinations, insomnia, restlessness

Cardiovascular System—Palpitations, tachycardia, vasodilation

Dermatologic System—Decreased sweating, rash

Gastrointestinal System—Dry mouth, nausea, constipation, diarrhea, decreased gastrointestinal motility, intestinal obstruction

Genitourinary System—Urinary hesitance and retention

Ocular System—Amblyopia, cycloplegia, decreased lacrimation, mydriasis, blurred vision

Other—Impotence, suppression of lactation

Dosage and Administration

Adults—The usual dose is one 5mg tablet or one teaspoon (5mg/5mL) two-to-three times a day. The maximum recommended dose is one 5mg tablet or one teaspoon (5mg/5mL) four times a day.

Children over 5 years-of-age—The usual dose is one 5mg or one teaspoon (5mg/5mL) two times a day. The maximum recommended dose is one 5mg tablet or one teaspoon (5mg/5mL) three times a day.

Overdosage

The symptoms of overdose with DITROPAN may include signs of central nervous system excitation (e.g., restlessness, tremor, irritability, convulsions, delirium, hallucinations), flushing, fever, nausea, vomiting, tachycardia, hypotension or hypertension, respiratory failure, paralysis, and coma.

DEXEDRINE

(Dextroamphetamine Sulfate)

Pharmacodynamics

Amphetamines are non-catecholamine, sympathomimetic amines with CNS stimulant activity. Peripheral actions include elevations of systolic and diastolic blood pressures and weak bronchodilator and respiratory stimulant action.

There is neither specific evidence that clearly establishes the mechanism whereby amphetamines produce mental and behavioral effects in children, nor conclusive evidence regarding how these effects relate to the condition of the central nervous system.

Pharmacokinetics

Tablet

- The single ingestion of two 5mg tablets produces an average peak dextroamphetamine blood level at 2 hours post-administration.

- The average half-life is about 10 hours.

- The average urinary recovery is 45% in 48 hours.

Spansule capsule

- Ingestion of a Spansule capsule containing 15mg dextroamphetamine sulfate produced a peak blood level on the average at 8 to 10 hours post-administration with peak urinary recovery at 12 to 24 hours.

Indications

1. Attention deficit disorder with hyperactivity

2. Narcolepsy

Pediatric Use—Long-term effects of amphetamines in pediatric patients have not been well established.

Contraindications

1. Advanced arteriosclerosis, symptomatic cardiovascular disease, moderate to severe hypertension, hyperthyroidism, known hypersensitivity or idiosyncrasy to the sympathomimetic amines, glaucoma

2. Agitated states

3. Patients with a history of drug abuse

4. During or within 14 days following the administration of monoamine oxidase inhibitors

Potential Side Effects

Central Nervous System—Over stimulation, restlessness, dizziness, insomnia, euphoria, dyskinesia, dysphoria, tremor, headache, exacerbation of motor and phonic tics and Tourette syndrome

Cardiovascular System—Palpitations, tachycardia, elevation of blood pressure

Gastrointestinal System—Dry mouth, unpleasant taste, diarrhea, constipation, other gastrointestinal disturbances, anorexia and weight loss

Allergies—Urticaria

Endocrine System—Impotence, changes in libido

Potential Drug Interactions

1. Gastrointestinal acidifying agents (reserpine, ascorbic acid, fruit juices, etc.) lower absorption of amphetamines. Urinary acidifying agents (ammonium chloride, sodium acid phosphate, etc.) increase the concentration of the ionized species of the amphetamine molecule, thereby increasing urinary excretion. Both groups of agents lower blood levels and efficacy of amphetamines.

2. Gastrointestinal alkalinizing agents (sodium bicarbonate, etc.) increase absorption of amphetamines. Urinary alkalinizing agents (acetazolamide, some thiazides) increase the concentration of the non-ionized species of the amphetamine molecule, thereby decreasing urinary excretion. Both groups of agents increase blood levels and therefore potentiate the actions of amphetamines.

3. Amphetamines inhibit adrenergic blockers.

4. Amphetamines may enhance the activity of tricyclic or sympathomimetic agents; d-amphetamine with NORPRAMIN cause striking and sustained increases in the concentration of d-amphetamine in the brain; cardiovascular effects can be potentiated.

5. MAOI antidepressants slow amphetamine metabolism. This slowing potentiates amphetamines, increasing their effect on the release of norepinephrine and other monoamines from adrenergic nerve endings; this can cause headaches and other signs of hypertensive crisis. A variety of neurological toxic effects and malignant hyperpyrexia can occur, sometimes with fatal results.

6. Amphetamines may counteract the sedative effect of antihistamines.

7. Amphetamines may antagonize the hypotensive effects of antihypertensives.

8. THORAZINE and HALDOL block dopamine and norepinephrine reuptake, thus inhibiting the central stimulant effects of amphetamines, and can be used to treat amphetamine poisoning.

9. Amphetamines may delay intestinal absorption of ZARONTIN.

10. The antiobesity and stimulatory effects of amphetamines may be inhibited by lithium carbonate.

11. Amphetamines enhance the adrenergic effect of norepinephrine.

12. Amphetamines may delay intestinal absorption of phenobarbital; co-administration of phenobarbital may produce a synergistic anticonvulsant action.

13. Amphetamines may delay intestinal absorption of DILANTIN; co-administration of DILANTIN may produce a synergistic anticonvulsant action.

Potential Laboratory Test Interactions

1. Amphetamines can cause a significant elevation in plasma corticosteroid levels. This increase is greatest in the evening.

2. Amphetamines may interfere with urinary steroid determinations.

Drug Abuse and Dependence

Dextroamphetamine sulfate is a Schedule II controlled substance. Amphetamines have been extensively abused. Tolerance, extreme psychological dependence, and severe social disability have occurred.

Withdrawal Symptoms

Abrupt cessation following prolonged high dosage administration results in extreme fatigue and mental depression; changes are also noted on the sleep EEG.

Dosage and Administration

Treatment of ADHD—Not recommended for children under 3 years-of-age. In children from 3 to 5 years-of-age, start with 2.5mg daily, by tablet; daily dosage may be raised in increments of 2.5mg at weekly intervals until optimal response is obtained.

In children 6 years-of-age and older, start with 5mg once or twice daily; daily dosage may be raised in increments of 5mg at weekly intervals until optimal response is obtained. Only in rare cases will it be necessary to exceed a total of 40mg per day.

Spansule capsules may be used for once-a-day dosage whenever appropriate.

With tablets, give first dose on awakening; additional doses (1 or 2) at intervals of 4-to-6 hours.

Treatment of Narcolepsy—Usual dose is 5 to 60mg per day in divided doses, depending on the individual response. Narcolepsy seldom occurs in children under 12 years-of-age; however, when it does, Dexedrine may be used. The suggested initial dose for patients aged 6-12 is 5mg daily; daily dose may be raised in increments of 5mg at weekly intervals until optimal response is obtained. In patients 12 years-of-age and older, start with 10mg daily; daily dosage may be raised in increments of 10mg at weekly intervals until optimal response is obtained. If bothersome adverse reactions appear (e.g., insomnia or anorexia), dosage should be reduced. Spansule capsules may be used for once-a-day dosage wherever appropriate. With tablets, give first dose on awakening, with additional doses (1 or 2) at intervals of 4-to-6 hours.

Overdosage

Toxic symptoms rarely developed with doses of less than 15mg; 30mg can produce severe reactions. Symptoms of overdosage include restlessness, tremor, hyperreflexia, rhabdomyolysis, rapid respiration, nausea, vomiting, diarrhea and abdominal cramps, arrhythmias, hypertension or hypotension and circulatory collapse, hyperpyrexia, confusion, fatigue, depression, assaultiveness, hallucinations, panic states. Fatal poisoning is usually preceded by convulsions and coma.

EFFEXOR

(Venlafaxine)

EFFEXOR is a structurally novel antidepressant for oral administration. It is chemically unrelated to tricyclic, tetracyclic, or other available antidepressant agents.

Pharmacodynamics

The mechanism of EFFEXOR is believed to be associated with its potentiation of neurotransmitter activity in the CNS (i.e., potent inhibitors of neuronal serotonin and norepinephrine reuptake and weak inhibitors of dopamine reuptake).

Pharmacokinetics

- EFFEXOR is well absorbed and extensively metabolized in the liver.

- Food has no significant effect on the absorption of EFFEXOR.

- Steady-state concentration of EFFEXOR in plasma is attained within 3 days of multiple-dose therapy.

- Elimination half-life is about 5 hours.

- Renal elimination of EFFEXOR and its metabolites is the primary route of excretion.

Indications

Treatment of depression

Pediatric Use—Safety and effectiveness in individuals less than 18 years-of-age have not been established.

Contraindications

1. In patients known to be hypersensitive to EFFEXOR

2. Concomitant use of monoamine oxidase inhibitors (MAOIs)

Potential Side Effects

Body as a whole—Accidental injury, neck pain, chest pain, abdominal pain, headache, asthenia, infection, chills, enlarged abdomen, allergic reaction, cyst, face edema, generalized edema, hangover effect, hernia, intentional injury, moniliasis, neck rigidity, overdose, chest pain substernal, pelvic pain, photosensitivity reaction, suicide attempt

Neurological system—Trismus, dizziness, vertigo, tremor, hypertonia, paresthesia, twitching, apathy, ataxia, circumoral paresthesia, CNS stimulation, hyperesthesia, hyperkinesia, hypertonia, hypotonia, incoordination, myoclonus, neuralgia, neuropathy, abnormal speech, stupor, torticollis, seizure

Psychiatric Disorders—Emotional lability, anxiety, nervousness, abnormal dreams, insomnia, somnolence, agitation, confusion, abnormal thinking, depersonalization, depression, hypomania or mania, euphoria, hallucinations, hostility, paranoid reaction, psychosis, psychotic depression

Cardiovascular System—Sustained increases in blood pressure, vasodilatation, tachycardia, postural hypotension, migraine, angina pectoris, extrasystoles, hypotension, peripheral vascular disorder (mainly cold feet and/or cold hands), syncope, and thrombophlebitis

Gastrointestinal System—Dry mouth, nausea, anorexia, dysphagia, constipation, diarrhea, vomiting, dyspepsia, flatulence, eructation, colitis, tongue edema, esophagitis, gastritis, gastroenteritis, gingivitis, glossitis, rectal hemorrhage, hemorrhoids, melena, stomatitis, stomach ulcer, mouth ulceration

Hematological and Lymphatic System—Ecchymosis, anemia, leukocytosis, leukopenia, lymphadenopathy, lymphocytosis, thrombocythemia, thrombocytopenia

Metabolic System—Peripheral edema, weight gain, weight loss, alkaline phosphatase increased, creatinine increased, diabetes mellitus, edema, glycosuria, hypercholesteremia, hyperglycernia, hyperlipernia, hyperuricemia, hypoglycemia, hypokalemia, increased SGOT, thirst

Muscular and Skeletal Systems—Arthritis, arthrosis, bone pain, bone spurs, bursitis, joint disorder, myasthenia, tenosynovitis

Respiratory System—Bronchitis, yawn, dyspnea, asthma, chest congestion, epistaxis, hyperventilation, laryngismus, laryngitis, pneumonia, voice alteration

Genitourinary System—Anorgasmia, dysuria, hematuria, metrorrhagia, impaired urination, vaginitis, urinary frequency, urinary retention, menstrual disorder, alburninuria, amenorrhea, kidney calculus, cystitis, leukorrhea, menorrhagia, nocturia, bladder pain, breast pain, kidney pain, polyuria, prostatitis, pyelonephritis, pyuria, urinary incontinence, urinary urgency, uterine fibroids enlarged, uterine hemorrhage, vaginal hemorrhage, vaginal moniliasis

Sexual Function—Abnormal ejaculation/orgasm, impotence, decreased libido, increased libido

Dermatological System—Acne, alopecia, brittle nails, contact dermatitis, dry skin, sweating, herpes simplex, herpes zoster, pruritus maculopapular rash, urticaria

Special Senses—Abnormal vision, mydriasis, blurred vision, ear pain, tinnitus taste perversion, cataract, conjunctivitis, corneal lesion, diplopia, dry eyes, exophthalmos, eye pain, otitis media, parosmia, photophobia, subconjunctival hemorrhage, taste loss, visual field defect

Potential Drug Interactions

1. In individuals receiving EFFEXOR in combination with an MAOI, or in individuals who have recently been discontinued from an MAOI and started on EFFEXOR, or who have recently had EFFEXOR therapy discontinued prior to initiation of an MAOI, adverse reactions, some of which may be serious, may occur. These reactions include tremor, myoclonus, diaphoresis, nausea, vomiting, flushing, dizziness, hyperthermia with features resembling neuroleptic malignant syndrome, seizures, and death.

2. Concomitant administration of TAGAMET and EFFEXOR result in inhibition of first-pass metabolism of EFFEXOR.

3. EFFEXOR is metabolized to its active metabolite by cytochrome P40ID6, the isoenzyme that is responsible for the genetic polymorphism seen in the metabolism of many antidepressants. Therefore, the potential exists for a drug interaction between EFFEXOR and drugs that inhibit cytochrome P40ID6 metabolism. Drug interactions that reduce the metabolism of EFFEXOR could potentially increase the plasma concentrations of EFFEXOR and lower the concentrations of the active metabolite.

Laboratory Tests

There are no specific laboratory tests recommended.

Dosage and Administration

In older adolescents and adults, the recommended starting dose for EFFEXOR is 75mg/day, administered in two or three divided doses, taken with food. Depending on tolerability and the need for further clinical effect, the dose may be increased with increment of 50 to 75mg/day at intervals of no less than 4 days up to 225mg/day, but more severely depressed individuals may need a higher dose, up to a maximum of 375mg/day.

In children 6 years and older, the total daily dose should be reduced by 50%.

It is generally agreed that acute episodes of major depression require several months or longer of sustained pharmacologic therapy. Whether the dose of antidepressant needed to induce remission is identical to the dose needed to maintain or sustain euthymia is unknown.

When discontinuing EFFEXOR after more than 1 week of therapy, it is generally recommended that the dose be tapered to minimize the risk of discontinuation symptoms. Patients who have received EFFEXOR for 6 weeks or more should have their dose tapered gradually over a 2-week period.

Overdosage

Symptoms: somnolence, generalized convulsions, and a prolongation of QTc, mild sinus tachycardia

ESKALITH and ESKALITH CR

(Lithium Carbonate and Lithium Carbonate Controlled Release Tablets)

Pharmacodynamics

Lithium alters sodium transport in nerve and muscle cells and effects a shift toward intraneuronal metabolism of catecholamines, but the specific biochemical mechanism of lithium action in mania is unknown.

Pharmacokinetics

- The half-life of elimination of lithium is approximately 24 hours.

- Lithium is primarily excreted in urine with insignificant excretion in feces. Renal excretion of lithium is proportional to its plasma concentration.

Indications

1. For treatment of manic episodes of Bipolar Disorder

2. Unlabeled use in aggression

Pediatric Use—Since information regarding the safety and effectiveness of lithium carbonate in children less than 12 years-of-age is not available, its use in such patients is not recommended.

Contraindications

In individuals with significant renal or cardiovascular disease, severe debilitation or dehydration, or sodium depletion, and to individuals receiving diuretics

Potential Side Effects

Central Nervous System Disorders—Slurred speech, dizziness, vertigo, headache, blackout spells, seizures incontinence of urine or feces, somnolence, psychomotor retardation, restlessness, confusion, stupor, coma, acute dystonia, downbeat nystagmus, pseudotumor cerebri (increased intracranial pressure and papilledema) with constriction of visual fields, EEG changes (diffuse slowing, widening of frequency spectrum, potentiation and disorganization of background rhythm)

Neuromuscular System Disorders—Tremor, muscle hyperirritability (fasciculations, twitching, clonic movements of whole limbs), ataxia, choreo-athetotic movements, hyperactive deep tendon reflexes

Cardiovascular System Disorders—Cardiac arrhythmia, hypotension, peripheral circulatory collapse, EKG Changes (reversible flattening, isoelectricity or inversion of T-waves)

Gastrointestinal System Disorders—Anorexia, nausea, vomiting, diarrhea, metallic taste

Genitourinary System Disorders—Albuminuria, oliguria, polyuria, glycosuria

Dermatological Disorders—Drying and thinning of hair, anesthesia of skin, chronic folliculitis, xerosis cutis, alopecia and exacerbation of psoriasis, generalized pruritus with or without rash, cutaneous ulcers

Autonomic Nervous System Disorders—Blurred vision, dry mouth

Endocrine System Disorders—euthyroid goiter and/or hypothyroidism (including myxedema) accompanied by lower Ts and T4, elevated iodine-131 uptake, rare cases of hyperthyroidism, transient hyperglycemia

Miscellaneous—Fatigue, lethargy, transient scotomata, dehydration, weight loss, excessive weight gain, tendency to sleep, leucocytosis, edematous swelling of ankles or wrists

Potential Drug Interactions

1. An encephalopathic syndrome (characterized by weakness, lethargy, fever, tremulousness and confusion, extrapyramidal symptoms, leucocytosis, elevated serum enzymes, BUN and FBS) followed by irreversible brain damage has occurred in a few individuals treated with lithium plus HALDOL.

2. Lithium may prolong the effects of neuromuscular blocking agents.

3. Indomethacin and piroxicam have been reported to increase significantly steady state plasma lithium levels. In some cases lithium toxicity has resulted from such interactions. There is also evidence that other non-steroidal, anti-inflammatory agents may have a similar effect.

4. Concomitant use of diuretics or angiotensin converting enzyme inhibitors with lithium may reduce the renal clearance of lithium and increase serum lithium levels with risk of lithium toxicity. When such combinations are used, the lithium dosage may need to be decreased, and more frequent monitoring of lithium plasma levels is recommended.

Laboratory Tests

When kidney function is assessed, for baseline data prior to starting lithium therapy or thereafter, routine urinalysis and other tests may be used to evaluate tubular function (e.g., urine specific gravity or osmolality following a period of water deprivation, or 24-hour urine volume) and glomerular function (e.g., serum creatinine or creatinine clearance).

Dosage and Administration

Treatment of Acute Mania—In older adolescents and adults, optimal response to lithium usually can be established and maintained with 1800mg/day. Immediate release capsules are usually given three or four times daily. Doses of controlled release tablets are usually given twice daily (approximately 12-hour intervals). Such doses will normally produce an effective serum lithium level ranging between 1.0 and 1.5mEq/L.

Regular monitoring of the individual's clinical state and of serum lithium levels is necessary. Serum levels should be determined twice per week during the acute phase, and until the serum level and clinical condition of the individual have been stabilized. Blood samples for serum lithium determination should be drawn immediately prior to the next dose when lithium concentrations are relatively stable (i.e., 8-12 hours after the previous dose.)

Most individuals on maintenance therapy are stabilized on 900mg daily, e.g., 450mg Eskalith CR twice daily or 300mg Eskalith three times daily. When switching from the immediate release Eskalith to Eskalith CR, initiate Eskalith CR dosage at the multiple of 450mg nearest to, but below, the original daily dose. For example, when the previous dosage of immediate release lithium is 1500mg, the dose for Eskalith CR should be 1350mg. When the two doses are unequal, give the larger dose in the evening. In the above example, with a total daily dosage of 1350mg, generally 450mg Eskalith CR should be given in the morning and 900mg Eskalith CR in the evening. If desired, the total daily dosage of 1350mg can be given in three equal 450mg Eskalith CR doses. These individuals should be monitored at 1-to-2 week intervals, and the dosage adjusted if necessary, until stable and satisfactory serum levels and clinical state are achieved.

Long-Term Control—The desirable serum lithium levels are 0.6 to 1.2mEq/L. Serum lithium levels in un-complicated cases receiving maintenance therapy during remission should be monitored at least every two months.

Overdosage

The likelihood of lithium toxicity increases with increasing serum lithium levels. Serum lithium levels greater than 1.5mEq/L carry a greater risk than lower levels. However, individuals sensitive to lithium may exhibit toxic signs at serum levels below 1.5mEq/L.

Diarrhea, vomiting, drowsiness, muscular weakness, and lack of coordination may be early signs of lithium toxicity and can occur at lithium levels below 2.0mEq/L. At higher levels, giddiness, ataxia, blurred vision, tinnitus, and a large output of dilute urine may be seen. Serum lithium levels above 3.0mEq/L may produce a complex clinical picture involving multiple organs and organ systems. Serum lithium levels should not be permitted to exceed 2.0mEq/L during the acute treatment phase.

HALDOL

(Haloperidol)

Pharmacodynamics

HALDOL blocks the effects of dopamine and increases its turnover rate; however, the precise mechanism of action is unknown.

Pharmacokinetics

- HALDOL Decanoate 50 and HALDOL Decanoate 100 reach peak plasma concentration about six days after administration, with an apparent half-life of about three weeks.

- Steady state plasma concentrations are achieved after the third or fourth dose.

Indications

1. For the treatment of psychotic disorders

2. For the treatment of Tourette syndrome

3. For the treatment of severe behavior problems in children of combative, explosive hyperexcitability

4. For short-term treatment of hyperactive children who show excessive motor activity with accompanying conduct disorders consisting of some or all of the following symptoms: impulsivity, difficulty sustaining attention, aggression, mood lability, and poor frustration tolerance.

Pediatric Use—HALDOL is not intended for children under 3 years old. In children between the ages of 3 and 12 years, therapy should begin at the lowest dose possible.

Contraindications

1. In severe toxic central nervous system depression or comatose states from any cause and in individuals who have Parkinson's disease

2. In individuals who are hypersensitive to this medication

Potential Side Effects

Neurological System—Headache, confusion, vertigo, grand mal seizures, extrapyramidal symptoms (EPS) including tardive dystonia, tardive dyskinesia, neuroleptic malignant syndrome (NMS), hyperpyrexia, and heat stroke

Psychiatric Disorders—Switch mania depression, exacerbation of psychotic symptoms including hallucinations, insomnia, restlessness, anxiety, euphoria, agitation, drowsiness, depression, lethargy

Cardiovascular System—Tachycardia, hypotension, hypertension, ECG changes including prolongation of the Q-T interval

Respiratory System—Laryngospasm, bronchospasm, increased depth of respiration

Hematological System—Mild and transient leukopenia and leukocytosis, minimal decreases in red blood cell counts, anemia, or a tendency toward lymphomonocytosis

Hepatic System—Impaired liver function and/or jaundice

Dermatological System—Maculopapular and acneiform skin reactions, photosensitivity, hair loss

Endocrine System—Lactation, breast engorgement, mastalgia, menstrual irregularities, gynecomastia, hyperglycernia, hypoglycemia, and hyponatremia

Gastrointestinal System—Dry mouth, anorexia, constipation, diarrhea, hypersalivation, dyspepsia, nausea, vomiting

Genitourinary System—Urinary retention, diaphoresis, priapism

Sexual Function—Impotence, increased libido

Special Senses—Cataracts, retinopathy, visual disturbances, blurred vision

Potential Drug Interactions

1. An encephalopathic syndrome (characterized by weakness, lethargy, fever, tremulousness and confusion, extrapyramidal symptoms, leukocytosis, elevated serum enzymes, BUN, and FBS) followed by irreversible brain damage has occurred in a few individuals treated with lithium plus HALDOL.

2. HALDOL may lower the convulsive threshold in individuals receiving anticonvulsant medications, with a history of seizures, or with EEG abnormalities.

3. Intraocular pressure may increase when anticholinergic drugs, including antiparkinsonism agents, are administered concomitantly with HALDOL.

4. HALDOL may be capable of potentiating CNS depressants such as anesthetics, opiates, and alcohol.

5. Severe neurotoxicity (rigidity, inability to walk or talk) may occur in individuals with thyrotoxicosis who are also receiving HALDOL.

Withdrawal Emergent Neurological Signs

Generally, individuals receiving short-term therapy experience no problems with abrupt discontinuation of HALDOL. However, some individuals on maintenance treatment may experience transient dyskinetic signs after abrupt withdrawal. The dyskinetic movements may be indistinguishable from "Tardive Dyskinesia" except for duration.

Dosage and Administration

Oral Administration

HALDOL is not intended for children under 3 years old.

In children between the ages of 3 and 12 years, therapy should begin at the lowest dose possible (0.5mg per day). If required, the dose should be increased by an increment of 0.5mg at 5 to 7 day intervals until the desired therapeutic effect is obtained. The total dose may be divided and given two-to-three times daily.

In general, for psychotic disorders, doses of 0.05mg/kg/day to 0.15mg/kg/day, and for non-psychotic behavior disorders and Tourette syndrome, 0.05mg/kg/day to 0.075mg/kg/day are recommended.

Initial dosage range in adults with moderate symptoms is 0.5mg to 2mg two-to-three times daily, and for severe symptoms, 3mg to 5mg two-to-three times daily.

In chronic or resistant cases, 3mg to 5mg two-to-three times daily may be necessary.

Intramuscular Administration

Intramuscular administration in doses of 2 to 5mg may be used for prompt control of an acutely agitated individual with moderately severe to very severe symptoms. Depending on the response of the individual, subsequent doses may be administered as often as every hour, although 4 to 8 hour intervals may be satisfactory.

Switchover Procedure

For an initial approximation of the total daily dose required, the parenteral dose administered in the preceding 24 hours may be used. Since this dose is only an initial estimate, it is recommended that careful monitoring of clinical signs and symptoms, clinical efficacy, sedation, and adverse effects be carried out periodically for the first several days following the initiation of switchover. In this way, dosage adjustments, either upward or downward, can be quickly accomplished. Depending on the individual's clinical status, the first oral dose should be given within 12-24 hours following the last intramuscular dose.

Maintenance Dosage

Upon achieving a satisfactory therapeutic response, the dosage should then be gradually reduced to the lowest effective maintenance level.

In some cases where compliance has been a problem, the long-acting injectable forms of HALDOL (HALDOL Decanoate 50 and HALDOL Decanoate 100) should be used. The recommended interval between doses is four weeks.

Overdosage

The symptoms of HALDOL overdosage include

1. Severe extrapyramidal reactions

2. Hypotension

3. Sedation

The individual may appear comatose with respiratory depression and hypotension, which could be severe enough to produce a shock-like state.

INDERAL

(Propranolol)

Pharmacodynamics

Inderal is a synthetic beta-adrenergic receptor blocking agent. It specifically competes with beta-adrenergic receptor stimulating agents for available receptor sites. When INDERAL blocks access to beta-receptor sites, the chronotropic, inotropic, and vasodilator responses to beta-adrenergic stimulation are decreased proportionately.

The mechanism of the antihypertensive effect of Inderal has not been established. Among the factors that may be involved in contributing to the antihypertensive action are

1. Decreased cardiac output

2. Inhibition of renin release by the kidneys

3. Diminution of tonic sympathetic nerve outflow from vasomotor centers in the brain

In angina pectoris, INDERAL generally reduces the oxygen requirement of the heart at any given level of effort by blocking the catecholamine-induced increases in the heart rate, systolic blood pressure, and the velocity and extent of myocardial contraction.

INDERAL may increase oxygen requirements by increasing left ventricular fiber length, end diastolic pressure, and systolic ejection period. The net physiologic effect of beta-adrenergic blockade is usually advantageous and is manifested during exercise by delayed onset of pain and increased work capacity.

INDERAL exerts its antiarrhythmic effects in concentrations associated with beta-adrenergic blockade, and this appears to be its principal antiarrhythmic mechanism of action. In dosages greater than required for beta blockade, INDERAL also exerts a quinidine-like or anesthetic-like membrane action, which affects the cardiac action potential.

*   The mechanism of the antimigraine effect of INDERAL has not been established.

*   The specific mechanism of INDERAL's anti-tremor effects has not been established.

*   The mechanism of INDERAL's anti-rages effects has not been established.

Pharmacokinetics

- INDERAL is almost completely absorbed from the gastrointestinal tract, but the liver immediately binds a portion.

- Peak effect occurs in one to one and one-half hours.

- The biologic half-life is approximately four hours.

Indications

1. Hypertension

2. Long-term treatment of angina pectoris

3. Cardiac arrhythmias

4. Migraine

5. Familial or hereditary essential tremor

6. Unlabeled use for controlling rages

Pediatric Use—Evaluation of the effects of INDERAL in children, relative to the drug's efficacy and safety, has not been systematically performed.

Contraindications

In the following conditions:

1. Cardiogenic shock

2. Sinus bradycardia and greater than first degree block

3. Bronchial asthma

4. Congestive heart failure unless the failure is secondary to a tachyarrhythmia treatable with INDERAL

Potential Side Effects

Most adverse effects have been mild, transient, and rarely required the withdrawal of therapy.

Cardiovascular System—Bradycardia, congestive heart failure, intensification of AV block, hypotension, paresthesia of hands, thrombocytopenic purpura, arterial insufficiency of the Raynaud type

Neurological System—Light-headedness, visual disturbances, slightly clouded sensorium, and decreased performance on neuropsychometrics

Psychiatric Disorders—Mental depression manifested by insomnia, lassitude, weakness, fatigue, reversible mental depression progressing to catatonia, emotional lability, hallucinations, vivid dreams, an acute reversible syndrome characterized by disorientation for time and place, short-term memory loss

Gastrointestinal System—Pharyngitis, nausea, vomiting, epigastric distress, abdominal cramping, diarrhea, constipation, mesenteric arterial thrombosis, ischemic colitis

Dermatological System—Alopecia, systemic lupus erythematosus, erythematous rash, fever combined with aching and sore throat, psoriasis form rashes

Respiratory System—Laryngospasm, respiratory distress, bronchospasm

Hematological System—Agranulocytosis, nonthrombocytopenic purpura, thrombocytopenic purpura

Sexual Function—Male impotence

Special Senses—Dry eyes

Potential Drug Interactions

1. Individuals receiving catecholamine-depleting drugs such as reserpine should be closely observed if INDERAL is added, as that may produce an excessive reduction of resting sympathetic nervous activity and cause hypotension, marked bradycardia, vertigo, syncopal attacks, or orthostatic hypotension.

2. Administration of a calcium-channel-blocking drug may depress myocardial contractility or atrioventricular conduction in individuals receiving INDERAL.

3. Adding nonsteroidal anti-inflammatory drugs may cause blunting of the antihypertensive effect of INDERAL.

4. Hypotension and cardiac arrest have been reported with the concomitant use of INDERAL and HALDOL.

5. Aluminum hydroxide gel greatly reduces intestinal absorption of INDERAL.

6. Ethanol slows the rate of absorption of INDERAL.

7. DILANTIN and LUMINAL accelerate INDERAL clearance

8. THORAZINE, when used concomitantly with INDERAL, results in increased plasma levels of both drugs

9. Antipyrine and lidocaine may reduce clearance when used concomitantly with INDERAL.

10. Thyroxine may result in a lower than expected T3 concentration when used concomitantly with INDERAL.

11. TAGAMET decreases the hepatic metabolism of INDERAL, delaying elimination and increasing blood levels.

12. Theophylline clearance is reduced when used concomitantly with INDERAL.

Dosage and Administration

In older adolescents, the initial oral dose is 80mg daily in divided doses. The dosage may be increased gradually to achieve optimum treatment response. The usual dose range is 160mg to 240mg per day. If a satisfactory response is not obtained within four to six weeks after reaching the maximum dose, INDERAL therapy should be discontinued gradually. A decreasing dose titration over a 7-to14-day period is recommended.

In older children, the usual dosage range is 2mg to 4mg/kg/day in two equally divided doses. Pediatric dosage calculated by weight (recommended) generally produces INDERAL plasma levels in a therapeutic range similar to that in adults. Doses above 16mg/kg/day should not be used in children.

INDERAL LA provides propranolol hydrochloride in a sustained-release capsule for administration once daily. If individuals are switched from INDERAL Tablets to INDERAL LA

Capsules, INDERAL Tablets should **not** be considered a simple mg-for-mg substitute for INDERAL LA. INDERAL LA has different kinetics and produces lower blood levels. Re-titration may be necessary, especially to maintain effectiveness at the end of the 24-hour dosing interval.

LUVOX

(Fluvoxamine Maleate)

Pharmacodynamics

LUVOX is a selective serotonin reuptake inhibitor (SSRI). The mechanism of action of LUVOX in Obsessive Compulsive Disorder is presumed to be linked to its specific serotonin reuptake inhibition in brain neurons.

Pharmacokinetics

- Oral bioavailability is not significantly affected by food.

- Approximately 80% of LUVOX is bound to plasma protein, mostly albumin.

- LUVOX is extensively metabolized by the liver and is mainly excreted in the urine.

- Maximum plasma concentrations at steady-state occurred within 3-8 hours of dosing.

- Steady state is usually achieved after about a week of dosing.

- The mean plasma half-life of LUVOX at steady state after multiple oral doses is about 16 hours.

Indications

1. Major Depressive Disorder

2. Obsessive Compulsive Disorder (OCD)

3. Panic Disorder

Pediatric Use—Safety and effectiveness of LUVOX in individuals below 18 years-of-age have not been established.

Contraindications

1. Co-administration of terfenadine, asternizole, or cisapride with LUVOX

2. In individuals with a history of hypersensitivity to LUVOX

Potential Side Effects

Body as a Whole—Accidental injury, malaise, allergic reaction, neck pain, neck rigidity, overdose, photosensitivity reaction

Neurological System—Amnesia, apathy, hyperkinesia, hypokinesia, myoclonus, akathisia, ataxia, CNS depression, convulsion/seizure, delirium, dyskinesia, dystonia, extrapyramidal syndrome, unsteady gait, hemiplegia, hypersomnia, hypotonia, incoordination, increased salivation, neuralgia, paralysis, stupor, twitching, and vertigo

Psychiatric Disorders—Manic/hypomanic reaction, psychotic reaction, agoraphobia, hysteria, delusion, depersonalization, hypochondriasis, drug dependence, emotional lability, euphoria, hallucinations, hostility, paranoid reaction, phobia, sleep disorder

Cardiovascular System—Hypertension, hypotension, syncope, tachycardia, angina pectoris, bradycardia, cardiomyopathy, cardiovascular disease, cold extremities, conduction delay, heart failure, myocardial infarction, pallor, irregular pulse, ST segment changes

Gastrointestinal System—Elevated liver transaminases, colitis, eructation, esophagitis, gastritis, gastroenteritis, gastrointestinal hemorrhage, gastrointestinal ulcer, gingivitis, glossitis, hemorrhoids, melena, rectal hemorrhage, and stomatitis

Endocrine System—Hypothyroidism, delayed menstruation, premenstrual syndrome, breast pain, female lactation

Hematological and Lymphatic Systems—Anemia, ecchymosis, leukocytosis, lymphadenopathy, thrombocytopenia

Metabolic and Nutritional Systems—Edema, weight gain, weight loss, dehydration, and hypercholesterolemia

Muscular and Skeletal Systems—Arthralgia, arthritis, bursitis, generalized muscle spasm, myasthenia, tendinous contracture, and tenosynovitis

Respiratory System—Increased cough, sinusitis, asthma, bronchitis, epistaxis, hoarseness, hyperventilation

Dermatological System—Acne, alopecia, dry skin, eczema, exfoliative dermatitis, furunculosis, seborrhea, skin discoloration, urticaria, toxic epidermal necrolysis, Stevens-Johnson syndrome, Henoch-Schönlein purpura, bullous eruption

Genitourinary System—Anuria, cystitis, dysuria, hematuria, menopause, menorrhagia, metrorrhagia, nocturia, polyuria, urinary incontinence, urinary tract infection, urinary urgency, impaired urination, vaginal hemorrhage, vaginitis, and priapism

Sexual Function—Increased libido

Special Senses—Abnormal accommodation, conjunctivitis, deafness, diplopia, dry eyes, ear pain, eye pain, mydriasis, otitis media, parosmia, photophobia, taste loss, visual field defect

Potential Drug Interactions

1. Individuals receiving LUVOX in combination with monoamine oxidase inhibitors (MAOI), or starting an MAOI shortly after LUVOX is discontinued may develop serious, sometimes fatal, reactions including hyperthermia, rigidity, myoclonus, autonomic instability with possible rapid fluctuations of vital signs, and mental status changes that include extreme agitation progressing to delirium and coma.

2. Benzodiazepines (e.g., alprazolam, midazolam, triazolam, etc.) metabolized by hepatic oxidation should be used with caution because the clearance of these drugs is likely to be reduced by LUVOX. If alprazolam is co-administered with LUVOX, the initial alprazolam dosage should be at least halved and titration to the lowest effective dose is recommended. No dosage adjustment is required for LUVOX.

3. The co-administration of LUVOX and diazepam should be avoided because LUVOX reduces the clearance of both diazepam and its active metabolite, N-desmethyldiazepam; there is a strong likelihood of substantial accumulation of both species during chronic co-administration.

4. The clearance of theophylline will be decreased approximately 3-fold when it is co-administered with LUVOX. Therefore, if theophylline is co-administered with LUVOX its dose should be reduced to one third of the usual daily maintenance dose and plasma concentrations of theophylline should be monitored. No dosage adjustment is required for LUVOX.

5. Lithium may enhance the serotonergic effects of LUVOX. Seizures have been reported with the co-administration LUVOX and lithium. Therefore, the combination should be used with caution.

6. Tryptophan may enhance the serotonergic effects of LUVOX. Severe vomiting has been reported with the co-administration of LUVOX and tryptophan.

7. Serum CLOZARIL level may increase when it is taken with LUVOX. Since CLOZARIL related seizures and orthostatic hypotension appear to be dose related, the risk of these adverse events might be higher when LUVOX and CLOZARIL are co-administered.

8. Significantly increased plasma TCA levels have been reported with the co-administration of LUVOX.

9. Elevated TEGRETOL levels and symptoms of toxicity have been reported with the co-administration of LUVOX and TEGRETOL.

10. Co-administration of LUVOX and INDERAL may cause several folds increase of INDERAL plasma concentration and may cause reduction in heart rate, reduction in the exercise diastolic pressure, and orthostatic hypotension. If Inderal or other beta-blocker is co-administered with LUVOX, a reduction in the initial beta-blocker dose and more cautious dose titration is recommended. No dosage adjustment is required for LUVOX.

11. Smokers had a 25% increase in the metabolism of LUVOX compared to nonsmokers.

Dosage and Administration

The recommended starting dose for LUVOX in older adolescents and adults is 50mg administered as a single daily dose at bedtime. The dose can be increased in 50mg increments every 4 to 7 days, as tolerated, until maximum therapeutic benefit is achieved, not to exceed 300mg per day. It is advisable that a total daily dose of more than 100mg should be given in two divided doses. If the doses are not equal, the larger dose should be given at bedtime.

In children 6 to 12 years, the initial dose of 25mg/day is recommended. A 25mg/day weekly increment up to 150-200mg/day may be considered after two weeks if no clinical improvement is observed. A dose exceeding 200mg/day may not add any more treatment effect. It may increase the risk of side effects.

In children younger than 6 years-of-age, LUVOX has been used unlabeled for "perseverative speech" "repetitive behaviors," or "difficulty with transitions." An initial dose of 25mg/day is recommended. A 25mg/day weekly increment up to 100-150mg/day may be considered after 4 weeks if no clinical improvement is observed. A dose exceeds 150mg/day usually does not add any more treatment effect. It tends to increase the risk of side effects.

Maintenance, Continuation, and Extended Treatment—While there are no systematic studies that answer the question of how long to continue LUVOX, it is generally agreed among experts that acute episodes of depression require several months or longer of sustained pharmacologic therapy. Whether the dose of antidepressant needed to induce remission is identical to the dose needed to maintain and/or sustain euthymia is unknown.

Since OCD and Anxiety/Panic Disorders are chronic conditions, it is reasonable to consider continuation for a responding individual with dosage adjustments made to maintain the individual on the lowest effective dosage, and the individual should be periodically reassessed to determine the need for further treatment.

Overdosage

Commonly observed symptoms and signs of LUVOX overdose included drowsiness, vomiting, diarrhea, dizziness, coma, tachycardia, bradycardia, hypotension, ECG abnormalities, liver function abnormalities, convulsions, and symptoms such as aspiration pneumonitis, respiratory difficulties, or hypokalemia that may occur secondary to loss of consciousness or vomiting, and coma.

NAVANE

(Thiothixene)

Pharmacodynamics

NAVANE is a thioxanthene derivative. It possesses certain chemical and pharmacological similarities to the piperazine phenothiazines and differences from the aliphatic group of phenothiazines.

Pharmacokinetics

Pharmacokinetic information is not currently available.

Indications

For the treatment of psychotic disorders

Pediatric Use—The use of NAVANE in children under 12 years-of-age is not recommended because safe conditions for its use have not been established.

Contraindications

1. Individuals with circulatory collapse, comatose states, central nervous system depression due to any cause, and blood dyscrasias

2. Individuals who have shown hypersensitivity to NAVANE

Potential Side Effects

Body as a Whole—Hyperpyrexia, increased weight, weakness or fatigue, and peripheral edema

Cardiovascular System—Tachycardia, hypotension, and syncope

Neurological System—Drowsiness, light-headedness, seizures, cerebral edema, cerebrospinal fluid abnormalities, extrapyramidal symptoms (pseudoparkinsonism, akathisia and dystonia), tardive dyskinesia, Neuroleptic Malignant Syndrome (NMS)

Psychiatric Disorders—Restlessness, agitation, insomnia, paradoxical exacerbation of psychotic symptoms

Hepatic System—Elevations of serum transaminase and alkaline phosphatase

Hematological and Lymphatic Systems—Leukopenia and leucocytosis, agranulocytosis, eosinophilia, hemolytic anemia, thrombocytopenia and pancytopenia

Dermatological System—Rash, pruritus, urticaria, photosensitivity, increased sweating

Endocrine System—Elevate prolactin levels, lactation, moderate breast enlargement, galactorrhea amenorrhea, false positive pregnancy tests, gynecomastia, hypoglycemia, hyperglycemia and glycosuria

Gastrointestinal System—Dry mouth, anorexia, nausea, vomiting, diarrhea, increase in appetite, polydipsia, constipation, increased salivation, adynamic ileus

Sexual Function—Impotence

Special Senses—Blurred vision, miosis, mydriasis, nasal congestion

Dosage and Administration

In adults with milder conditions, an initial dose of 2mg three times daily is recommended. If indicated, a subsequent increase to 15mg/day total daily dose is often effective.

In more severe conditions, an initial dose of 5mg twice daily is recommended. The usual optimal dose is 20 to 30mg daily. If indicated, an increase to 60mg total daily dose is often effective. Exceeding a total daily dose of 60mg rarely increases the beneficial response. Some individuals have been successfully maintained on once-a-day NAVANE therapy.

Overdosage

Manifestations of overdosage include muscular twitching, drowsiness, and dizziness. Symptoms of gross overdosage may include CNS depression, rigidity, weakness, torticollis, tremor, salivation, dysphagia, hypotension, gait disturbance, or coma.

NORPRAMIN

(Desipramine)

Pharmacodynamics

NORPRAMIN is an antidepressant drug of the tricyclic type. While the precise mechanism of action of the tricyclic antidepressants is unknown, a leading theory suggests that they restore normal levels of neurotransmitters by blocking the re-uptake of these substances from the synapse in the central nervous system. Evidence indicates that the secondary amine tricyclic antidepressants, including NORPRAMIN, may have greater activity in blocking the re-uptake of norepinephrine.

Tertiary amine tricyclic antidepressants, such as amitriptyline, may have greater effect on serotonin reuptake.

Pharmacokinetics

- NORPRAMIN is rapidly absorbed from the gastrointestinal tract.

- NORPRAMIN is metabolized in the liver, and approximately 70% is excreted in the urine.

Indications

For the treatment of depression

Pediatric Use—NORPRAMIN is not recommended for use in children since safety and effectiveness in the pediatric age group have not been established.

Contraindications

1. In conjunction with, or within 2 weeks of, treatment with an MAOI

2. During the acute recovery period following myocardial infarction.

3. Prior hypersensitivity to the drug

Potential Side Effects

Body as a Whole—Weight gain or loss, perspiration, flushing, parotid swelling, drowsiness, dizziness, weakness and fatigue, headache, fever, alopecia, elevated alkaline phosphatase

Neurological Disorders—Numbness, tingling, paresthesias of extremities, incoordination, ataxia, tremors, peripheral neuropathy, extrapyramidal symptoms, seizures, alterations in EEG patterns, tinnitus. Symptoms attributed to Neuroleptic Malignant Syndrome have been reported during desipramine use with and without concomitant neuroleptic therapy.

Psychiatric Disorders—Confusional states (especially in the elderly) with hallucinations, disorientation, delusions, anxiety, restlessness, agitation, insomnia and nightmares, hypomania, exacerbation of psychosis

Cardiovascular System—Hypotension, hypertension, palpitations, heart block, myocardial infarction, stroke, arrhythmias, premature ventricular contractions, tachycardia, ventricular tachycardia, ventricular fibrillation, sudden death

Gastrointestinal System—Dry mouth, constipation, paralytic ileus, anorexia, nausea and vomiting, epigastric distress, peculiar taste, abdominal cramps, diarrhea, stoma-titis, black tongue, increased pancreatic enzymes

Hepatic System—Hepatitis, jaundice (simulating obstructive), altered liver function, elevated liver function tests

Dermatological System—Skin rash, petechiae, urticaria, itching, photosensitization, edema of face and tongue, general edema, drug fever, cross-sensitivity with other tricyclic drugs

Hematological and Lymphatic Systems—Bone marrow depressions including agranulocytosis, eosinophilia, purpura, thrombocytopenia

Endocrine System—Gynecomastia in males, breast enlargement and galactorrhea in females, testicular swelling, elevation or depression of blood sugar levels, syndrome of inappropriate antidiuretic hormone secretion

Genitourinary System—Urinary retention, urinary frequency, nocturia, delayed micturition, dilation of urinary tract

Sexual Function—Increased or decreased libido, impotence, painful ejaculation

Special Senses—Blurred vision, disturbance of accommodation, mydriasis, increased intraocular pressure

Potential Drug Interactions

1. Certain drugs, particularly the psychostimulants and the phenothiazines, increase plasma levels of concomitantly administered NORPRAMIN through competition for the same metabolic enzyme systems. Hence, the sedative effects of NORPRAMIN and benzodiazepines (e.g., chlordiazepoxide or diazepam) are additive. Both the sedative and anticholinergic effects of the major tranquilizers are also additive to those of NORPRAMIN.

2. Concurrent administration of TAGAMET and NORPRAMIN can produce clinically significant increases in the plasma concentrations of the NORPRAMIN. Conversely, NORPRAMIN plasma level decreases upon discontinuation of cimetidine, which may result in the loss of the therapeutic efficacy of the NORPRAMIN.

3. Other substances, particularly barbiturates and alcohol, induce liver enzyme activity and thereby reduce NORPRAMIN plasma levels. Similar effects have been reported with tobacco smoke. On the other hand, individuals taking NORPRAMIN may exaggerate their response to alcoholic beverages.

4. An individual who is stable on a given dose of NORPRAMIN may become abruptly toxic when given one of the cytochrome P450 2D6 inhibiting drugs (quinidine, cimetidine, many other antidepressants, phenothiazines, and the type 1C antiarrhythmics propafenone and flecainide). Concomitant use of NORPRAMIN with these drugs may require lower doses than usually prescribed for either the NORPRAMIN or the other drug. Furthermore, whenever one of these other drugs is withdrawn from co-therapy, an increased dose of NORPRAMIN may be required. It is desirable to monitor NORPRAMIN plasma levels whenever it is going to be co-administered with another drug known to be an inhibitor of P450 2D6.

5. Individuals with thyroid disease or taking thyroid medication with NORPRAMIN may experience cardiovascular toxicity, including arrhythmias.

6. NORPRAMIN may block the antihypertensive effect of guanethidine and similarly acting compounds.

Withdrawal Symptoms

Abrupt cessation of NORPRAMIN treatment after prolonged therapy may produce nausea, headache, and malaise.

Laboratory Tests

Leukocyte and differential counts should be performed in any individual who develops fever and sore throat during therapy; the drug should be discontinued if there is evidence of pathologic neutrophil depression.

Dosage and Administration

It has been found in some studies that NORPRAMIN has a more rapid onset of action than TOFRANIL. Earliest therapeutic effects may occasionally be seen in 2 to 5 days, but full treatment benefit usually requires 2-to-3 weeks to obtain. An optimal range of therapeutic plasma levels has not been established for NORPRAMIN.

Treatment of Depression—In adults, dosage should be initiated at a lower level and increased according to tolerance and clinical response. The usual adult dose is 100 to 200mg per day. In more severely ill patients, dosage may be further increased gradually to 300mg/day if necessary. Dosages above 300mg/day are not recommended.

In adolescents, the usual dose is 25 to 100mg daily. Dosage should be initiated at a lower level and increased according to tolerance and clinical response to a usual maximum of 100mg daily. In more severely ill patients, dosage may be further increased to 150mg/day. Doses above 150mg/day are not recommended in these age groups.

Initial therapy may be administered in divided doses or a single daily dose. Maintenance therapy may be given on a once-daily schedule for individual convenience and compliance.

Overdosage

Critical manifestations of overdose include cardiac dysrhythmias, severe hypotension, convulsions, and CNS depression including coma, and changes in the electrocardiogram, particularly in QRS axis or width. Other signs of overdose may include confusion, disturbed concentration, transient visual hallucinations, dilated pupils, agitation, hyperactive reflexes, stupor, drowsiness, muscle rigidity, vomiting, hypothermia, hyperpyrexia.

ORAP

(Pimozide)

Pharmacodynamics

ORAP is an orally active antipsychotic agent of the diphenylbutylpiperidine series, which shares with other antipsychotics the ability to blockade dopaminergic receptors on neurons in the central nervous system. Although its exact mode of action has not been established, the ability of ORAP to suppress motor and phonic tics in Tourette syndrome is thought to be a function of its dopaminergic blocking activity. However, receptor blockade is often accompanied by a series of secondary alterations in central dopamine metabolism and function, which may contribute to both ORAP's therapeutic and untoward effects. In addition, pimozide, in common with other antipsychotic drugs, has various effects on other central nervous system receptor systems, which are not fully characterized.

Pharmacokinetics

- More than 50% of a dose of ORAP is absorbed after oral administration.

- ORAP appears to undergo significant first pass metabolism.

- Peak serum levels occur generally six to eight hours (range 4-12 hours) after dosing.

- ORAP is extensively metabolized in the liver.

- The major route of elimination of ORAP and its metabolites is through the kidney.

- The mean serum elimination half-life of ORAP is approximately 55 hours.

- Effects of food, disease, or concomitant medication upon the absorption, distribution, metabolism, and elimination of ORAP are not known.

Indications

For the suppression of motor and phonic tics in individuals with Tourette syndrome who have failed to respond satisfactorily to standard treatment. ORAP is not intended as a treatment of first choice nor is it intended for the treatment of tics that are merely annoying or cosmetically troublesome. ORAP should be reserved for use in Tourette syndrome patients whose development or daily life function is severely compromised by the presence of motor and phonic tics.

Pediatric Use—Although Tourette syndrome most often has its onset between the ages of 2 and 15 years, information on the use and efficacy of ORAP in patients less than 12 years-of-age is limited. Because its use and safety have not been evaluated in other childhood disorders, ORAP is not recommended for use in any condition other than Tourette syndrome.

Contraindication

1. In the treatment of simple tics or tics other than those associated with Tourette syndrome

2. In individuals taking drugs that may cause motor and phonic tics (e.g., RITALIN and DEXEDRINE) until such patients have been withdrawn from these drugs to determine whether or not the drugs, rather than Tourette syndrome, are responsible for the tics

3. In individuals with the following conditions: congenital long QT syndrome, a history of cardiac arrhythmias, taking other drugs that prolong the QT interval of the electrocardiogram

4. In individuals with severe toxic central nervous system depression or comatose states from any cause

5. In individuals with hypersensitivity to ORAP

Potential Side Effects

Body as a Whole—Headache, asthenia, chest pain, periorbital edema

Neurological System—Drowsiness, sedation, dizziness, akathisia, rigidity, speech disorder, handwriting change, akinesia, hyperkinesia, somnolence, abnormal dreaming, torticollis, limb tremor, seizure, Parkinsonism, fainting, dyskinesia, tardive dyskinesia, hyperpyrexia Neuroleptic Malignant Syndrome

Psychiatric Disorders—Depression, excitement, nervousness, adverse behavior effect, insomnia

Cardiovascular System—Postural hypotension, hypotension, hypertension, tachycardia, palpitations, ECG changes (prolongation of the QT interval, flattening, notching, and inversion of the T wave, and the appearance of U-waves)

Gastrointestinal System—Dry mouth, diarrhea, nausea, anorexia, vomiting, constipation, eructations, thirst, appetite increase, dysphagia, increased salivation

Endocrine System—Menstrual disorder, breast secretions

Hematological and Lymphatic System—Hemolytic anemia

Musculoskeletal System—Muscle cramps, muscle tightness, stooped posture, myalgia

Dermatological System—Rash, sweating, skin irritation

Special Senses—Visual disturbance, blurred vision, taste change, sensitivity of eyes to light, decreased accommodation, spots before eyes, cataracts

Genitourinary System—Nocturia, urinary frequency

Sexual Function—Loss of libido, impotence

Potential Drug Interaction

1. Because ORAP prolongs the QT interval of the ECG, an additive effect on QT interval would be anticipated if administered with drugs such as phenothiazines, tricyclic antidepressants or antiarrhythmic agents, which prolong the QT interval. Also, the use of macrolide antibiotics in patients with prolonged QT intervals has been rarely associated with ventricular arrhythmias. Such concomitant administration should not be undertaken.

2. ORAP may be capable of potentiating CNS depressants, including analgesics, sedatives, anxiolytics, and alcohol.

3. ORAP should be administered with caution to individuals receiving anticonvulsant medication, with a history of seizures, or with EEG abnormalities, because it may lower the convulsive threshold. If indicated, adequate anticonvulsant therapy should be maintained concomitantly.

Withdrawal Symptoms

Some individuals on maintenance treatment may experience transient dyskinetic signs after abrupt withdrawal. In some of these cases, the dyskinetic movements are indistinguishable from Tardive Dyskinesia except for duration. It is not known whether gradual withdrawal of ORAP will reduce the rate of occurrence of withdrawal emergent neurological signs, but until further evidence becomes available, it seems reasonable to gradually withdraw use of ORAP.

Laboratory Tests

Sudden, unexpected deaths have occurred in experimental studies of conditions other than Tourette syndrome. These deaths occurred while patients were receiving dosages in the range of 1mg per kg. One possible mechanism for such deaths is prolongation of the QT interval predisposing patients to ventricular arrhythmia. An electrocardiogram should be performed before ORAP treatment is initiated and periodically thereafter, especially during the period of dose adjustment. Any indication of prolongation of QT interval beyond an absolute limit of 0.47 seconds (children) or 0.52 seconds (adults) or more than 25% above the patient's original baseline should be considered a basis for stopping further dose increase and considering a lower dose.

Since hypokalemia has been associated with ventricular arrhythmias, potassium insufficiency secondary to diuretics, diarrhea, or other cause, it should be corrected before ORAP therapy is initiated and normal potassium maintained during therapy.

Dosage and Administration

The suppression of tics by ORAP requires a slow and gradual introduction of the drug. The individual's dose should be carefully adjusted to a point where the suppression of tics and the relief afforded is balanced against the untoward side effects of the drug. An ECG should be done at baseline and periodically thereafter, especially during the period of dose adjustment.

In older adolescents and adults, treatment with ORAP should be initiated with a dose of 1-to-2mg a day in divided doses. The dose may be increased thereafter every other day or every third day with increment dose of 0.5mg/day. Most individual are maintained at less than 0.2mg/kg per day, or 10mg/day, whichever is less. Doses greater than 0.2mg/kg/day or 10mg/day are not recommended.

Reliable dose response data for the effects of ORAP on tic manifestation in Tourette syndrome patients below the age of twelve are limited. In these children, treatment should be initiated at a dose of 0.05mg/kg preferably taken once at bedtime. The dose may be increased every third to fifth day to a maximum of 0.2mg/kg not to exceed 10mg/ day.

Periodic attempts should be made to reduce the dosage of ORAP to see whether or not tics persist at the level and extent first identified. In attempts to reduce the dosage of ORAP, consideration should be given to the possibility that increases of tic intensity and frequency may represent a transient, withdrawal related phenomenon rather than a return of disease symptoms. Specifically, one-to-two weeks should be allowed to elapse before one concludes that an increase in tic manifestations is a function of the underlying disease syndrome rather than a response to drug withdrawal. A gradual withdrawal is recommended in any case.

Overdosage

In general, the signs and symptoms of overdosage with ORAP would be an exaggeration of known pharmacologic effects and adverse reactions, the most prominent of which would be electrocardiographic abnormalities, severe extrapyramidal reactions, hypotension, and comatose state with respiratory depression.

PAMELOR

(Nortriptyline)

Pharmacodynamics

PAMELOR inhibits the activity of such diverse agents as histamine, 5-hydroxytryptamine, and acetylcholine. It increases the pressor effect of norepinephrine but blocks the pressor response of phenethylamine. PAMELOR interferes with the transport, release, and storage of catecholamines. PAMELOR may have a combination of stimulant and depressant properties.

Pharmacokinetics

Pharmacokinetic information is not currently available.

Indications

For the relief of symptoms of depression

Pediatric Use—This drug is not recommended for use in children since safety and effectiveness in the pediatric age group have not been established.

Contraindications

1. Concurrent use of PAMELOR with an MAOI

2. In individuals hypersensitive to PAMELOR

3. During the acute recovery period after myocardial infarction.

Potential Side Effects

Body as a Whole—Weight gain or loss, weakness, fatigue, headache

Neurological Disorders—Numbness, tingling, paresthesias of extremities, dizziness, incoordination, ataxia, tremors, peripheral neuropathy, extrapyramidal symptoms, seizures, alteration in EEG patterns

Psychiatric Disorders—Confusioned states, drowsiness, hallucinations, disorientation, delusions, anxiety, restlessness, agitation, hostility, insomnia, panic, nightmares, activation of hypomania or mania, exacerbation of psychosis

Cardiovascular System—Hypotension, hypertension, tachycardia, palpitation, myocardial infarction, arrhythmias, heart block, stroke, perspiration, flushing

Gastrointestinal System—Dry mouth and, (rarely) associated sublingual adenitis, nausea and vomiting, anorexia, epigastric distress, diarrhea, peculiar taste, stomatitis, abdominal cramps, constipation, paralytic ileus, black tongue, jaundice (simulating obstructive), altered liver function

Special Senses—Blurred vision, disturbance of accommodation, mydriasis, tinnitus

Genitourinary System—Urinary retention, delayed micturition, dilation of the urinary tract, urinary frequency, and nocturia

Dermatological System—Skin rash, petechiae, urticaria, itching, photosensitization (avoid excessive exposure to sunlight), edema (general or of face and tongue), drug fever, cross-sensitivity with other tricyclic drugs, alopecia

Hematological and Lymphatic Systems—Bone marrow depression including agranulocytosis; eosinophilia; purpura; thrombocytopenia

Endocrine System—Gynecomastia in males, breast enlargement and galactorrhea in females; testicular swelling, elevation or depression of blood sugar levels, syndrome of inappropriate ADH (anti-diuretic hormone) secretion.

Sexual Function—Increased or decreased libido, impotence

Potential Drug Interactions

1. PAMELOR given to individuals with hyperthyroid disorders or to those receiving thyroid medication may cause cardiac arrhythmias.

2. The concomitant administration of quinidine and PAMELOR may result in a significantly longer plasma half-life and lower clearance of PAMELOR.

3. Administration of reserpine with PAMELOR may produce a "stimulating" effect in some depressed patients.

4. Concurrent administration of TAGAMET and PAMELOR can produce clinically significant increases in the plasma concentrations of the PAMELOR.

5. An individual who is stable on a given dose of PAMELOR may become abruptly toxic when given one of the cytochrome P450 2D6 inhibiting drugs (quinidine, cimetidine, many other antidepressants, phenothiazines, and the SRIs) as concomitant therapy. Concomitant use of PAMELOR with drugs that can inhibit cytochrome P450 2D6 may require lower doses than usually prescribed for either the PAMELOR or the other drug. Furthermore, whenever one of these other drugs is withdrawn from co-therapy, an increased dose of PAMELOR may be required. It is desirable to monitor PAMELOR plasma levels whenever PAMELOR is going to be co-administered with another drug known to be an inhibitor of P450 2D6.

Withdrawal Symptoms

Though these are not indicative of addiction, abrupt cessation of treatment after prolonged therapy may produce nausea, headache, and malaise.

Dosage and Administration

In older adolescents and adults, begin with a dosage of 25mg three or four times daily; dosage should begin at a low level and be increased as required. As an alternate regimen, the total daily dosage may be given once a day. When doses above 100mg daily are administered, plasma levels of nortriptyline should be monitored and maintained in the optimum range of 50-150ng/mL. Doses above 150mg/day are not recommended.

Following remission, maintenance medication may be required for a longer period of time at the lowest dose that will maintain remission. If an individual develops minor side effects, the dosage should be reduced. The drug should be discontinued promptly if adverse effects of a serious nature or allergic manifestations occur.

Overdosage

Critical manifestations of overdose include cardiac dysrhythmias, severe hypotension, shock, congestive heart failure, pulmonary edema, convulsions, and CNS depression, including coma. Changes in the electrocardiogram, particularly in QRS axis or width, are clinically significant indicators of PAMELOR toxicity. Other signs of overdose may include confusion, restlessness, disturbed concentration, transient visual hallucinations, dilated pupils, agitation, hyperactive reflexes, stupor, drowsiness, muscle rigidity, vomiting, hypothermia, and hyperpyrexia.

PAXIL

(Paroxetine)

PAXIL is an orally administered antidepressant with a chemical structure unrelated to other selective serotonin reuptake inhibitors or to tricyclic, tetracyclic or other available antidepressant agents.

Pharmacodynamics

The antidepressant action of paroxetine and its efficacy in the treatment of obsessive-compulsive disorder (OCD) and panic disorder (PD) is presumed to be linked to potentiation of serotonergic activity in the central nervous system resulting from inhibition of neuronal reuptake of serotonin into platelets.

Pharmacokinetics

- PAXIL is completely absorbed after oral dosing of a solution of the hydrochloride salt.

- Steady-state PAXIL concentrations are achieved by approximately 10 days.

- Approximately 93% to 95% of PAXIL is bound to plasma protein.

- PAXIL is extensively metabolized after oral administration.

- Approximately ⅔ of oral solution dose of PAXIL is excreted in the urine and about ⅓ is excreted in the feces (probably via the bile) over a 10-day postdosing period.

- PAXIL distributes throughout the body, including the CNS, with only 1% remaining in the plasma.

Indications

1. Major depressive disorder

2. Obsessive compulsive disorder

3. Panic disorder with or without agoraphobia

4. Unlabeled use in "perseverative speech," "repetitive behaviors," and "difficulty with transition"

Pediatric Use—Safety and effectiveness in the pediatric population have not been established.

Contraindications

In individuals taking monoamine oxidase inhibitors

Potential Side Effects

Body as a Whole—Chills, malaise, asthenia, allergic reaction, carcinoma, face edema, moniliasis, and neck pain

Neurological System—Amnesia, CNS stimulation, vertigo, akinesia, alcohol abuse, ataxia, convulsion, dystonia, hyperkinesia, hypertonia, cogwheel rigidity, oculogyric crisis, hypesthesia, incoordination, dizziness, tremor, paralysis

Psychiatric Disorders—Impaired concentration, somnolence, insomnia, depression, emotional lability, abnormal thinking, depersonalization, hallucinations, hostility, lack of emotion, nervousness manic reaction, neurosis, paranoid reaction

Cardiovascular System—Hypertension, syncope, tachycardia, bradycardia, conduction abnormalities, abnormal electrocardiogram, hematoma, hypotension, migraine, peripheral vascular disorder

Gastrointestinal System—Bruxism, colitis, dry mouth, nausea, decreased appetite, constipation, dysphagia, eructation, gastroenteritis, gingivitis, glossitis, increased salivation, abnormal liver function tests, mouth ulceration, rectal hemorrhage, ulcerative stomatitis

Hematological and Lymphatic Systems—Anemia, leukopenia, lymphadenopathy, purpura

Metabolic System—Edema, weight gain, weight loss, hyperglycernia, peripheral edema, SGOT increased, increased SGPT, thirst

Musculoskeletal System—Arthralgia, arthritis

Respiratory System—Increased cough, rhinitis, asthma, bronchitis, dyspnea, epistaxis, hyperventilation, pneumonia, respiratory flu, sinusitis, voice alteration

Dermatological System—Pruritus, acne, alopecia, dry skin, sweating, ecchymosis, eczema, furunculosis, urticaria

Special Senses—Tinnitus, abnormality of accommodation, conjunctivitis, ear pain, eye pain, mydriasis, otitis media, taste loss, visual field defect

Genitourinary System—Abortion, amenorrhea, breast pain, cystitis, dysmenorrhea, dysuria, hematuria, menorrhagia, nocturia, polyuria, urethritis, urinary incontinence, urinary retention, urinary urgency, vaginitis

Sexual Function—Impotence, ejaculatory disturbance, and other male genital disorders

Potential Drug Interactions

1. In individuals receiving PAXIL in combination with a monoamine oxidase inhibitor (MAOI), there may be serious, sometimes fatal, reactions including hyperthermia, rigidity, myoclonus, autonomic instability with possible rapid fluctuations of vital signs, and mental status changes that include extreme agitation progressing to delirium and coma. These reactions may also happen in individuals who have recently discontinued PAXIL and have been started on an MAOI. It is recommended that PAXIL not be used in combination with an MAOI, or within 14 days of discontinuing treatment with an MAOI. At least 2 weeks should be allowed after stopping PAXIL before starting an MAOI.

2. An interaction between PAXIL and tryptophan may occur when they are co-administered and may cause headache, nausea, sweating and dizziness.

3. TAGAMET inhibits many cytochrome P450 enzymes when it is administered concurrently with PAXIL; dosage adjustment of PAXIL should be guided by clinical effect.

4. Phenobarbital induces many cytochrome P460 enzymes. No initial PAXIL dosage adjustment is considered necessary when co-administered with phenobarbital, but any subsequent adjustment should be guided by clinical effect.

5. DILANTIN level may increase when PAXIL and DILANTIN are co-administered.

6. Many drugs, including most antidepressants (PAXIL, other SSRIs and many tricyclics), are metabolized by the cytochrome P450 isozyme P4502D6. Concomitant use of PAXIL with other drugs metabolized by cytochrome P4502D6 including certain antidepressants and phenothiazines may require lower doses than usually prescribed for either PAXIL or the other drug. Serotonin syndrome may develop in some individuals with concomitant use of serotonergic drugs and with drugs that may have impaired PAXIL metabolism. The symptoms of serotonin syndrome include agitation, confusion, diaphoresis, hallucinations, hyperreflexia, myoclonus, shivering, tachycardia and tremor.

7. Because PAXIL is highly bound to plasma protein, administration of PAXIL to an individual taking another drug that is highly protein bound may cause increased free concentrations of the other drug, potentially resulting in adverse events.

8. Severe hypotension may develop when Paxil is added to chronic metoprolol treatment.

Withdrawal Symptoms

Abrupt discontinuation may lead to symptoms such as dizziness, sensory disturbances, agitation or anxiety, nausea and sweating; these events are generally self-limiting.

Dosage and Administration

In the treatment of depression, obsessive-compulsive disorder, or anxiety/panic disorders, older adolescents and adults may begin with 20mg/day administered in the morning. Usually individuals may notice improvement in 1 to 4 weeks. A 10mg/day weekly increment up to a maximum of 50mg/day may be considered after 4 weeks if no clinical improvement is observed. Doses above 20mg/day may be administered on a once a day (morning) or twice daily schedule.

In children 6 to 12 years, the initial dose of 10mg/day is recommended. A 5mg/day (using PAXIL Oral Solution) weekly increment up to 30mg/day may be considered after 4 weeks if no clinical improvement is observed. A dose exceeding 30mg/day may not add any more treatment effect. It tends to increase the risk of side effects.

In children younger than 6 years-of-age, PAXIL has been used off-label for "perseverative speech," "repetitive behaviors," or "difficulty with transitions." An initial dose of 0.5 to 1mg/day (using PAXIL Oral Solution) is recommended. A 0.5-1mg/day weekly increment up to 15mg/day may be considered after 4 weeks if no clinical improvement is observed. A dose exceeding 15mg/day usually does not add any more treatment effect. It tends to increase the risk of side effects.

Panic Disorder—Usual Initial Dosage: PAXIL should be administered as a single daily dose, usually in the morning. The target dose of PAXIL in the treatment of panic disorder is 40mg/day. Individuals should be started on 10mg/day. Dose changes should occur in 10mg/week increments and at intervals of at least one week. Individuals are dosed in a range of 10 to 60mg/day of PAXIL The maximum dosage should not exceed 60mg/day.

Maintenance Treatment—While there are no systematic studies that answer the question of how long to continue PAXIL, it is generally agreed among experts that acute episodes of depression require several months or longer of sustained pharmacologic therapy. Whether the dose of antidepressant needed to induce remission is identical to the dose needed to maintain or sustain euthymia is unknown.

Because OCD and Anxiety/Panic Disorders are chronic conditions, it is reasonable to consider continuation for a responding individual with dosage adjustments made to maintain the individual on the lowest effective dosage, and the individual should be periodically reassessed to determine the need for further treatment.

Overdosage

Signs and symptoms of overdose with PAXIL included nausea, vomiting, drowsiness, sinus tachycardia, and dilated pupils. There were no reports of ECG abnormalities, coma, or convulsions following overdosage with Paxil alone.

PROZAC

(Fluoxetine)

Prozac is an antidepressant for oral administration; it is chemically unrelated to tricyclic, tetracyclic, or other available antidepressant agents.

Pharmacodynamics

The antidepressant and anti-obsessive-compulsive action of PROZAC is presumed to be linked to its inhibition of CNS neuronal uptake of serotonin into platelets.

Pharmacokinetics

- Following a single oral 40mg dose, peak plasma concentrations of PROZAC are observed after 6 to 8 hours.

- Food does not appear to affect the systemic bioavailability of PROZAC. Thus, PROZAC may be administered with or without food.

- PROZAC is extensively metabolized in the liver. The primary route of elimination appears to be hepatic metabolism to inactive metabolites excreted by the kidney.

- The relatively slow elimination of PROZAC (elimination half-life of 1 to 3 days after acute administration and 4 to 6 days after chronic administration) and its active metabolite, norfluoxetine (elimination half-life of 4 to 16 days after acute and chronic administration), leads to significant accumulation of these active species in chronic use and delayed attainment of steady state, even when a fixed dose is used.

Indications

1. Depression

2. Obsessive-compulsive disorder

3. Tic disorders

4. Eating disorders

5. Anxiety disorders

Pediatric Use—Safety and effectiveness in children have not been established.

Contraindications

1. Individuals known to be hypersensitive to it

2. Use in combination with an MAOI, or within 14 days of discontinuing therapy with an MAOI

Potential Side Effects

Body as a Whole—Chills, fever, cyst, face edema, hangover effect, drowsiness and fatigue or asthenia, jaw pain, neck pain, neck rigidity, and pelvic pain

Neurological System—Tremor, abnormal gait, acute brain syndrome, akathisia, amnesia, apathy, ataxia, buccoglossal syndrome, CNS stimulation, headache, dizziness, seizure or convulsion, hyperkinesia, hypesthesia, incoordination, neuralgia, neuropathy, vertigo

Psychiatric Disorders—Insomnia, abnormal dreams, agitation, delusions, depersonalization, emotional lability, euphoria, hallucinations, hostility, manic reaction, paranoid reaction, psychosis

Cardiovascular System—Angina pectoris, arrhythmia, hemorrhage, hypertension, vasodilatation, hypotension, postural hypotension, syncope, migraine and tachycardia

Gastrointestinal System—Increased or decreased appetite with anorexia or nausea, stomatitis, dysphagia, esophagitis, gastritis, gingivitis, glossitis, abnormal liver function tests, melena, and dry mouth or thirst

Endocrine System—Hypothyroidism

Hematological and Lymphatic Systems—Aplastic anemia and lymphadenopathy

Metabolic System—Weight loss, generalized edema, hypoglycemia, peripheral edema, and weight gain

Musculoskeletal System—Arthritis, bone pain, bursitis, tenosynovitis, and twitching

Respiratory System—Bronchitis, rhinitis, yawn, asthma, epistaxis, hiccup, hyperventilation, and pneumonia

Dermatological System—Acne, alopecia, contact dermatitis, dry skin, herpes simplex, maculopapular rash, urticaria

Special Senses—Amblyopia, conjunctivitis, ear pain, eye pain, mydriasis, photophobia, abnormal vision, tinnitus

Genitourinary System—amenorrhea, breast pain, cystitis, dysuria, fibrocystic breast, leukorrhea, menopause, menorrhagia, ovarian disorder, urinary incontinence, urinary retention, urinary urgency, impaired urination, vaginitis

Sexual Function—Decreased libido, abnormal ejaculation

Potential Drug Interactions

1. Because PROZAC's metabolism involves the cytochrome P450IID6 system, concomitant therapy with drugs also metabolized by this enzyme system (such as the tricyclic antidepressants) may lead to drug interactions. These concomitant medications should be initiated at the low end of the dose range if an individual is receiving PROZAC concurrently or has taken it in the previous 5 weeks. If PROZAC is added to the treatment regimen of an individual already receiving a drug metabolized by P450IID6, the need for decreased dose of the original medication should be considered. Drugs with a narrow therapeutic index represent the greatest concern (e.g., TEGRETOL, and tricyclic antidepressants).

2. PROZAC in combination with tryptophan may cause adverse reactions including agitation, restlessness, and gastrointestinal distress.

3. Both increased and decreased lithium levels have been observed when lithium was used concomitantly with PROZAC.

4. The half-life of concurrently administered VALIUM may be prolonged.

5. PROZAC may increase plasma DILANTIN concentration and cause DILANTIN toxicity.

Dosage and Administration

Because of the long elimination half-lives of PROZAC and its major active metabolite, changes in dose will not be fully reflected in plasma for several weeks, affecting both strategies for titration to final dose and withdrawal from treatment.

In the treatment of depression or obsessive-compulsive disorder, older adolescents and adults may begin with 20mg/day administered in the morning. A 10mg/day weekly increment may be considered after several weeks if no clinical improvement is observed. Doses above 20mg/day may be administered once a day (morning) or twice daily. The full therapeutic effect may be delayed until 5 weeks of treatment or longer. A dose range of 20 to 60mg/day is recommended; however, doses of up to 80mg/day have been well tolerated in open studies of OCD. The maximum PROZAC dose should not exceed 80mg/day.

In children 6 years or older, the initial dose of 10mg/day is recommended. A 5mg/day (using PROZAC Oral Solution) weekly increment may be considered after several weeks if no clinical improvement is observed. A dose range of 20 to 40mg/day is recommended, however, doses of up to 50mg/day have been well tolerated in some children with OCD. A dose exceeding 40-50mg/day may not add any more treatment effect, but tends to increase the risk of side effects.

In children younger than 6 years-of-age, PROZAC has been used unlabeled for "perseverative speech," "repetitive behaviors," or "difficulty with transitions." An initial dose of 0.5 to 1mg/day (using PROZAC Oral Solution) is recommended. A 0.5-1mg/day weekly increment may be considered after several weeks if no clinical improvement is observed. A dose range of 2 to 15mg/day is recommended. The dose exceeds 15-20mg/day usually does not add any more treatment effect. It tends to increase the risk of side effects.

Maintenance—While there are no systematic studies that answer the question of how long to continue PROZAC, it is generally agreed among experts that acute episodes of depression require several months or longer of sustained pharmacologic therapy. Whether the dose of antidepressant needed to induce remission is identical to the dose needed to maintain and/or sustain euthymia is unknown.

Because OCD is a chronic condition, it is reasonable to consider continuation for a responding individual with dosage adjustments made to maintain the individual on the lowest effective dosage, and the individual should be periodically reassessed to determine the need for further treatment.

Overdosage

Nausea and vomiting were prominent in overdoses involving PROZAC. Other prominent symptoms of overdose included agitation, restlessness, hypomania, and other signs of CNS excitation.

REMERON

(Mirtazapine)

Pharmacodynamics

REMERON works by its central presynaptic alpha2-adrenergic antagonist effects, which results in increased release of norepinephrine and serotonin. It is also a potent antagonist of 5HT2 and 5HT3 serotonin receptors and H1 histamine receptors and a moderate peripheral alpha1-adrenergic and muscarinic antagonist.

Pharmacokinetics

- Protein binding is about 85%.
- REMERON is extensively metabolized in the liver by cytochrome p-450.
- Bioavailability is about 50%.
- Half-life is 20-40 hours.
- Time to peak serum concentration is about 2 hours.
- REMERON is eliminated extensively via renal system (75%) and about 15% via feces.

Indications

For the treatment of depression

Pediatric Use—Safety and effectiveness in pediatric patients have not been established.

Potential Side Effects

Body as a Whole—Malaise, headache, infection, pain, chest pain, abdominal pain, abdominal syndrome, weight gain, chills, fever, face edema, ulcer, photosensitivity reaction, neck rigidity, neck pain, enlarged abdomen

Neurological System—Hypertonia, hypesthesia, apathy, hypokinesia, vertigo, dizziness, twitching, hyperkinesia, paresthesia, ataxia, delirium, dyskinesia, extrapyramidal syndrome, coordination abnormal, dysarthria, hallucinations, manic reaction, neurosis, dystonia, hostility, increased reflexes, emotional lability, euphoria, and paranoid reaction

Psychiatric Disorders—Depression, agitation, anxiety, nervousness, amnesia, insomnia, somnolence, delusions, depersonalization, activation of mania/hypomania

Cardiovascular System—Hypertension, vasodilatation, palpitation, tachycardia, postural hypotension, angina pectoris, myocardial infarction, miocardia, ventricular extrasystoles, syncope, migraine, hypotension

Gastrointestinal System—Increased appetite, nausea, dyspepsia, anorexia, diarrhea, flatulence, vomiting, eructation, glossitis, cholecystitis, nausea and vomiting, gum hemorrhage, stomatitis, colitis, abnormal liver function tests

Metabolic System—Non-fasting cholesterol increases, thirst, dehydration, weight loss

Musculoskeletal System—myasthenia, arthralgia, arthritis, and tenosynovitis

Respiratory System—Increased cough, sinusitis, pharyngitis, epistaxis, bronchitis, asthma, pneumonia

Dermatological System—Pruritus, rash, sweating, acne, exfoliative dermatitis, dry skin, herpes simplex, alopecia

Special Senses—Rhinitis, amblyopia, tinnitus, taste perversion, eye pain, abnormality of accommodation, conjunctivitis, deafness, keratoconjunctivitis, lacrimation disorder, glaucoma, hyperacusis, ear pain

Genitourinary System—Urinary tract infection, kidney calculus, cystitis, dysuria, urinary incontinence, urinary retention, vaginitis, hematuria, breast pain, amenorrhea, dysmenorrhea, leukorrhea, breast enlargement, and urinary urgency

Sexual Function—Impotence, increased libido, or decreased libido

Potential Drug Interactions

Serious, and sometimes fatal, reactions (e.g., nausea, vomiting, flushing, dizziness, tremor, myoclonus, rigidity, diaphoresis, hyperthermia, autonomic instability with rapid fluctuations of vital signs, seizures, and mental status changes ranging from agitation to coma) may occur in individuals receiving REMERON in combination with an MAOI or in individuals who have recently discontinued REMERON and then are started on an MAOI.

Laboratory Tests

There are no routine laboratory tests recommended. But if an individual develops a sore throat, fever, stomatitis, or other signs of infection, a complete blood cell count (CBC) should be done. If a low white blood cell (WBC) count (agranulocytosis) is found, treatment with REMERON should be discontinued and the individual should be closely monitored.

Dosage and Administration

In adults, the initial dose is 15mg nightly; titrate up to 15-45mg/day with dosage increases no more frequently than every 1-2 weeks. There is an inverse relationship between dose and sedation.

Overdosage

Signs and symptoms in association with overdose include disorientation, drowsiness, impaired memory, and tachycardia. There were no reports of ECG abnormalities, coma, or convulsions following overdose with REMERON alone.

REVIA

(Naltrexone)

Pharmacodynamics

REVIA is a pure opioid antagonist. It markedly attenuates or completely blocks, reversibly, the subjective effects of intravenously administered opioids. REVIA blocks the effects of opioids by competitive binding (i.e., analogous to competitive inhibition of enzymes) at opioid receptors. When co-administered with morphine, on a chronic basis, REVIA blocks the physical dependence to morphine, heroin, and other opioids.

Pharmacokinetics

- REVIA is well absorbed orally and is subject to significant first pass metabolism with oral bioavailability estimates ranging from 5 to 40%.

- Following oral administration, REVIA undergoes rapid and nearly complete absorption with approximately 96% of the dose absorbed from the gastrointestinal tract. Peak plasma levels of REVIA occur within one hour of dosing.

- Both parent drug and metabolites are excreted primarily by the kidneys.
- The mean elimination half-life value for REVIA is 4 hours.

Indications

1. For the treatment of alcohol dependence and for the blockade of the effects of exogenously administered opioids

2. Unlabeled use for the treatment of self-injurious behaviors

3. Unlabeled use for the treatment of social withdrawal

4. Unlabeled use for the treatment of ADHD

Pediatric Use -The safe use of REVIA in subjects younger than 18 years has not been established.

Contraindications

1. Individuals receiving opioid analgesics

2. Individuals currently dependent on opioids

3. Individuals in acute opioid withdrawal

4. Any individual who has failed the NARCAN challenge test or who has a positive urine screen for opioids

5. Any individual with a history of sensitivity to REVIA

6. Any individual with acute hepatitis or liver failure

Potential Side Effects

Body as Whole—Increased energy, low energy, chills, abdominal pain/cramps, headache, weight loss, weight gain, yawning, somnolence, fever, dry mouth, pounding head, inguinal pain, swollen glands, side pains, cold feet, hot spells

Psychiatric Disorders—Feeling down, irritability, dizziness, difficulty sleeping, anxiety, nervousness, depression, paranoia, fatigue, restlessness, confusion, disorientation, hallucinations, nightmares, bad dreams

Respiratory System—Nasal congestion, itching, rhinorrhea, sneezing, sore throat, excess mucus or phlegm, sinus trouble, heavy breathing, hoarseness, cough, shortness of breath

Cardiovascular System—Nose bleeds, phlebitis, edema, increased blood pressure, non-specific ECG changes, palpitations, tachycardia

Gastrointestinal System—Loss of appetite, nausea and/or vomiting, diarrhea, constipation, increased thirst, elevations of serum transaminases (SGOT, SGPT), increased appetite, excessive gas, hemorrhoids, diarrhea, and ulcer

Muscular and Skeletal Systems—Joint and muscle pain, twitching

Genitourinary System—Increased frequency of or discomfort during urination

Sexual Function—Delayed ejaculation, decreased potency, increased or decreased sexual interest

Dermatological System—Skin rash, oily skin, pruritus, acne, athlete's foot, cold sores, alopecia

Special Senses—Eyes-blurred, burning, light sensitive, swollen, aching, strained; ears-clogged, aching, tinnitus (ringing in the ears)

Potential Drug Interactions

1. Lethargy and somnolence have been reported following doses of REVIA and MELLARIL.

2. Individuals taking REVIA may not benefit from opioid containing medicines, such as cough and cold preparations, antidiarrheal preparations, and opioid analgesics. In an emergency situation when opioid analgesia must be administered to an individual receiving REVIA, the amount of opioid required may be greater than usual, and the resulting respiratory depression may be deeper and more prolonged.

Withdrawal Symptoms

Severe opioid withdrawal syndromes precipitated by the accidental ingestion of REVIA have been reported in opioid-dependent individuals. Symptoms of withdrawal have usually appeared within five minutes of ingestion of REVIA and have lasted for up to 48 hours. Mental status changes including confusion, somnolence and visual hallucinations have occurred. Significant fluid losses from vomiting and diarrhea have required intravenous fluid administration.

Laboratory Tests

REVIA causes hepatocellular injury in a substantial proportion of individuals exposed at higher doses. A high index of suspicion for drug-related hepatic injury is critical if the occurrence of liver damage induced by REVIA is to be detected at the earliest possible time. Evaluations using appropriate batteries of tests to detect liver injury are recommended at a frequency appropriate to the clinical situation and the dose of REVIA.

Dosage and Administration

Only dosage and administration for the treatment of self-injurious behaviors, social withdrawal, and ADHD are included here. In the treatment of self-injurious behaviors in older adolescents and adults, the dose is 0.5-2mg/kg/day in divided doses (two-to-three times daily).

Overdosage

There is limited clinical experience with REVIA overdosage in humans. In one study, subjects who received 800mg daily REVIA for up to one week showed no evidence of toxicity.

RISPERDAL

(Risperidone)

Pharmacodynamics

The mechanism of action of RISPERDAL is unknown. However, it has been proposed that this drug's antipsychotic activity is mediated through a combination of dopamine type 2 (D2) and serotonin type 2 (5HT2) antagonism.

Pharmacokinetics

- Risperidone is extensively metabolized in the liver.

- Food does not affect either the rate or extent of absorption of RISPERDAL. Thus, RISPERDAL can be given with or without meals.

- The mean peak plasma concentration of RISPERDAL occurs at about 1 hour.

- The half-life of RISPERDAL is three hours in extensive metabolizers and 20 hours in poor metabolizers.

- Steady-state concentrations of RISPERDAL are reached in 1 day in extensive metabolizers and in about 5 days in poor metabolizers.

Pediatric Use—Safety and effectiveness in children have not been established.

Indications

1. Management of psychotic disorders

2. Unlabeled use in controlling frequent and severe tantrums with aggression or aggressive behaviors in individuals with ASD or other developmental disorders

Contraindications

RISPERDAL is contraindicated in patients with a known hypersensitivity to the product.

Potential Side Effects

Body as a Whole—Fatigue, edema, rigors, malaise, influenza-like symptoms

Neurological System—Increased sleep duration, dysarthria, vertigo, stupor, paresthesia, confusion, seizures

Psychiatric Disorders—Increased dream activity, diminished sexual desire, nervousness, impaired concentration, depression, apathy, catatonic reaction, euphoria, increased libido, amnesia

Gastrointestinal Disorders—Anorexia, reduced salivation, flatulence, diarrhea, increased appetite, stomatitis, melena, dysphagia, hemorrhoids, gastritis

Respiratory System Disorders—Hyperventilation, bronchospasm, pneumonia, stridor

Dermatological System—Increased pigmentation, photosensitivity, increased sweating, acne, decreased sweating, alopecia, hyperkeratosis, pruritus, skin exfoliation

Cardiovascular System—Palpitation, hypertension, hypotension, AV block, myocardial infarction, prolonged QT interval

Metabolic and Nutritional System—Hyponatremia, weight increase, creatine phosphokinase increase, thirst, weight decrease, diabetes mellitus

Genitourinary System—Polyuria, polydipsia, urinary incontinence, hematuria, dysuria

Muscular and Skeletal System—Myalgia

Liver and Biliary System—Increased SGOT, increased SGPT

Hematological System—Epistaxis, purpura, anemia, hypochromic anemia

Vision Disorders—Abnormal accommodation, or xerophthalmia

Reproductive Disorders in Females—Menorrhagia, orgasmic dysfunction, dry vagina, non-puerperal lactation, amenorrhea, female breast pain, leukorrhea, mastitis, dysmenorrhea, female perineal pain, intermenstrual bleeding, vaginal hemorrhage

Reproductive Disorders in Male—Erectile dysfunction, ejaculation failure

Potential Drug Interaction

1. When RISPERDAL is taken in combination with other centrally acting drugs and alcohol, because of its potential for inducing hypotension, RISPERDAL may enhance the hypotensive effects of other therapeutic agents with this potential.

2. RISPERDAL may antagonize the effects of levodopa and dopamine agonists

3. Chronic administration of TEGRETOL with RISPERDAL may increase the clearance of RISPERDAL

4. Chronic administration of CLOZARIL with RISPERDAL may decrease the clearance of RISPERDAL.

Dosage and Administration

Initial Dose—RISPERDAL should be administered on a twice daily schedule, generally beginning with 1mg twice daily initially, with increases in increments of 1mg twice/day on the second and third day, as tolerated, to a target dose of 3mg twice/day by the third day. For dosages above 3mg twice/day, slower titration may be medically appropriate.

Antipsychotic efficacy had been demonstrated in a dose range of 4 to 16mg/day, however, maximum effect was generally seen in a range of 4 to 6mg/day. Doses above 6mg/day are not more efficacious than lower doses, are associated with more extrapyramidal symptoms and other adverse effects, and are not generally recommended.

Maintenance Therapy—While it is unclear how long the individual with schizophrenia being treated with RISPERDAL should remain on it, it is recommended that responding individuals be continued on RISPERDAL, but at the lowest dose needed to maintain remission. Individuals should be periodically reassessed to determine the need for maintenance treatment. In individuals with ASD and using RISPERDAL to control frequent temper outbursts with aggressions, there is no data to support maintenance therapy. Periodical reinitiation of treatment may be more appropriate.

Reinitiation of Treatment in Patients Previously Discontinued—Although there are no data to specifically address reinitiation of treatment, it is recommended that when restarting individuals who have had an interval off RISPERDAL, the initial titration schedule should be followed.

Switching from Other Antipsychotics. There are no systematically collected data to specifically address switching from other antipsychotics to RISPERDAL or concerning concomitant administration with other antipsychotics. In general, it may be more appropriate to begin titration of RISPERDAL while gradually discontinuing the other antipsychotic. In all cases, the period of overlapping antipsychotic administration should be minimized. The need for continuing existing EPS medication should be reevaluated periodically.

Overdosage

In general, symptoms of overdosage include: drowsiness and sedation, tachycardia, hypotension, extrapyramidal symptoms, hyponatremia, hypokalemia, prolonged QT and widened QRS, seizure, cardiopulmonary arrest, and rare fatality associated with multiple drug overdose.

RITALIN and RITALIN-SR

(Methylphenidate and Methylphenidate Hydrochloride Sustained-Release Tablets)

Pharmacodynamics

RITALIN is a mild central nervous system stimulant. The mode of action in humans is not completely understood, but RITALIN presumably activates the brain stem arousal system and cortex to produce its stimulant effect. There is neither specific evidence that clearly establishes the mechanism whereby RITALIN produces its mental and behavioral effects in children, nor conclusive evidence regarding how these effects relate to the condition of the central nervous system.

Pharmacokinetics

- RITALIN-SR is more slowly but as extensively absorbed as are the regular tablets.

- The time to peak rate in children is about 5 hours (1-8 hours) for the SR tablets and 2 hours (0.5-4 hours) for the regular tablets.

Indications

1. Attention Deficit- Hyperactivity Disorders

2. Narcolepsy

Pediatric Use—Safety and efficacy of RITALIN in children under six years have not been established and sufficient data on safety and efficacy of long-term use of RITALIN in children are not yet available.

Contraindications

1. Marked anxiety, tension, and agitation are contraindications to RITALIN, since the drug may aggravate these symptoms.

2. RITALIN is contraindicated in individuals known to be hypersensitive to the drug.

3. RITALIN is contraindicated for individuals with glaucoma, motor tics, or with a diagnosis or family history of Tourette syndrome.

Potential Side Effects

Neurological System—dizziness, headache, visual disturbances, dyskinesia, drowsiness

Psychiatric Disorders—Nervousness, insomnia, Tourette syndrome, toxic psychosis, transient depressed mood, exacerbated symptoms of behavior disturbance and thought disorder in psychotic children

Dermatological System—Hypersensitivity including skin rash, urticaria, fever, arthralgia, exfoliative dermatitis, erythema multiforme with histopathological findings of necrotizing vasculitis, and thrombocytopenic purpura

Gastrointestinal System—Anorexia, nausea, abdominal pain, abnormal liver function

Cardiovascular System—Palpitations, both up and down blood pressure and pulse changes, tachycardia, angina, cardiac arrhythmia

Endocrinological System—Weight loss during prolonged therapy

Potential Drug Interactions

1. RITALIN may decrease the hypotensive effect of guanethidine. Use cautiously with pressor agents and MAO inhibitors.

2. RITALIN may inhibit the metabolism of Coumadin anticoagulants, anticonvulsants (LIMINAL, DILANTIN, MYSOLINE), phenylbutazone, and tricyclic drugs (TOFRANIL, ANAFRANIL, NORPRAMIN). Downward dosage adjustments of these drugs may be required when given concomitantly with RITALIN.

3. RITALIN may lower the convulsive threshold in individuals with prior history of seizures, prior EEG abnormalities in absence of seizures, and, very rarely, in absence of history of seizures and no prior EEG evidence of seizures. Safe concomitant use of anticonvulsants and Ritalin has not been established. In the presence of seizures, the drug should be discontinued.

Drug Dependence

Chronically abusive use can lead to marked tolerance and psychic dependence with varying degrees of abnormal behavior. Frank psychotic episodes can occur, especially with parenteral abuse.

Withdrawal Symptoms

Careful supervision is required during drug withdrawal, since severe depression as well as the effects of chronic overactivity can be unmasked.

Laboratory Tests

Periodic CBC, differential, platelet counts, and liver function tests are advised during prolonged therapy.

Dosage and Administration

Regular Tablets—Administer in divided doses 2 or 3 times daily, preferably 30 to 45 minutes before meals. Individuals who have significant suppressed appetite from taking RITALIN should take it after meals. In adults, average dosage is 20 to 30mg daily. Some individuals may require 40 to 60mg daily. In others, 10 to 15mg daily will be adequate. In children, RITALIN should be initiated in small doses (5mg twice daily), with gradual weekly increments of 5 to 10mg. Daily dosage above 60mg is not recommended. The average dosage can be calculated based on body weight at the rate of 0.3-2.0mg/kg/day. Individuals who are unable to sleep if medication is taken late in the day should take the last dose before 6 p.m.

SR Tablets—RITALIN-SR tablets have a duration of action of approximately 8 hours. Therefore, RITALIN-SR tablets may be used in place of regular RITALIN tablets when the 8-hour dosage of

RITALIN-SR corresponds to the titrated 8-hour dosage of regular RITALIN. *RITALIN-SR tablets must be swallowed whole and never crushed or chewed.*

- If improvement is not observed after appropriate dosage adjustment over a one-month period, the drug should be discontinued.

- If paradoxical aggravation of symptoms or other adverse effects occur, reduce dosage, or, if necessary, discontinue the drug.

- RITALIN should be periodically discontinued to assess the child's condition. Improvement may be sustained when the drug is either temporarily or permanently discontinued.

- RITALIN treatment should not and need not be indefinite and usually may be discontinued after puberty.

Overdosage

Signs and symptoms of acute overdosage may include agitation, tremors, hyperreflexia, muscle twitching, convulsions (may be followed by coma), euphoria, confusion, hallucinations, delirium, sweating, flushing, headache, hyperpyrexia, tachycardia, palpitations, cardiac arrhythmias, hypertension, mydriasis, and dryness of mucous membranes.

SERAX®

(Oxazepam)

Pharmacodynamics

SERAX produce CNS depression at the subcortical level, except at high doses, whereby it works at the cortical level. SERAX facilitates the action of GABA.

Pharmacokinetics

- The absorption of SERAX is almost complete.

- Protein binding is 85% to 99%.

- Peak plasma level is reached about 3 hours after oral administration.

- The mean elimination half-life is approximately 8 hours (range 6 to 11 hours).

- A single, major inactive metabolite, a glucuronide, is excreted in the urine.

Indications

1. Anxiety disorders or the short-term relief of the symptoms of anxiety

2. Anxiety associated with depression

3. Anxiety, tension, agitation, and irritability in older individuals

4. Alcoholics with acute tremulousness, inebriation, or with anxiety associated with alcohol withdrawal

Pediatric Use—Safety and effectiveness in children less than 6 years-of-age have not been established. Absolute dosage for children 6 to 12 years-of-age is not established.

Contraindications

1. History of previous hypersensitivity reaction to SERAX

2. Past or current psychoses.

Potential Side Effects

Side effects caused by SERAX are few and infrequent.

Neurological System—Transient mild drowsiness, dizziness, vertigo, headache, ataxia, slurred speech, tremor

Psychiatric Disorders—Mild paradoxical reactions (excitement, stimulation of affect), lethargy

Potential Drug Interactions

The effects of alcohol or other CNS-depressant medications may be additive to those of SERAX, possibly requiring adjustment of dosage or elimination of such agents.

Drug Abuse and Dependence

SERAX may produce psychological and physical dependence.

Withdrawal Symptoms

Symptoms of convulsions, tremor, abdominal and muscle cramps, vomiting, sweating, dysphoria, and insomnia have occurred following abrupt discontinuance of SERAX. The more severe withdrawal symptoms have usually been limited to those individuals who received excessive doses over an extended period of time. After extended therapy, abrupt discontinuation should be avoided and a gradual dosage tapering schedule be followed.

Laboratory Tests

Although rare, leukopenia and hepatic dysfunction including jaundice have been reported during therapy. Periodic blood counts and liver-function tests are advisable.

Dosage and Administration

Because of the flexibility of this product and the range of emotional disturbances responsive to it, dosage should be individualized for maximum beneficial effects. In children, the dose is 1mg/kg/day. In older adolescents and adults, the dosage for anxiety disorders is 10-30mg 3-4 times daily, for use as a hypnotic dosage is 15-30mg.

Overdosage

Overdosage of SERAX is usually manifested by varying degrees of central nervous system depression ranging from drowsiness to coma. In mild cases, symptoms include drowsiness, mental confusion, and lethargy. In more serious cases, and especially when other medications or alcohol were ingested, symptoms may include ataxia hypotonia, hypotension, hypnotic state, coma, and very rarely, death.

SEROQUEL

(Quetiapine fumarate)

Pharmacodynamics

SEROQUEL is an antipsychotic drug belonging to a new chemical class, the dibenzothiazepine derivatives. SEROQUEL is an antagonist at multiple neurotransmitter receptors in the brain: serotonin $5HT_{1A}$ and $5HT_2$, dopamine D_1 and D_2, histamine H_1, and adrenergic a_1 and a_2 receptors.

The mechanism of action of SEROQUEL is unknown. However, it has been proposed that this drug's antipsychotic activity is mediated through a combination of dopamine type 2 (D_2) and serotonin type 2 ($5-HT_2$) antagonism. Antagonism at receptors other than dopamine and $5HT_2$ with similar receptor affinities may explain some of the other effects of SEROQUEL. SEROQUEL's antagonism of histamine H_1 receptors may explain the somnolence observed with this drug, and antagonism of adrenergic at receptors may explain the orthostatic hypotension observed.

Pharmacokinetics

- SEROQUEL is rapidly absorbed after oral administration, reaching peak Plasma concentrations in 1.5 hours.

- The bioavailability of SEROQUEL is marginally affected by administration with food.

- It is 83% bound to plasma proteins at therapeutic concentrations.

- Steady state concentrations are usually achieved within two days of dosing.

- Elimination of SEROQUEL is mainly via hepatic metabolism.

- Terminal half-life is about 6 hours.

- The liver extensively metabolizes SEROQUEL.

Indications

1. Management of psychotic disorders

2. Unlabeled use in controlling rages and frequent temper outbursts with aggression or destruction

Pediatric Use—The safety and effectiveness of SEROQUEL in pediatric patients have not been established.

Contraindications

SEROQUEL is contraindicated in individuals with a known hypersensitivity to this medication or any of its ingredients.

Potential Side Effects

Body as a Whole—Flu syndrome, weight gain, headache, asthenia, abdominal pain, back pain, fever, neck pain, pelvic pain, suicide attempt, malaise, photosensitivity reaction, chills, face edema, moniliasis

Neurological System—Hypertonia, dysarthria, dizziness, dyskinesia, tardive dyskinesia, vertigo, involuntary movements, confusion, amnesia, hyperkinesia, incoordination, abnormal gait, myoclonus, ataxia, stupor, bruxism, catatonic reaction, hemiplegia, seizure

Psychiatric Disorders—Somnolence, abnormal dreams, abnormal thinking, psychosis, hallucinations, paranoid reaction, manic reaction, apathy, depersonalization, delusions

Gastrointestinal System—Dysphagia anorexia, constipation, dry mouth, dyspepsia, increased salivation, increased appetite, increased gamma glutamyl transpeptidase, gingivitis, dysphagia, flatulence, gastroenteritis, gastritis, hemorrhoids, stomatitis, thirst, tooth caries, fecal incontinence, gastroesophageal reflux, gum hemorrhage, mouth ulceration, rectal hemorrhage, tongue edema

Hepatic System—Increased SGPT, total cholesterol and triglycerides

Cardiovascular System—Orthostatic hypotension, palpitation, tachycardia, syncope, vasodilatation, prolonged QT interval, migraine, bradycardia, cerebral ischemia, irregular pulse, T-wave abnormality, bundle branch block, cerebrovascular accident, deep thrombophlebitis, T-wave inversion

Respiratory System—Pharyngitis, rhinitis, increased cough, dyspnea, aspiration pneumonia, pneumonia, epistaxis, asthma

Metabolic and Nutritional System—Peripheral edema, weight loss, alkaline phosphatase increased, hyperlipemia, alcohol intolerance, dehydration, hyperglycemia, creatinine increased, hypoglycemia

Dermatological System—Rash, sweating, pruritus, acne, eczema, contact dermatitis, maculopapular rash, seborrhea, skin ulcer

Muscular and Skeletal Systems—Pathological fracture, myasthenia, twitching, arthralgia, arthritis, leg cramps, bone pain

Hematological and Lymphatic Systems—Leukopenia, leukocytosis, anemia, ecchymosis, eosinophilia, hypochromic anemia, lymphadenopathy, cyanosis

Endocrine System—Hypothyroidism, diabetes mellitus

Urogenital System—Dysmenorrhea, vaginitis, urinary incontinence, urinary retention, metrorrhagia, dysuria, vaginal moniliasis, cystitis, urinary frequency, amenorrhea, female lactation, leukorrhea, vaginal hemorrhage, vulvovaginitis orchitis

Sexual Function—Impotence, abnormal ejaculation, increased libido

Special Senses—Ear pain, conjunctivitis, abnormal vision, dry eyes, tinnitus, taste perversion, blepharitis, eye pain

Potential Drug Interactions

1. The elimination SEROQUEL was enhanced in the presence of DILANTIN. Higher maintenance doses of SEROQUEL may be required when it is co-administered with DILANTIN and other enzyme inducers such as TEGRETOL and LUMINAL.

2. The mean oral clearance of ATIVAN may be reduced in the presence of SEROQUEL.

3. SEROQUEL may enhance the effects of certain antihypertensive agents.

4. SEROQUEL may antagonize the effects of levodopa and dopamine agonists.

5. MELLARIL may increase the oral clearance of SEROQUEL.

6. Administration of multiple daily doses of TAGAMET may decrease the mean oral clearance of SEROQUEL.

Laboratory Tests

SEROQUEL may cause cataracts. Examination of the lens by methods adequate to detect cataract formation, such as slit lamp exam or other appropriately sensitive methods, is recommended at initiation of treatment or shortly thereafter, and at 6-month intervals during chronic treatment.

Dosage and Administration

For treatment of schizophrenia or other psychotic disorders in older adolescents and adults, SEROQUEL should generally be administered with an initial dose of 25mg twice daily with increments of 25-50mg twice or three times daily on the second and third day, as tolerated, to a target dose range of 300 to 400mg daily by the fourth day in divided doses. Further dosage adjustments, if indicated, should generally occur at intervals of not less than 2 days, as steady state for SEROQUEL would not be achieved for approximately 1-2 days in the typical individuals. When dosage adjustments are necessary, dose increments/decrements of 25-50mg twice daily are recommended. Doses above 300mg/day most likely would not be more efficacious than the 300mg/day dose.

When SEROQUEL is used unlabeled to manage rages or frequent temper outbursts with aggressions and destructive behaviors, begin with 50-100mg twice daily. If necessary, dose increments of 25-50mg/day up to 300-400mg/day in divided doses may be used.

Maintenance Treatment

Responding individuals should be continued on SEROQUEL, but at the lowest dose needed to maintain remission. Patients should be periodically reassessed to determine the need for maintenance treatment.

Reinitiation of Treatment

When restarting individuals who have had an interval of less than one week off SEROQUEL, titration of SEROQUEL is not required and the maintenance dose may be reinitiated. When restarting therapy of patients who have been off SEROQUEL for more than one week, the initial titration schedule should be followed.

Switching from Other Antipsychotics

There are no systematically collected data to specifically address switching from other antipsychotics to SEROQUEL.

Overdosage

Signs and symptoms include those resulting from an exaggeration of the drug's known pharmacological effects, i.e., drowsiness and sedation, tachycardia, and hypotension.

Management and Treatment of Overdosage

There is no specific antidote to SEROQUEL. Therefore appropriate supportive measures should be instituted in case of acute overdosage. An airway should be established and maintained with adequate oxygenation and ventilation. Gastric lavage (after intubation, if patient is unconscious) and administration of activated charcoal together with a laxative should be considered. The possibility of obtundation, seizure, or dystonic reaction of the head and neck following overdose may create a risk of aspiration with induced emesis.

Cardiovascular monitoring should commence immediately and should include continuous electrocardiographic monitoring to detect possible arrhythmias. If antiarrhythmic therapy is administered, disopyramide, procainamide and quinidine carry a theoretical hazard of additive QT-prolonging effects when administered in patients with acute overdosage of SEROQUEL.

It is reasonable to expect that the alpha adrenergic-blocking properties of bretylium might be additive to those of SEROQUEL, resulting in problematic hypotension. Hypotension and circulatory collapse should be treated with appropriate measures such as intravenous fluids and/or sympathomimetic agents (epinephrine and dopamine should not be used, since beta stimulation may worsen hypotension in the setting of Quetiapine-induced alpha blockade). In cases of severe extrapyramidal symptoms, anticholinergic medication should be administered. Close medical supervision and monitoring should continue until the patient recovers.

SERZONE

(Nefazodone)

SERZONE is an antidepressant for oral administration with a chemical structure unrelated to selective serotonin reuptake inhibitors, tricyclics, tetracyclics, or monoamine oxidase inhibitors (MAOIs).

Pharmacodynamics

SERZONE inhibits neuronal uptake of serotonin and norepinephrine. SERZONE occupies central 5-HT2 receptors and acts as an antagonist at this receptor. It also antagonizes alpha-adrenergic receptors, a property which may be associated with postural hypotension.

Pharmacokinetics

- SERZONE is rapidly and completely absorbed but is subject to extensive metabolism, so that its absolute bioavailability is low, about 20%, and variable.

- Food delays the absorption of SERZONE and decreases the bioavailability of SERZONE by approximately 20%.

- Peak plasma concentrations occur at about one hour.

- The half-life of SERZONE is about 2-4 hours.

- Steady-state plasma concentration of SERZONE is attained within 4 to 5 days of initiation of dosing.

- SERZONE is widely distributed in body tissues, including the central nervous system.

- SERZONE is extensively (>99%) bound to plasma proteins

Indications

SERZONE is labeled for treatment of depression.

Pediatric Use—Safety and effectiveness in individuals below 18 years-of-age have not been established.

Contraindications

1. Co-administration of terfenadine, asternizole or cisapride with SERZONE is contraindicated.

2. SERZONE is contraindicated in individuals with known hypersensitivity to nefazodone or other phenylpiperazine antidepressants.

Potential Side Effects

Body as a Whole—Asthenia, headache, flu syndrome, migraine, sweating, chills, fever, neck rigidity, abdominal pain, back pain, chest pain, neck pain, breast pain, allergic reaction, malaise, photosensitivity reaction, face edema, hangover effect, enlarged abdomen, hernia, pelvic pain, and halitosis

Neurological System—Dizziness, memory impairment, paresthesia, abnormal dreams, decreased concentration, ataxia, incoordination, psychomotor retardation, tremor, hypertonia, myalgia, cramp, hypesthesia, CNS stimulation, vertigo, twitching, abnormal gait, neuralgia, dysarthria, myoclonus

Psychiatric Disorders—Activation of mania/hypomania, somnolence, confusion, insomnia, agitation, anxiety, depression, dysphoria, emotional lability, depersonalization, hallucinations, suicide attempt, apathy, euphoria, hostility, suicidal thoughts, abnormal thinking, decreased attention, derealization, paranoid reaction, suicide

Cardiovascular System—Bradycardia, palpitation, postural hypotension, vasodilatation, tachycardia, hypertension, syncope, ventricular extrasystoles, and angina pectoris

Dermatological System—Pruritus, rash, dry skin, acne, alopecia, urticaria, maculopapular rash, vesiculobullous rash, eczema.

Gastrointestinal System—Gastroenteritis, dry mouth, nausea, anorexia, vomiting, constipation, dyspepsia, diarrhea, increased appetite, eructation, periodontal abscess, abnormal liver function tests, gingivitis, colitis, gastritis, mouth ulceration, stomatitis, esophagitis, peptic ulcer, and rectal hemorrhage

Hematological and Lymphatic Systems—Ecchymosis, anemia, leukopenia, and lymphadenopathy

Metabolic and Nutritional Systems—Weight gain, peripheral edema, thirst, weight loss, gout, dehydration, increased lactic dehydrogenase, increased SGOT, and increased SGPT

Muscular and Skeletal Systems—Arthralgia, arthritis, tenosynovitis, muscle stiffness, and bursitis

Respiratory System—Dyspnea and bronchitis, pharyngitis, increased cough, asthma, pneumonia, laryngitis, voice alteration, epistaxis, hiccup

Genitourinary System—Urinary frequency, urinary tract infection, urinary retention, dysmenorrhea, dysuria, vaginitis, cystitis, urinary urgency, metrorrhagia, amenorrhea, polyuria, vaginal hemorrhage, breast enlargement, menorrhagia, urinary incontinence, hematuria, nocturia, and kidney calculus

Sexual Function—decreased libido, increased libido, impotence, abnormal ejaculation

Special Senses—Blurred vision, abnormal vision, visual field defect, eye pain, tinnitus, taste perversion, sinusitis, rhinitis, dry eye, ear pain, abnormality of accommodation, diplopia, conjunctivitis, mydriasis, keratoconjunctivitis, hyperacusis, and photophobia

Potential Drug Interactions

1. In individuals receiving SERZONE in combination with a monoamine oxidase inhibitor (MAOI), there may be serious, sometimes fatal, reactions including hyperthermia, rigidity, myoclonus, autonomic instability with possible rapid fluctuations of vital signs, and mental status changes that include extreme agitation progressing to delirium and coma. These reactions may also occur in individuals who have recently discontinued SERZONE and have been started on an MAOI.

2. When triazolam or alprazolam is administered concomitantly with SERZONE, there may be substantial and clinically important increases in plasma concentrations of these compounds.

3. When HALDOL is co-administered with SERZONE, at steady state, clearance of Haldol may be decreased by 35% with no significant increase in peak Haldol plasma concentrations or time of peak, but dosage adjustment of Haldol may be necessary when co-administered with SERZONE.

Dosage and Administration

Initial Treatment

In older adolescents and adults, the recommended starting dose for SERZONE is 200mg/day administered in two divided doses. After one-to-two weeks, if necessary, the dose can be increased 100-200mg/day on a twice-daily schedule at intervals of no less than 1 week up to 600mg/day. Several weeks on treatment may be required to obtain a full antidepressant response.

In children 6 years and older, the recommended initial dose for is 100mg/day on a twice daily schedule. After two weeks, if necessary, the dose can be increased 50-100mg/day on a twice-daily schedule at intervals of no less than 1 week up to 300-400mg/day. Several weeks on treatment may be required to obtain a full antidepressant response.

Maintenance

SERZONE treatment for acute episodes of depression should continue for up to six months or longer. However, it is unclear whether the dose of SERZONE needed to induce remission is identical to the dose needed to maintain euthymia.

Overdosage

Commonly reported symptoms from overdose of SERZONE include nausea, vomiting, and somnolence.

SINEQUAN

(Doxepin)

Pharmacodynamics

The mechanism of action of SINEQUAN is not definitely known. The current hypothesis is that the clinical effects are due, at least in part, to influences on the adrenergic activity at the synapses so that deactivation of norepinephrine by reuptake into the nerve terminals is prevented.

Pharmacokinetics

- Peak effect of anti-depression may take more than 2 weeks, anxiolytic effects may occur sooner

- About 80% to 85% SINEQUAN binds to serum protein

- Elimination half-life is 6-8 hours

- SINEQUAN is eliminated primarily through the renal system

Indications

1. Psychoneurotic individuals with depression or anxiety

2. Depression or anxiety associated with alcoholism

3. Depression or anxiety associated with organic disease

4. Psychotic depressive disorders with associated anxiety

Pediatric Use—The use of SINEQUAN in children under 12 years-of-age is not recommended because safe conditions for its use have not been established.

Contraindications

Glaucoma, a tendency to urinary retention, or known hypersensitivity to the drug

Potential Side Effects

Body as a Whole—Chills, fatigue, weakness, flushing

Neurological Disorders—Drowsiness, dizziness, disorientation, headache, numbness, paresthesias, ataxia, extrapyramidal symptoms, tardive dyskinesia, tremor, seizures

Psychiatric Disorders—Confusion, hallucinations

Cardiovascular System—Hypotension, hypertension, or tachycardia

Respiratory System—Exacerbation of asthma

Hematologic System—Eosinophilia, agranulocytosis, leukopenia, thrombocytopenia, purpura

Gastrointestinal System—Nausea, vomiting, indigestion, taste disturbances, diarrhea, constipation, anorexia, dry mouth, aphthous stomatitis

Hepatic System—Jaundice

Endocrine System—Weight gain, testicular swelling, gynecomastia in males, enlargement of breasts and galactorrhea in females, raising or lowering of blood sugar levels, inappropriate antidiuretic hormone secretion

Genitourinary System—Urinary retention

Sexual Function—Raised or lowered libido

Dermatologic System—Skin rash, sweating, edema, photosensitization, pruritus, alopecia

Special Sense—Tinnitus, blurred vision

Potential Drug Interactions

1. Medications that inhibit the activity of isoenzyme of cytochrome P450 2D6 may significantly change plasma concentration of SINEQUAN. The medications that inhibit P450 2D6 include quinidine, TAGAMET, many other antidepressants, phenothiazines, and all the serotonin reuptake inhibitors (SRIs). Concomitant use of SINEQUAN with medications that can inhibit cytochrome P450 2D6 may require lower doses than usually prescribed for either SINEQUAN or the other medication. Furthermore, whenever one of these other medications is withdrawn from co-therapy, an increased dose of SINEQUAN may be required.

2. Serious side effects and even death have been reported following the concomitant use of certain drugs with MAO inhibitors. Therefore, MAO inhibitors should be discontinued at least two weeks prior to the cautious initiation of therapy with SINEQUAN.

3. Alcohol ingestion may increase the risk of overdosage with SINEQUAN

Withdrawal Symptoms

The possibility of development of withdrawal symptoms upon abrupt cessation of treatment after prolonged SINEQUAN administration should be borne in mind.

Dosage and Administration

For treatment of mild to moderate depression, a starting daily dose of 75mg is recommended. Dosage may subsequently be increased or decreased at appropriate intervals and according to individual response. The usual optimum dose range is 75mg/day to 150mg/day.

For treatment of severe depression, higher doses may be required with subsequent gradual increase to 300mg/day if necessary. Additional therapeutic effect is rarely obtained by exceeding a dose of 300mg/day.

In individual, with very mild depression accompanying organic disease, lower doses (25-50mg/day) may be adequate.

The total daily dosage of SINEQUAN may be given on a divided or once-a-day dosage schedule. If the once-a-day schedule is employed, the maximum recommended dose is 150mg/day. This dose may be given at bedtime. The anti-anxiety effect is apparent before the antidepressant effect. Optimal antidepressant effect may not be evident for two-to-three weeks.

Overdosage

Critical manifestations of overdose include: cardiac dysrhythmias, severe hypotension, convulsions, and CNS depression, including coma. Changes in the electrocardiogram, particularly in QRS axis or width, are clinically significant indicators of SINEQUAN toxicity.

Other signs of overdose may include: confusion, disturbed concentration, transient visual hallucinations, dilated pupils, agitation, hyperactive reflexes, stupor, drowsiness, muscle rigidity, vomiting, hypothermia, hyperpyrexia. Deaths may occur from SINEQUAN overdose.

SYMMETREL

(Amantadine)

SYMMETREL has pharmacological actions as both an anti-Parkinson and an antiviral drug. Only its use as anti-Parkinson drug will be described here.

Pharmacodynamics

The mechanism of action of amantadine in the treatment of Parkinson's disease and drug-induced extra-pyramidal reactions is not known. It may relate to an increase in dopamine release in the brain.

Pharmacokinetics

- SYMMETREL is well absorbed orally.

- Maximum plasma concentrations are directly related to dose for doses up to 200mg/day. Doses above 200mg/day may result in a greater than proportional increase in maximum plasma concentrations.

- It is primarily excreted unchanged in the urine by glomerular filtration and tubular secretion.

- The time to peak concentration is 3.3 ± 1.5 hours (range: 1 to 8 hours).

- The half-life is 9 to 21 hours.

- There appears to be a relationship between plasma amantadine concentrations and toxicity.

Indications

1. For the treatment of Parkinsonism and drug- induced extrapyramidal reactions

2. For the prophylaxis and treatment of signs and symptoms of infection caused by various strains of influenza A virus

Pediatric Use—The safety and efficacy of SYMMETREL in newborn infants and infants below the age of one year have not been established.

Contraindications

Individuals with known hypersensitivity to the drug

Potential Side Effects

Neurological System—Dizziness, lightheadedness, ataxia, headache, slurred speech, confusion, amnesia, hyperkinesia

Psychiatric Disorders—Insomnia, depression, anxiety and irritability, hallucinations, confusion, somnolence, nervousness, dream abnormality, agitation, fatigue, psychosis, euphoria, abnormal thinking

Cardiovascular System—Peripheral edema, orthostatic hypotension, congestive heart failure, hypertension

Respiratory System—Dry nose, dyspnea

Gastrointestinal System—Nausea, anorexia, vomiting, dry mouth, constipation, diarrhea

Genitourinary System—Urinary retention

Dermatological System—Skin rash

Sexual Function—Decreased libido

Ocular System—Visual disturbance, including punctuate subepithelial or other corneal opacity, corneal edema, decreased visual acuity, sensitivity to light, and optic nerve palsy

Potential Drug Interactions

1. Co-administration of MELLARIL may worsen the tremor in elderly individuals with Parkinson's disease, however, it is not known if other phenothiazines produce a similar response.

2. The administration of urine acidifying drugs may increase the elimination of the drug from the body.

3. The dose of anticholinergic drugs or of SYMMETREL should be reduced if atropine-like effects appear when these drugs are used concurrently.

Withdrawal Symptoms

Sporadic cases of possible neuroleptic malignant syndrome have been reported in association with dose reduction or withdrawal of SYMMETREL therapy.

Dosage and Administration

Use in drug-induced extra-pyramidal reactions

In adults, the usual dose of SYMMETREL is 100mg twice a day when used alone. Occasionally, individuals whose responses are not optimal with SYMMETREL at 200mg daily may benefit from an increase up to 300mg daily in divided doses. In children 12 years and older, half of the adult dosage may be considered.

After two weeks of good control of the extra-pyramidal reactions, the drug should be tapered off to determine the continued need for it. If such reactions recur, SYMMETREL can be re-instituted.

Overdosage

Central nervous system effects include insomnia, anxiety, aggressive behavior, hypertonia, hyperkinesia, tremor, confusion, disorientation, depersonalization, fear, delirium, hallucinations, psychotic reactions, lethargy, somnolence and coma. Seizures may be exacerbated in individuals with prior history of seizure disorders. Hyperthermia may also develop.

Drug overdose has resulted in cardiac, respiratory, renal or central nervous system toxicity. Cardiac dysfunction includes arrhythmia, tachycardia, and hypertension. Pulmonary edema and respiratory distress (including adult respiratory distress syndrome-ARDS) have been reported. Renal dysfunction including increased BUN, decreased creatinine clearance, and renal insufficiency can occur.

Deaths have been reported from overdose with SYMMETREL. The lowest reported acute lethal dose was 2 grams. Acute toxicity may be attributable to the anticholinergic effects of amantadine.

TENEX

(Guanfacine Hydrochloride)

Pharmacodynamics

TENEX is an orally active antihypertensive agent whose principal mechanism of action appears to be stimulation of central alpha-adrenergic receptors. By stimulating these receptors, TENEX reduces sympathetic nerve impulses from the vasomotor center to the heart and blood vessels. This results in a decrease in peripheral vascular resistance and a reduction in heart rate.

Pharmacokinetics

- Peak plasma concentrations occur from 1 to 4 hours with an average of 2 hours after single oral doses or at steady state.

- The average elimination half-fife is approximately 17 hours (range 10-30 hours). Younger individuals tend to have shorter elimination half-lives (13-14 hours) while older individuals tend to have half-lives at the upper end of the range.

- Steady state blood levels were attained within 4 days in most subjects.

Indications

1. For the management of hypertension, TENEX may be given alone or in combination with other antihypertensive agents, especially thiazide-type diuretics

2. Unlabeled use to treat ADHD and tic disorders

Pediatric Use—Safety and effectiveness in children less than 12 years-of-age have not been demonstrated. Therefore, the use of Tenex in this age group is not recommended.

Contraindications

Hypersensitivity to guanfacine hydrochloride

Potential Side Effects

Body as a Whole—Chest pain, asthenia, edema, malaise, tremor

Neurological System—Paresthesias, vertigo, dizziness

Psychiatric Disorders—Agitation, anxiety, confusion, depression, insomnia, nervousness, somnolence

Cardiovascular System—Bradycardia, palpitations, syncope, tachycardia

Gastrointestinal System—Abdominal pain, constipation, diarrhea, dyspepsia, nausea, dry mouth

Liver and Biliary System—Abnormal liver function

Muscular and Skeletal Systems—Arthralgia, leg cramps, leg pain, myalgia

Respiratory System—Dyspnea

Dermatological System—Alopecia, dermatitis, exfoliative dermatitis, pruritus, rash, sweating

Special Senses—Alterations in taste, blurred vision, iritis, conjunctivitis, rhinitis, tinnitus

Sexual Function—Impotence

Urinary System—Nocturia, increased urinary frequency or incontinence

Potential Drug Interactions

TENEX may potentiate the effects of other CNS-depressant medications.

Withdrawal Symptoms

Abrupt cessation of therapy with orally active central alpha-adrenergic agonists may be associated with symptoms of "nervousness and anxiety" and, less commonly, increases in blood pressure to levels significantly greater than those prior to therapy. The frequency of rebound hypertension is low, but it can occur. When rebound occurs, it does so after 2-4 days, which is delayed compared with CATAPRES. This is consistent with the longer half-life of TENEX. In most cases, after abrupt withdrawal of TENEX, blood pressure returns to pretreatment levels slowly (within 2-4 days) without ill effects.

Dosage and Administration

In the unlabeled use for treatment of ADHD, the recommended initial dose of TENEX when given alone is 1mg daily for older children, adolescents, and adults, 0.5mg for younger children given in the morning. Further increments of 0.5mg per day may be made at weekly interval if necessary until the desired response is achieved. The dose of TENEX must be adjusted according to the individual's blood pressure and clinical responses. At the optimal dosage with positive response, TENEX can then be taken twice or three times daily. Higher daily doses have been used, but adverse reactions increase significantly with doses above 3mg/day.

Overdosage

Symptoms include drowsiness, lethargy, bradycardia and hypotension.

TOFRANIL

(Imipramine)

TOFRANIL, the original tricyclic antidepressant, is a member of the dibenzazepine group of compounds.

Pharmacodynamics

The mechanism of action of TOFRANIL is not definitely known. The clinical effect is hypothesized as being due to potentiation of adrenergic synapses by blocking uptake of norepinephrine at nerve endings. The mode of action of the drug in controlling childhood enuresis is thought to be apart from its antidepressant effect.

Pharmacokinetics

- TOFRANIL is well absorbed.

- TOFRANIL is metabolized in the liver and has a significant first-pass metabolism.

- Eliminate half-life is 6-18 hours.

- Peak antidepressant effect is reached after 2 weeks.

- Almost all compounds following metabolism are excreted in urine.

Indications

1. For the relief of symptoms of depression

2. May be useful as temporary adjunctive therapy in reducing enuresis in children aged 6 years and older, after possible organic causes have been excluded by appropriate tests

Pediatric Use—The effectiveness of TOFRANIL in children for conditions other than nocturnal enuresis has not been established. The safety and effectiveness of TOFRANIL as temporary adjunctive therapy for nocturnal enuresis in children less than 6 years-of-age has not been established. The safety of the drug for long-term, chronic use as adjunctive therapy for nocturnal enuresis in children has not been established.

Contraindications

1. The concomitant use of monoamine oxidase inhibiting compounds is contraindicated.

2. The drug is contraindicated during the acute recovery period after a myocardial infarction.

3. Patients with a known hypersensitivity to TOFRANIL should not be given the drug.

Potential Side Effects

Body as Whole—Weight gain or loss, weakness and fatigue, tiredness

Neurological System—Numbness, tingling, paresthesias of extremities, headache, incoordination, ataxia, proneness to falling, tremors, peripheral neuropathy, extrapyramidal symptoms, seizures, alterations in EEG patterns, tinnitus

Psychiatric Disorders—Confusional states with hallucinations, disorientation, delusions, drowsiness, dizziness, nervousness, anxiety, restlessness, agitation, insomnia and nightmares, hypomania, exacerbation of psychosis

Cardiovascular System—Orthostatic hypotension, hypertension, tachycardia, palpitation, flushing, myocardial infarction, arrhythmias, heart block, ECG changes, precipitation of congestive heart failure, stroke, syncope, collapse

Dermatological System—Skin rash, petechiae, urticaria, itching, photosensitization, perspiration, alopecia, edema (general or of face and tongue), drug fever, cross-sensitivity with desipramine

Hematologic and Lymphatic System—Bone marrow depression including agranulocytosis, eosinophilia, purpura, thrombocytopenia

Gastrointestinal System—Nausea and vomiting, anorexia, epigastric distress, diarrhea, peculiar taste, stomatitis, abdominal cramps, black tongue, jaundice (simulating obstructive), altered liver function dry mouth, constipation, paralytic ileus, sublingual adenitis

Genitourinary System—Urinary frequency, urinary retention, delayed micturition, dilation of the urinary tract

Endocrine System—Gynecomastia in the male, breast enlargement and galactorrhea in the female, increased or decreased libido, impotence, testicular swelling, elevation or depression of blood sugar levels, inappropriate antidiuretic hormone (ADH) secretion syndrome

Special Senses—Blurred vision, disturbances of accommodation, mydriasis

Potential Drug Interactions

1. An individual who is stable on a given dose of TOFRANIL may become abruptly toxic when given one of the cytochrome P450 2D6 inhibiting drugs (e.g., quinidine; cimetidine, many other antidepressants including SRIs, phenothiazines) as concomitant therapy. Concomitant use of TOFRANIL with drugs that can inhibit cytochrome P450 2D6 may require lower doses than usually prescribed for either the TOFRANIL or the other drug. Furthermore, whenever one of these other drugs is withdrawn from co-therapy, an increased dose of TOFRANIL may be required. It is desirable to monitor TOFRANIL plasma levels whenever TOFRANIL is going to be co-administered with another drug known to be an inhibitor of P450 2D6.

2. The plasma concentration of TOFRANIL may increase when it is given concomitantly with hepatic enzyme inhibitors (e.g., TAGAMET, PROZAC) and decrease by concomitant administration with hepatic enzyme inducers (e.g., barbiturates, DILANTIN), and adjustment of the dosage of TOFRANIL may therefore be necessary.

3. When TOFRANIL is administered concomitantly with anticholinergic drugs including antiparkinsonism agents, the atropine-like effects may become more pronounced (e.g., paralytic ileus).

4. Avoid the use of preparations such as decongestants and local anesthetics that contain any sympathornimetic amine (e.g., epinephrine, norepinephrine), since TOFRANIL may potentiate the effects of catecholamines.

5. TOFRANIL may potentiate the effects of agents that lower blood pressure.

6. TOFRANIL may potentiate the effects of CNS depressant drugs.

7. In individuals with hyperthyroidism or on thyroid medication, concomitant administration may cause cardiovascular toxicity.

8. In individuals receiving CATAPRES or similar agents, TOFRANIL may block the pharmacologic effects of these drugs.

9. RITALIN may inhibit the metabolism of TOFRANIL, and downward dosage adjustment of TOFRANIL may become necessary.

Withdrawal Symptoms

Abrupt cessation of treatment after prolonged therapy may produce nausea, headache, and malaise.

Laboratory Tests

Individuals who develop a fever and a sore throat during therapy with TOFRANIL should have leukocyte and differential blood counts performed.

The therapeutic ranges for treatment of depression are imipramine and desipramine (the active metabolite): 150-250ng/mL, and desipramine: 150-300ng/mL.

Dosage and Administration

An ECG recording should be taken prior to the initiation of larger-than-usual doses of TOFRANIL and at appropriate intervals thereafter until steady state is achieved.

Depression—In adults, begin with 75mg/ day in divided doses, then gradually increase to 150mg/ day. Dosages over 200mg/day are not recommended. In adolescents, begin with 30-40mg/day in divided doses, then gradually increased to 100mg/day. For children, the daily dose of TOFRANIL should not exceed 2.5mg/kg.

TOFRANIL-PM capsules may be used when total daily dosage is established at 75mg or higher. The total daily dosage can be administered on a once-a-day basis, preferably at bedtime. Following remission, maintenance medication may be required for a longer period of time, at the lowest dose that will maintain remission.

For Treatment of Childhood Enuresis—Initially, an oral dose of 25mg/day should be tried in children aged 6 and older. Medication should be given one hour before bedtime. If a satisfactory response does not occur within one week, increase the dose to 50mg nightly in children under 12 years; children over 12 may receive up to 75mg nightly. A daily dose greater than 75mg does not enhance efficacy and tends to increase side effects. In early night bedwetters, the drug is more effective given earlier and in divided amounts, i.e., 25mg in mid-afternoon, repeated at bedtime.

Consideration should be given to instituting a drug-free period following an adequate therapeutic trial with a favorable response. Dosage should be tapered off gradually rather than abruptly discontinued; this may reduce the tendency to relapse. Children who relapse when the drug is discontinued do not always respond to a subsequent course of treatment.

Overdosage

Critical manifestations of overdose include cardiac dysrhythmias, severe hypotension, convulsions, and CNS depression including coma. Changes in the electrocardiogram, particularly in QRS axis or width, are clinically significant indicators of TOFRANIL toxicity. Other CNS manifestations may include drowsiness, stupor, ataxia, restlessness, agitation, hyperactive reflexes, muscle rigidity, athetoid and choreiform movements. Cardiac abnormalities may include tachycardia and signs of congestive failure. Respiratory depression, cyanosis, shock, vomiting, hyperpyrexia, mydriasis, and diaphoresis may also be present.

TRANXENE

(Clorazepate Dipotassium)

Pharmacodynamics

Pharmacologically, TRANXENE has the characteristics of the benzodiazepines. It has depressant effects on the central nervous system.

Pharmacokinetics

- The primary metabolite, desmethyldiazepam, quickly appears in the blood stream.

- The serum half-life is about 2 days.

- The drug is metabolized in the liver and excreted primarily in the urine.

Indications

1. For the treatment of anxiety disorders or for the short-term relief of the symptoms of anxiety

2. As adjunctive therapy in the management of partial seizures

3. For the symptomatic relief of acute alcohol withdrawal

Pediatric Use—Because of the lack of sufficient clinical experience, TRANXENE is not recommended for use in children less than 9 years-of-age.

Contraindications

Known hypersensitivity to the drug or with acute narrow angle glaucoma

Potential Side Effects

Neurological System—Drowsiness, dizziness, headache, mental confusion, ataxia, tremor, slurred speech

Psychiatric Disorders—Nervousness, insomnia, fatigue, irritability, depression

Hepatic System—Abnormal liver function

Gastrointestinal System—Various gastrointestinal complaints, dry mouth

Genitourinary System—Abnormal kidney function test, genitourinary complaints

Cardiovascular System—Decreased systolic blood pressure

Hematological System—Decrease in hematocrit

Dermatological System—Transient skin rashes

Special Senses—Blurred vision, diplopia

Potential Drug Interactions

1. TRANXENE prolongs the sleeping time after hexobarbital or after ethyl alcohol.

2. TRANXENE increases the inhibitory effects of THORAZINE.

3. TRANXENE increases sedation with concurrent hypnotic medications.

4. The actions of the benzodiazepines may be potentiated by barbiturates, narcotics, phenothiazines, monoamine oxidase inhibitors or other antidepressants.

Withdrawal Symptoms

Withdrawal symptoms have occurred following abrupt discontinuance of TRANXENE. Withdrawal symptoms include convulsions, delirium, tremor, abdominal and muscle cramps, vomiting, sweating, nervous-ness, insomnia, irritability, diarrhea, and memory impairment. The more severe withdrawal symptoms have usually been limited to those patients who had received excessive doses over an extended period of time. Consequently, after extended therapy, abrupt discontinuation of TRANXENE should generally be avoided and a gradual dosage tapering schedule followed.

Laboratory Tests

Individuals taking TRANXENE for prolonged periods should have blood counts and liver function tests periodically.

Dosage and Administration

For the treatment of anxiety in older adolescents and adults, TRANXENE is administered orally in divided doses. The usual daily dose is 30mg. The dose should be adjusted gradually within the range of 15 to 60mg daily. TRANXENE may also be administered in a single dose daily at bedtime; the recommended initial dose is 15mg. After the initial dose, the response of the individual may require adjustment of subsequent dosage. Drowsiness may occur at the initiation of treatment and with dosage increment.

As an adjunct to antiepileptic drugs in older adolescents and adults, the maximum recommended initial dose is 7.5mg three times a day. Dosage should be increased by no more than 7.5mg every week and should not exceed 90mg/day.

In children 9-12 years-of-age, the maximum recommended initial dose is 7.5mg two times a day. Dosage should be increased by no more than 7.5mg every week and should not exceed 60mg/day.

TRANXENE-SD (22.5mg) tablets may be administered as a single dose every 24 hours. This tablet is intended as an alternate dosage form for the convenience of individuals stabilized on a dose of 7.5mg tablets three times a day. TRANXENE-SD tablets should not be used to initiate therapy.

TRANXENE-SD HALF STRENGTH (11.25mg) tablets may be administered as a single dose every 24 hours. This tablet is intended as an alternate dosage form for the convenience of patients stabilized on a dose of 3.75mg tablets three times a day. TRANXENE-SD HALF STRENGTH should not be used to initiate therapy.

Overdosage

Overdosage is usually manifested by varying degrees of CNS depression ranging from slight sedation to coma. Sedation in varying degrees is the most common physiological manifestation of TRANXENE overdosage. If deep coma occurs, is usually associated with the ingestion of other drugs in addition to TRANXENE.

WELLBUTRIN

(Bupropion)

Wellbutrin, an antidepressant of the aminoketone class, is chemically unrelated to tricyclic, tetracyclic, or other known antidepressant agents.

Pharmacodynamics

The neurochemical mechanism of the antidepressant effect of WELLBUTRIN is not known. Compared to classical tricyclic antidepressants, it is a weak blocker of the neuronal uptake of serotonin and norepinephrine; it also inhibits the neuronal re-uptake of dopamine to some extent.

Pharmacokinetics

- Following oral administration of WELLBUTRIN, peak plasma concentrations are usually achieved within 2 hours, followed by a biphasic decline.

- The average half-life of the second (post-distributional) phase is approximately 14 hours, with a range of 8 to 24 hours.

Indications

1. For the treatment of depression

2. Unlabeled use in the treatment of ADHD

Contraindications

1. In individuals with a seizure disorder

2. In individuals with a current or prior diagnosis of bulimia or anorexia nervosa because of a higher incidence of seizures noted in such individuals treated with WELLBUTRIN

3. The concurrent administration of WELLBUTRIN and an MAOI is contraindicated

Potential Side Effects

Body as a Whole—Weight gain, weight loss, flu-like symptoms (fatigue, fever, chills), excessive sweating, nonspecific pain

Neurological system—Headache, migraine, dizziness, ataxia/ incoordination, seizure, myoclonus, dyskinesia, akinesia/bradykinesia, akathisia, dystonia, tremor, coma, delirium, dream abnormalities, sleep disturbances, paresthesia, pseudoparkinsonism, unmasking of tardive dyskinesia, mydriasis, vertigo, and dysarthria

Psychiatric Disorders—Confusion, disturbed concentration, euphoria, activation of mania/ hypomania, agitation, hostility, delusion, hallucinations, anxiety, and depression, memory impairment, depersonalization, psychosis, dysphoria, mood instability, paranoia, formal thought disorder, and frigidity

Cardiovascular system—Edema, hypertension, orthostatic hypotension, palpitations, tachycardia, cardiac arrhythmias, third degree heart block, syncope, chest pain, EKG abnormalities (premature beats and non-specific ST-T changes), and shortness of breath/dyspnea

Respiratory system—Bronchitis and shortness of breath/dyspnea

Endocrine system—Inappropriate antidiuretic hormone secretion, gynecomastia

Hematological and Lymphatic Systems—Ecchymosis, leukocytosis, leukopenia

Muscular and Skeletal Systems—Arthralgia, arthritis, myalgia, muscle spasms, muscle rigidity, and rhabdomyolysis

Gastrointestinal System—Dry mouth, increased salivary flow, increased appetite, dyspepsia, anorexia, nausea, vomiting, stomatitis, esophagitis, hepatitis, constipation, diarrhea, toothache, bruxism, gum irritation, and oral edema, dysphagia, thirst, and liver damage/jaundice

Genitourinary System—Impotence, urinary frequency, urinary retention, nocturia, increased libido, decreased sexual function, vaginal irritation, testicular swelling, urinary tract infection, painful erection, and retarded ejaculation

Dermatological System—Nonspecific rashes, Stevens-Johnson syndrome, angioedema, exfoliative dermatitis, urticaria, pruritus, alopecia, dry skin

Special Senses—Tinnitus, blurred vision, visual disturbance

Potential Drug Interactions

No systematic data have been collected on the consequences of the concomitant administration of WELLBUTRIN and other drugs.

Dosage and Administration

For Treatment of Depression

No single dose of WELLBUTRIN should exceed 150mg. WELLBUTRIN should be administered three times daily, preferably with at least 6 hours between successive doses. Increases in dose should not exceed 100mg/day in a 3-day period.

In older adolescents and adults, dosing begins at 200mg/day, given as 100mg twice daily. This dose may be increased to 300mg/day, given as 100mg three times daily, no sooner than 3 days after beginning therapy. Avoiding bedtime doses may minimize insomnia.

The full antidepressant effect of WELLBUTRIN may not be evident until 4 weeks of treatment or longer. An increase in dosage, up to a maximum of 450mg/day, given in divided doses of not more than 150mg each, may be considered for individuals in whom no clinical improvement is noted after several weeks of treatment at 300mg/day. WELLBUTRIN should be discontinued in individuals who do not demonstrate an adequate response after an appropriate period of treatment at 450mg/day.

For treatment of ADHD

In school age children, the dosage is 3 to 6mg/kg/day in divided doses.

Maintenance

The lowest dose that maintains remission is recommended. Although it is not known how long the individual should remain on WELLBUTRIN, it is generally recognized that acute episodes of depression require several months or longer of antidepressant drug treatment. When WELLBUTRIN is used for the treatment of ADHD with good response, it should be discontinued after 4 months so that the need for continuation of treatment can be evaluated.

Overdosage

Signs of acute toxicity included labored breathing, salivation, arched back, ptosis, ataxia, convulsions (in about one-third of all cases with overdosage), hallucinations, loss of consciousness, and tachycardia. Fever, muscle rigidity, rhabdomyolysis, hypotension, stupor, coma, and respiratory failure may occur WELLBUTRIN is part of multiple drug overdoses.

Deaths associated with overdoses of WELLBUTRIN alone have been reported rarely in individuals ingesting massive doses of WELLBUTRIN. Multiple uncontrolled seizures, bradycardia, cardiac failure, and cardiac arrest usually occur prior to death.

XANAX

(Alprazolam)

Pharmacodynamics

XANAX, a benzodiazepine, presumably exerts its effect by binding at stereo specific receptors at several sites within the central nervous system. Their exact mechanism of action is unknown. Clinically, it causes a dose-related central nervous system depressant activity varying from mild impairment of task performance to hypnosis.

Pharmacokinetics

- Following oral administration, XANAX is readily absorbed from the GI tract.

- Peak concentrations in the plasma occur in one-to-two hours following administration.

- Mean plasma elimination half-life of XANAX is about 11 hours (range: 6-27 hours) in healthy adults.

- XANAX is bound (80 percent) to human serum protein.

Indications

For the management of anxiety disorder, panic disorder with or without agoraphobia, and the short-term relief of symptoms of anxiety

Pediatric Use—Safety and effectiveness of XANAX in individuals below 18 years-of-age have not been established.

Contraindications

1. In individuals with known sensitivity to this medication or other benzodiazepines

2. In individuals with acute narrow angle glaucoma

Potential Side Effects

Body as a Whole—Weakness, fatigue, tiredness, sleepiness, chest pain, edema

Neurological System—Ataxia, loss of coordination, dystonia, syncope, seizures, dizziness, light-headedness, akathisia, abnormal involuntary movement, transient amnesia or memory impairment, seizures, sedation, slurred speech, dysarthria, paresthesia

Psychiatric Disorders—Agitation, irritability, disinhibition, talkativeness, concentration difficulties, drowsiness, depression, headache, confusion, insomnia, anxiety, nervousness, depression, activation of hypomania or mania, derealization, hallucinations, depersonalization, dream abnormalities, fear, warm feeling

Gastrointestinal System—Dry mouth, increased salivation, decreased salivation, abdominal distress, increased appetite, decreased appetite, anorexia, constipation, diarrhea, nausea, vomiting

Cardiovascular System—Tachycardia, palpitations, hypotension, vasomotor disturbances

Hepatic System—Jaundice, elevated bilirubin, elevated hepatic enzymes, hepatitis, hepatic failure

Muscular and Skeletal Systems—Rigidity, tremor, muscular twitching, musculoskeletal weakness, muscle tone disorders, muscular cramps, muscle stiffness

Dermatologic System—Dermatitis, allergies, pruritus, sweating, rash, Stevens-Johnson syndrome

Respiratory System—Nasal congestion, hyperventilation, upper respiratory infection

Endocrine System—Weight gain, weight loss, hyperprolactinemia, gynecomastia, galactorrhea

Genitourinary System—Urinary incontinence, urinary retention, micturition difficulties

Sexual Function—Increased libido, change in libido, menstrual irregularities, sexual dysfunction

Special Senses—Blurred vision, diplopia, tinnitus, taste alterations

Potential Drug Interactions

1. XANAX interacts with medications that inhibit metabolism via cytochrome P450 3A and may increase plasma concentration levels of XANAX. Consequently, XANAX should be avoided in individuals receiving very potent inhibitors of CYP 3A (Azole antifungal agents, ketoconazole and itraconazole, PROZAC, LUVOX, SERZONE, ZOLOFT, PAXIL, oral contraceptives).

2. XANAX produces additive CNS depressant effects when co-administered with other psychotherapeutic medications, anticonvulsants, antihistamines, ethanol and other drugs which themselves produce CNS depression.

3. The steady state plasma concentrations of TOFRANIL and NORPRAMIN have been reported to be increased an average of 30% and 20%, respectively, by the concomitant administration of XANAX in doses up to 4mg/day.

Drug/Laboratory Test Interactions

Although interactions between benzodiazepines and commonly employed clinical laboratory tests have occasionally been reported, there is no consistent pattern for a specific drug or specific test.

Drug Abuse and Dependence

Psychological dependence is a risk with XANAX. The risk of psychological dependence increases at doses greater than 4mg/day and with longer-term use (more than 12 weeks). Because the management of panic disorder often requires the use of average daily doses of XANAX above 4mg, the risk of dependence among panic disorder individuals may be higher than that among those treated for less severe anxiety. This risk is further increased in individuals with a history of alcohol or drug abuse. Some individuals have experienced considerable difficulty in tapering and discontinuing XANAX, especially those receiving higher doses for extended periods.

Inter-dose Symptoms—Early morning anxiety and emergence of anxiety symptoms between doses of XANAX have been reported in individuals with panic disorder taking prescribed maintenance doses of XANAX. These symptoms may reflect the development of tolerance or a time interval between doses which is longer than the duration of clinical action of the administered dose. In either case, it is presumed that the prescribed dose is not sufficient to maintain plasma levels above those needed to prevent relapse, rebound or withdrawal symptoms over the entire course of the inter-dosing interval.

Withdrawal Symptoms

Withdrawal reactions may occur when dosage reduction occurs for any reason. This includes purposeful tapering, but also inadvertent reduction of dose (e.g., the individual forgets to take the medication). Withdrawal symptoms similar in character to those noted with sedative/hypnotics and alcohol have occurred following discontinuance of XANAX. The symptoms can range from mild dysphoria and insomnia to a major syndrome that may include abdominal and muscle cramps, vomiting, sweating, tremors and convulsions. In most cases reported, only a single withdrawal seizure was reported; however, multiple seizures and status epilepticus were reported as well.

While the severity and incidence of withdrawal phenomena appear to be related to dose and duration of treatment, withdrawal symptoms have been reported after only brief therapy with XANAX at doses within the recommended range for the treatment of anxiety. Signs and symptoms of withdrawal are often more prominent after rapid decrease of dosage or abrupt discontinuance.

The risk of withdrawal seizures may be increased at doses above 4mg/day. Individuals with a history of seizure disorders should not be abruptly discontinued from XANAX. It is recommended that all individuals on XANAX who require a dosage reduction be gradually tapered under close supervision. When necessary, immediate management of withdrawal symptoms requires re-institution of treatment at doses of XANAX sufficient to suppress symptoms.

Controlled Substance Class

XANAX is a controlled substance and has been assigned to Schedule IV.

Laboratory Tests:

Laboratory tests are not ordinarily required in otherwise healthy patients. However, when treatment with XANAX is protracted, periodic blood counts, urinalysis, and blood chemistry analyses are recommended.

Dosage and Administration

Anxiety Disorders and Transient Symptoms of Anxiety—Treatment should begin with a dose of 0.25 to 0.5mg given three times daily. The dose may be increased to achieve a maximum therapeutic effect, at intervals of 3-to-4 days, to a maximum daily dose of 4mg, given in divided doses. The lowest possible effective dose should be employed and the need for continued treatment reassessed frequently.

In all individuals, dosage should be reduced gradually when discontinuing therapy or when decreasing the daily dosage. It is suggested that the daily dosage be decreased by no more than 0.5mg every three days. Some individuals may require an even slower dosage reduction.

Panic Disorder—Treatment may be initiated with a dose of 0.5mg three times daily. Depending on the response, the dose may be increased at intervals of 3-to-4 days in increments of no more than 1mg per day. To lessen the possibility of inter-dose symptoms, the times of administration should be distributed as evenly as possible throughout the waking hours, that is, on a three or four times per day schedule.

The necessary duration of treatment for panic disorder individuals responding to XANAX is unknown. After a period of extended freedom from attacks, a carefully supervised tapered discontinuation may be attempted, but in some individuals this may be difficult to accomplish without recurrence of symptoms and/or the manifestation of withdrawal phenomena. Nonetheless, reduction of dose must be undertaken under close supervision and must be gradual.

If significant withdrawal symptoms develop, the previous dosing schedule should be re-instituted and, only after stabilization, should a less rapid schedule of discontinuation be attempted. In general, the dose should be reduced by no more than 0.5mg every three days, though some individuals may benefit from an even more gradual discontinuation.

Overdosage

Manifestations of XANAX overdose include somnolence, confusion, impaired coordination, diminished reflexes, and coma. Death has been reported in association with overdoses of XANAX.

ZOLOFT

(Sertraline)

ZOLOFT is an antidepressant.

Pharmacodynamics

The mechanism of action of ZOLOFT is presumed to be linked to its inhibition of CNS neuronal uptake of serotonin into platelets.

Pharmacokinetics

- Following oral once-daily dosing over the range of 50 to 200mg for 14 days, mean peak plasma concentrations of ZOLOFT occur between 4 and 8 hours post-dosing.

- When ZOLOFT is administered with food, the time to reach peak plasma concentration decreases from 8 hours post-dosing to 5 hours.

- ZOLOFT is highly bound to serum proteins (98%).

- The average terminal elimination half-life of plasma LUVOX is about 26 hours.

- Steady-state ZOLOFT plasma levels are usually achieved after approximately one week of once-daily dosing.

- ZOLOFT undergoes extensive first pass metabolism. Liver impairment can significantly affect the elimination of ZOLOFT.

Indications

1. Treatment of depression

2. Treatment of OCD

Pediatric Use—Safety and effectiveness in children have not been established.

Contraindications

Concomitant use in individuals taking monoamine oxidase inhibitors (MAOIs) is contraindicated.

Potential Side Effects

Body as Whole—Asthenia, malaise, generalized edema, rigors, weight decrease, weight increase

Neurological System—Confusion, ataxia, abnormal coordination, abnormal gait, hyperesthesia, hyperkinesia, hypokinesia, migraine, nystagmus, vertigo, neuroleptic malignant syndrome-like events

Psychiatric Disorders—Abnormal dream, aggressive reaction, amnesia, apathy, delusion, depersonalization, depression, aggravated depression, emotional lability, euphoria, hypomania or mania hallucination, neurosis, paranoid reaction, psychosis, suicide ideation and attempt, teeth grinding, abnormal thinking

Autonomic Nervous System—Flushing, mydriasis, increased saliva, cold clammy skin

Cardiovascular System—Postural dizziness, hypertension, hypotension, dependent edema, periorbital edema, peripheral edema, peripheral ischemia, syncope, tachycardia

Respiratory System—Bronchospasm, coughing, dyspnea, epistaxis

Gastrointestinal System—Dysphagia, eructation

Hematologic and Lymphatic Systems— Lymphadenopathy, purpura

Muscular and Skeletal Systems—Arthralgia, arthrosis, dystonia, muscle cramps, muscle weakness

Reproductive System—Dysmenorrhea and intermenstrual bleeding In females

Genitourinary System—Dysuria, face edema, nocturia, polyuria, urinary incontinence

Dermatologic System—Acne, alopecia, pruritus, erythematous rash, maculopapular rash, dry skin

Special Senses—Abnormal accommodation, conjunctivitis, diplopia, earache, eye pain, xerophthalmia

Potential Drug Interactions

1. Serious, sometimes fatal, reactions may develop in individuals receiving ZOLOFT in combination with a monoamine oxidase inhibitor (MAOI). These reactions may also develop in individuals who have recently discontinued ZOLOFT and have been started on an MAOI.

2. The administration of ZOLOFT to an individual taking another drug that is tightly bound to protein, (e.g., warfarin, digitoxin) may cause a shift in plasma concentrations potentially resulting in an adverse effect.

3. ZOLOFT may inhibit TCA metabolism. Plasma TCA concentrations may need to be monitored, and the dose of TCA may need to be reduced if a TCA is co-administered with ZOLOFT.

Dosage and Administration

In older adolescents and adults, ZOLOFT treatment should be initiated with a dose of 50mg once daily either in the morning or evening. Individuals not responding to a 50mg/day dose may benefit from dose increment of 50mg/day weekly up to a maximum of 200mg/day.

In children 6 to 12 years, an initial dose of 25mg/day is recommended. A 25mg/day weekly increment up to 100-150mg/day may be considered after 2 weeks if no clinical improvement is observed. A dose exceeding 200mg/day may not add any more treatment effect, but it may increase the risk of side effects.

Maintenance—While there are no systematic studies that answer the question of how long to continue ZOLOFT, it is generally agreed among experts that acute episodes of depression require several months or longer of sustained pharmacologic therapy. Whether the dose of antidepressant needed to induce remission is identical to the dose needed to maintain and/or sustain euthymia is unknown.

Since OCD and Anxiety/Panic Disorders are chronic conditions, it is reasonable to consider continuation for a responding individual with dosage adjustments made to maintain the individual on the lowest effective dosage, and the individual should be periodically reassessed to determine the need for further treatment.

Overdosage

Symptoms of overdose with ZOLOFT alone included somnolence, nausea, vomiting, tachycardia, ECG changes, anxiety, and dilated pupils. Treatment was primarily supportive and included monitoring and use of activated charcoal, gastric lavage, or cathartics and hydration.

ZYPREXA

(Olanzapine)

ZYPREXA is an antipsychotic agent that belongs to the thienobenzodiazepine class.

Pharmacodynamics

1. ZYPREXA is a selective monoaminergic antagonist with high affinity binding to the following receptors: serotonin 5HT2A/2C, dopamine D1-4, muscarinic MI-5, histamine H1, and adrenergic receptors. ZYPREXA binds weakly to $GABA_A$, BZD, and P adrenergic receptors.

2. The mechanism of action of ZYPREXA is unknown. However, it has been proposed that this medication's antipsychotic activity is mediated through a combination of dopamine and serotonin type 2 (5HT2) antagonism.

3. ZYPREXA's antagonism of muscarinic M1-5 receptors may explain its anticholinergic effects.

4. ZYPREXA's antagonism of histamine H1 receptors may explain the somnolence observed.

5. ZYPREXA's antagonism of adrenergic receptors may explain the orthostatic hypotension observed.

Pharmacokinetics

- ZYPREXA is well absorbed and reaches peak concentrations in approximately 6 hours following an oral dose.

- It is eliminated extensively by first pass metabolism, with approximately 40% of the dose metabolized before reaching the systemic circulation.

- Food does not affect the rate or extent of ZYPREXA absorption.

- Its half-life ranges from 21 to 54 hours (mean of 30 hr), and the manufacturer reports plasma clearance ranges from 12 to 47 L/hr (mean of 25 L/hr).

- Administration of ZYPREXA once daily leads to steady-state concentrations in about one week that are approximately twice the concentrations after single doses.

Indications

For the management of psychotic disorders

Contraindications

Known hypersensitivity to olanzapine

Potential Side Effects

Body as a Whole—Flu-like syndrome, chills, fever, face edema, hangover effect, malaise, moniliasis, neck pain, pelvic pain

Neurological System—Tardive dyskinesia, abnormal gait, antisocial reaction, ataxia, CNS stimulation, coma, delirium, hypoesthesia, hypotonia, incoordination, seizure, stupor, vertigo, withdrawal syndrome

Psychiatric Disorders—Somnolence, obsessive compulsive symptoms, phobias, depersonalization

Cardiovascular System—Cerebrovascular accident, hemorrhage, migraine, palpitation, tachycardia, vasodilatation, orthostatic hypotension, ventricular extrasystoles

Gastrointestinal System—Increased salivation, nausea, vomiting, thirst, aphthous stomatitis, dysphagia, eructation, esophagitis, dysphagia, fecal incontinence, flatulence, gastritis, gastroenteritis, gingivitis, glossitis, hepatitis, melena, mouth ulceration, oral moniliasis, periodontal abscess, rectal hemorrhage, stomatitis, and tongue edema

Endocrine System—Diabetes mellitus, goiter, weight gain, hyperprolactinemia, galactorrhea, amenorrhea, gynecomastia

Hepatic System—Increased SGPT, SGOT, and GGT

Hematologic and Lymphatic Systems—Cyanosis, leukocytosis, lymphadenopathy, increased eosinophil count

Metabolic and Nutritional Disorders—Weight loss, alkaline increased phosphatase, bilirubinemia, dehydration, hyperglycernia, hyperkalemia, hyperuricemia, hyperglycernia, hypokalemia, hyponatremia, ketosis, water intoxication

Muscular and Skeletal System—Arthritis, back and hip pain, bursitis, leg cramps, rheumatoid arthritis

Respiratory System—Dyspnea, apnea, asthma, epistaxis, hemoptysis, hyperventilation, voice alteration

Dermatologic System—Alopecia, contact dermatitis, dry skin, eczema, hirsutism, seborrhea, skin ulcer, urticaria, photosensitivity reaction

Genitourinary System—Hematuria, metrorrhagia, urinary incontinence, urinary tract infection

Sexual Function—Increased libido, impotence

Potential Drug Interactions

1. Given the primary CNS effects of ZYPREXA, caution should be used when olanzapine is taken in combination with other centrally acting drugs and alcohol.

2. Because of its potential for inducing hypotension, ZYPREXA may enhance the effects of certain antihypertensive agents.

3. ZYPREXA may antagonize the effects of levodopa and dopamine agonists.

4. Agents that induce CYPlA2 or glucuronyl transferase enzymes, such as omeprazole and rifampin, may cause an increase in olanzapine clearance. Inhibitors of CYPIA2 (e.g., fluvoxamine) could potentially inhibit olanzapine elimination.

5. TEGRETOL may cause an increase in the clearance of ZYPREXA.

6. The co-administration of either VALIUM or ethanol with ZYPREXA may potentiate the orthostatic hypotension.

Laboratory Tests

Periodic assessment of transaminases is recommended in individuals with significant hepatic disease.

Dosage and Administration

Usual Dose in Adults—ZYPREXA should be administered on a once a-day schedule without regard to meals, generally beginning with 5 to 10mg initially, with a target dose of 10mg/day within several days. Further dosage adjustments, if indicated, should generally occur at intervals of not less than 1 week, since steady state for ZYPREXA would not be achieved for approximately 1 week. When dosage adjustments are necessary, dose increments/ decrements of 5mg/day are recommended.

Antipsychotic efficacy was demonstrated in a dose range of 10 to 15mg/day in clinical trials. However, doses above 10mg/day were not demonstrated to be more efficacious than the 10mg/day dose. An increase to a dose greater than the target dose of 10mg/day (i.e., to a dose of 15mg/day or greater) is recommended only after clinical assessment. The safety of doses above 20mg/day has not been evaluated in clinical trials.

Maintenance Treatment—While there is no body of evidence available to answer the question of how long the individual treated with ZYPREXA should remain on it, the effectiveness of maintenance treatment is well established for many other antipsychotic drugs. It is recommended that responding individuals be continued on ZYPREXA, but at the lowest dose needed to maintain remission. Individuals should be periodically reassessed to determine the need for maintenance treatment.

Overdosage

Symptoms of overdosage include drowsiness and slurred speech. There are usually no observable adverse changes in laboratory analyses or ECG. Vital signs were usually within normal limits following overdoses.

Much of the above information was obtained from the *Physicians' Desk Reference* (PDR), published by the Medical Economics Company, and *Drug Information Handbook for Psychiatry*, published by Lexi-Comp, Inc.

Appendix I

Antiepileptic Drugs (AEDs)

Benzodiazepines

VALIUM

(Diazepam)

ATIVAN

(Lorazepam)

KLONOPIN

(Clonazepam)

TRANXENE

(Clorazepate)

These medications have been described in Chapter 10, which discusses how benzodiazepines are predominantly used as anti-anxiety medications but also have antiepileptic effects.

- Both VALIUM and ATIVAN are used intravenously in status epilepticus. VALIUM is not used as a chronic anticonvulsant because it has a reputation for causing sedation.

- ATIVAN is being used in some chronic seizure disorders, but adequate studies are not available.

- TRANXENE is used as adjunctive therapy in complex partial seizures.

DEPAKOTE®

(Divalproex Sodium)

Pharmacodynamics

DEPAKOTE is comprised of sodium valproate and valproic acid. DEPAKOTE dissociates to the valproate ion in the gastrointestinal tract. The mechanisms by which valproate exerts its therapeutic effects have not been established. It has been suggested that its activity in epilepsy is related to increased brain concentrations of gamma-aminobutyric acid (GABA), an inhibitory neurotransmitter, in brain neurons, or to enhance the action of GABA, or to mimic its action at postsynaptic receptor sites.

Pharmacokinetics

- The rate of valproate ion absorption may vary with the formulation administered (liquid, solid, or sprinkle), conditions of use (e.g., fasting or postprandial) and the method of administration (e.g., whether the contents of the capsule are sprinkled on food or the capsule is taken intact). These differences have minor clinical importance under the steady state conditions achieved in chronic use in the treatment of epilepsy.

- Co-administration of DEPAKOTE with food causes no clinical problems.

- Protein binding depends on dose of the medication and varies from 80% to 90%.

- Mean elimination half-life for DEPAKOTE monotherapy ranged from 9 to 16 hours following oral dosing regimens of 250 to 1000mg; when DEPAKOTE is used with other enzyme-inducing medications, half-life is about 8 to 9 hours.

- Steady-state blood level is reached in about 4 days.

- DEPAKOTE is metabolized almost entirely by the liver. Children between three months and ten years have 50% higher clearances than do adults. Over the age of 10 years, children have pharmacokinetic parameters that approximate those of adults.

Indications

1. Use as sole and adjunctive therapy in the treatment of simple and complex absence seizures, and adjunctively in individuals with multiple seizure types including absence and tonic-clonic seizures

2. For treatment of manic episodes associated with bipolar disorder

3. For prophylaxis of migraine headaches

4. Unlabeled use in rages with aggressive or destructive behaviors

Pediatric Use—The safety and effectiveness of DEPAKOTE for the treatment of acute mania has not been studied in individuals below the age of 18 years. The safety and effectiveness of DEPAKOTE for the prophylaxis of migraines has not been studied in individuals below the age of 16 years.

Contraindications

In individuals with

1. Hepatic disease or significant hepatic dysfunction

2. Known hypersensitivity to the drug or its components

Potential Side Effects

Body as a Whole—Asthenia, malaise, chest pain, back pain, chills, fever, infection, neck pain, pain (unspecified), neck rigidity, accidental injury, allergic reaction, face edema, edema of the extremities

Neurological System—Abnormal gait, ataxia, incoordination, headache, dizziness, tremor, catatonic reaction, amnesia, confusion, dysarthria, hypertonia, hypokinesia, paresthesia, increased reflexes, tardive dyskinesia, vertigo, nystagmus, "spots before eyes," speech disorder

Psychiatric Disorders—Abnormal dreams, insomnia, somnolence, agitation, thinking abnormalities, hallucinations, depression, emotional upset, emotional lability, nervousness, psychosis, aggression, hyperactivity, and behavioral deterioration

Cardiovascular System—Hypertension, hypotension, palpitations, postural hypotension, tachycardia, vascular anomaly, vasodilation

Gastrointestinal System—Indigestion, nausea, dyspepsia, vomiting, anorexia, increased appetite, weight loss, weight gain, dry mouth, flatulence, gastrointestinal disorder, stomatitis, abdominal pain, fecal incontinence, constipation, diarrhea, glossitis, pharyngitis, periodontal abscess

Hematologic and Lymphatic Systems—Thrombocytopenia, inhibition of the secondary phase of platelet aggregation, ecchymosis, petechiae, bruising, hematoma formation, frank hemorrhage, lymphocytosis, macrocytosis, hypofibrinogenemia, leukopenia, eosinophilia, anemia including macrocytic with or without folate deficiency, bone marrow suppression, acute intermittent porphyria

Metabolic and Endocrine Systems—Hyperammonemia, hyponatremia, inappropriate ADH secretion, peripheral edema, hyperglycemia, irregular menses, dysmenorrhea, secondary amenorrhea, breast enlargement, galactorrhea, parotid gland swelling, abnormal thyroid function tests, acute pancreatitis including fatalities

Hepatic System—Minor elevations of transaminases (e.g., SGOT and SGPT) and LDH, laboratory test results include increases in serum bilirubin and abnormal changes in other liver function tests

Muscular and Skeletal Systems—Arthralgia, arthrosis, leg cramp, twitching, myalgia

Respiratory System—Dyspnea, rhinitis, increased cough, sinusitis

Dermatologic System—Alopecia, rash, photosensitivity, generalized pruritus, erythema multiforme, Stevens-Johnson syndrome, discoid lupus erythematosis, dry skin, furunculosis, maculopapular rash, lupus erythematosus, seborrhea

Genitourinary System—Dysuria, urinary incontinence, enuresis, cystitis, metrorrhagia, and vaginal hemorrhage

Special Senses—Abnormal vision, diplopia, amblyopia, conjunctivitis, dry eyes, eye pain, deafness, ear disorder, ear pain, tinnitus, hearing loss, taste perversion

Potential Drug Interactions

1. DEPAKOTE may displace certain protein-bound medications (e.g., DILANTIN, TEGRETOL).

2. DEPAKOTE may produce CNS depression, especially when combined with another CNS depressant (e.g., alcohol).

3. Medications (e.g., DILANTIN, TEGRETOL, and MYSOLINE) that affect the level of expression of hepatic enzymes may increase the clearance of DEPAKOTE. Thus, individuals on DEPAKOTE monotherapy will generally have longer half-lives and higher concentrations than individuals receiving polytherapy with other AEDs.

4. Co-administration of aspirin with DEPAKOTE may cause a decrease in the protein binding and an inhibition of metabolism of DEPAKOTE, hence increased risk of toxicity.

5. Co-administration of FELBATOL with DEPAKOTE may produce an increase in mean valproate peak concentration. A decrease in DEPAKOTE dosage may be necessary when FELBATOL therapy is initiated.

6. Serum levels of TEGRETOL may decrease upon co-administration of DEPAKOTE and TEGRETOL.

7. The concomitant use of DEPAKOTE and KLONOPIN may induce absence status in individuals with a history of absence type seizures.

8. Plasma clearance and volume of distribution for free VALIUM may be reduced in the presence of DEPAKOTE.

9. DEPAKOTE inhibits the metabolism, decreases the total clearance, and increases the elimination half-life of MYSOLINE.

10. The elimination half-life of LAMICTAL may be increased with DEPAKOTE co-administration. The dose of LAMICTAL should be reduced when co-administered with DEPAKOTE.

11. DEPAKOTE inhibits the metabolism of LUMINAL and causes severe CNS depression, with or without significant elevations of barbiturate or valproate serum concentrations. Serum barbiturate concentrations should be obtained, if possible, and the barbiturate dosage decreased, if appropriate. MYSOLINE, which is metabolized to a barbiturate, may be involved in a similar interaction with DEPAKOTE.

12. DEPAKOTE displaces DILANTIN from its plasma albumin binding sites and inhibits its hepatic metabolism. Total plasma clearance of DILANTIN may be increased in the presence of DEPAKOTE. In individuals with epilepsy, there have been reports of break-through seizures occurring with the combination of DEPAKOTE and DILANTIN. The dosage of DILANTIN should be adjusted as required by the clinical situation.

Potential Laboratory Test Interactions

DEPAKOTE may alter thyroid function tests.

Laboratory Tests

1. Because of reports of thrombocytopenia, inhibition of the secondary phase of platelet aggregation, and abnormal coagulation parameters, (e.g., low fibrinogen), platelet counts and coagulation tests are recommended before initiating therapy and at periodic intervals.

2. Hepatic failure resulting in fatalities has occurred in individuals receiving DEPAKOTE. These incidents usually occur during the first six months of treatment. Serious or fatal hepatotoxicity may be preceded by non-specific symptoms such as malaise, weakness, lethargy, facial edema, anorexia, and vomiting. Liver function tests should be performed prior to therapy and at frequent intervals thereafter, especially during the first six months.

3. Since DEPAKOTE may interact with concurrently administered drugs which are capable of enzyme induction, periodic plasma concentration determinations of valproate and con-comitant medications are recommended during the early course of therapy.

4. The established serum therapeutic range of DEPAKOTE is 50-100µg/mL for seizure control, 50-125µg/mL for bipolar disorder. Risk of toxicity increases at levels greater than 125µg/mL.

Dosage and Administration

Since DEPAKOTE may cause GI upset, it should be taken with large amounts of water, milk, or food. DEPAKOTE solution should not be taken with carbonated beverages as it may cause mouth and throat irritation. DEPAKOTE Sprinkle capsules may be swallowed whole or opened and sprinkled on small amount of soft food and used immediately.

Treatment of Seizure Disorders

In older adolescents and adults, the recommended initial dose is 10-15mg/kg/day in one-to-three divided doses, increasing at weekly intervals by 5-10mg/kg/day until seizures are controlled or side effects preclude further increases. The maximum recommended dosage is 60mg/kg/day in two-to-three divided doses. Children receiving more than one AED may require doses up to 100mg/kg/day in three-to-four divided doses.

A good correlation has not been established between daily dose, serum concentration, and therapeutic effect. However, therapeutic valproate serum concentrations for most individuals with epilepsy will range from 50 to 100mg/mL. Some individuals may be controlled with lower or higher serum concentrations.

Anti-epilepsy drugs should not be abruptly discontinued in individuals for whom the medication is administered to prevent major seizures because of the strong possibility of precipitating status epilepticus with attendant hypoxia and threat to life. In epileptic individuals previously receiving DEPAKENE therapy, DEPAKOTE tablets should be initiated at the same daily dose and dosing schedule. After the individual is stabilized on DEPAKOTE, a dosing schedule of two or three times a day may be considered.

Treatment of Mania

In older adolescents and adults with mania, the recommended initial dose is 750mg daily in divided doses. The dose should be increased as rapidly as possible to achieve the lowest therapeutic dose that produces the desired clinical effect or the desired range of plasma concentrations. Maximum concentrations were generally achieved within 14 days. The maximum recommended dosage is 60mg/kg/day.

There is no body of evidence available from controlled trials to guide a clinician in the longer-term management of an individual who improves during DEPAKOTE treatment of an acute manic episode. While it is generally agreed that pharmacological treatment beyond an acute response in mania is desirable, both for maintenance of the initial response and for prevention of new manic episodes, there are no systematically obtained data to support the benefits of DEPAKOTE in such longer-term treatment.

Treatment of Migraine

The starting dose is 250mg twice daily. Some individuals may benefit from doses up to 1000mg/day.

Treatment of rages

There is no systematic study of using DEPAKOTE to treat rages. The clinicians are recommended to follow the above suggestion of dosage and administration for the treatment of acute mania.

Overdosage

Overdosage with DEPAKOTE may result in somnolence, deep sleep, restlessness, visual hallucination, heart block, and deep coma. Fatalities have been reported.

DEPAKENE®

(Valproic Acid)

DEPAKENE dissociates to the valproate ion in the gastrointestinal tract. Its pharmacologic properties are similar to that of DEPAKOTE.

DILANTIN® KAPSEALS®

(Extended Phenytoin Sodium Capsules)

DILANTIN-125®

(Phenytoin Oral Suspension)

INFANTABS® DILANTIN

Pharmacodynamics

The primary site of action appears to be the motor cortex where spread of seizure activity is inhibited, possibly by increasing efflux or decreasing influx of sodium ions across neuron cell membranes during generation of nerve impulses.

DILANTIN stabilizes the threshold against hyperexcitability caused by excessive stimulation or environmental changes capable of reducing membrane sodium gradient. This includes the reduction of post-tetanic potentiation at synapses. Loss of post-tetanic potentiation prevents cortical seizure foci from detonating adjacent cortical areas. DILANTIN reduces the maximal activity of brain stem centers responsible for the tonic phase of tonic-clonic (grand mal) seizures.

Pharmacokinetics

- Absorption of the extended phenytoin sodium capsules is characterized by a slow and extended rate with peak blood concentrations expected in 4-to-12 hours as contrasted to prompt phenytoin sodium capsules and the phenytoin oral suspension that have a rapid rate of absorption with peak blood concentration expected in 1½ to 3 hours.

- Fresh fruits containing vitamin C may increase urinary excretion of hydantoin and decrease the anticonvulsant effect of DILANTIN.

- The plasma half-life after oral administration of DILANTIN averages 22 hours, with a range of 7 to 42 hours.

- Steady-state therapeutic levels are achieved 7 to 10 days (5-7 half-lives) after initiation of therapy.

- Because DILANTIN is hydroxylated in the liver by an enzyme system that is saturable at high plasma levels, small incremental doses may increase the half-life and produce very substantial increases in serum levels, when these are in the upper range. The steady-state level may be disproportionately increased, with resultant intoxication, from an increase in dosage of 10% or more.

- As DILANTIN is highly protein bound, free phenytoin levels may be altered in individuals whose protein binding characteristics differ from normal.

- Most of the medication is excreted in the bile as inactive metabolites, which are then reabsorbed from the intestinal tract and excreted in the urine. Urinary excretion of DILANTIN and its metabolites occurs partly with glomerular filtration but more importantly by tubular secretion.

Indications

For the control of generalized tonic-clonic (grand mal), simple partial and complex partial seizures, and for the prevention and treatment of seizures occurring during or following neurosurgery or head trauma

Contraindications

1. Hypersensitive to DILANTIN, other hydantoins, or any component

2. Heart block or sinus bradycardia

Potential Side Effects

Central Nervous System—Nystagmus, ataxia, slurred speech, decreased coordination, mental confusion, dizziness, insomnia, transient nervousness, motor twitching, headaches, sensory peripheral polyneuropathy

Gastrointestinal System—Nausea, vomiting, constipation, toxic hepatitis, liver damage

Dermatologic System—Measles-like rashes, bullous, purpuric dermatitis, Stevens-Johnson syndrome, and toxic epidermal necrolysis

Hematologic and Lymphatic Systems—Thrombocytopenia, eosinophilia, leukopenia, granulocytopenia, agranulocytosis, pancytopenia with or without bone marrow suppression, macrocytosis, megaloblastic anemia, benign lymph node hyperplasia, pseudolymphoma, lymphoma, Hodgkin's Disease

Endocrine and Metabolic Systems—Porphyria, hyperglycemia

Connective Tissue System—Coarsening of the facial features, enlargement of the lips, gingival hyperplasia, hypertrichosis

Muscular and skeletal Systems—Osteomalacia

Cardiovascular System—Periarteritis nodosa

Immunologic System—Arthralgias, systemic lupus erythematosus, immunoglobulin abnormalities

Potential Drug Interactions

1. Medications that may increase DILANTIN serum levels include alcohol, CHLOROMYCETIN (an antibiotic), VALIUM, TAGAMET, RITALIN, THORAZINE, DESYREL, GLUCOTROL, and estrogens.

2. Medications that may decrease DILANTIN levels include TEGRETOL and chronic alcohol abuse.

3. Medications that may either increase or decrease DILANTIN serum levels include LUMINAL, DEPAKOTE, and DEPAKENE.

4. Medications whose efficacy is impaired by DILANTIN include corticosteroids, coumarin anticoagulants, digitoxin, estrogens, oral contraceptives, quinidine, theophylline, and vitamin D.

5. Ingestion times of DILANTIN and antacid preparations containing calcium should be staggered in individuals with low serum phenytoin levels to prevent absorption problems.

Potential Laboratory Test Interactions:

1. DILANTIN may produce lower than normal values for dexamethasone or metyrapone tests.

2. DILANTIN may cause increased serum levels of glucose, alkaline phosphatase, and gamma glutamyl transpeptidase (GGT).

Withdrawal Symptoms

Abrupt withdrawal of DILANTIN in epileptic individuals may precipitate status epilepticus. When, in the judgment of the clinician, the need for dosage reduction, discontinuation, or substitution of alternative AED arises, this should be done gradually. However, in the event of an allergic or hypersensitivity reaction, rapid substitution of alternative therapy may be necessary. In this case, alternative therapy should be an AED not belonging to the hydantoin chemical class.

Laboratory Tests

DILANTIN serum level determinations may be necessary to achieve optimal dosage adjustments. The clinically effective serum level (therapeutic range) is usually 10-20µg/mL. There may be wide interpatient variability in DILANTIN serum levels with equivalent dosages. Individuals with unusually low levels may be noncompliant or hypermetabolizers of DILANTIN.

Unusually high levels result from liver disease, congenital enzyme deficiency, or drug interactions which result in metabolic interference. The individual with large variations in DILANTIN plasma levels, despite standard doses, presents a difficult clinical problem. Serum level determinations in such individuals may be particularly helpful.

Dosage and Administration

DILANTIN or KAPSEALS is formulated with the sodium salt of DILANTIN. The free acid form of DILANTIN is used in DILANTIN-125 Suspension and DILANTIN INFANTABS. Because there is approximately an 8% increase in drug content with the free acid form over that of the sodium salt, dosage adjustments and serum level monitoring may be necessary when switching from a product formulated with the free acid to a product formulated with the sodium salt and vice versa.

With recommended dosage, a period of seven to ten days may be required to achieve steady-state blood levels with DILANTIN, and changes in dosage (increase or decrease) should not be carried out at intervals shorter than seven to ten days. When serum level determinations are necessary, they should be obtained at least seven to ten days after treatment initiation. The serum levels should be obtained just prior to the individual's next scheduled dose.

Optimum seizure control without clinical signs of toxicity occurs more often with serum levels between 10 and 20µg/mL, although some mild cases of tonic-clonic (grand mal) epilepsy may be controlled with lower serum levels (5-10µg/mL) of DILANTIN. However, serum levels below 5µg/mL are not likely to be effective.

Older adolescents and adults, who have received no previous treatment, may be started with a loading dose of 15-20mg/kg in a single or divided dose, followed by 100-150mg/dose at 30-minute intervals up to a maximum of 1500mg/24 hours. The maintenance dose can be 300mg/day or 5-6mg/kg/day in three divided doses or one-to-two divided doses using extended release.

In children 10-16 years, the maintenance dose is 6-7mg/kg/day every eight hours. In young children, the dosage should begin with 5mg/kg/day in two or three equally divided doses, with subsequent dosage individualized to a maximum of 300mg daily. A recommended daily maintenance dosage is usually 4 to 8mg/kg. If the daily dosage cannot be divided equally, the larger dose should be given before retiring.

Overdosage

The initial symptoms of overdosage are nystagmus, ataxia, and dysarthria. Other signs are tremor, hyperreflexia, lethargy, slurred speech, nausea, vomiting. The individuals may become comatose and hypotensive. Death is due to respiratory and circulatory depression.

There are marked variations among individuals with respect to DILANTIN plasma levels where toxicity may occur. Nystagmus, on lateral gaze, usually appears at 20μg/mL, ataxia at 30μg/mL, dysarthria and lethargy appear when the plasma concentration is over 40μg/mL, but as a concentration as high as 50μg/mL has been reported without evidence of toxicity.

FELBATOL

(Felbamate)

Pharmacodynamics

The mechanism by which FELBATOL exerts its anticonvulsant activity is unknown. Protection against maximal electroshock-induced seizures suggests that FELBATOL may reduce seizure spread, an effect possibly predictive of efficacy in generalized tonic-clonic or partial seizures. Protection against pentylenetetrazol-induced seizures suggests that FELBATOL may increase seizure threshold, an effect considered to be predictive of potential efficacy in absence seizures. FELBATOL has weak inhibitory effects on GABA-receptor binding and benzodiazepine receptor binding.

Pharmacokinetics

- FELBATOL is rapidly and almost completely absorbed after oral administration.

- There was no effect of food on absorption of the tablet; the effect of food on absorption of the suspension has not been evaluated.

- Peak serum concentration is reached within three hours.

- Elimination half-life is about 20-23 hours, which is unaltered after multiple doses.

- 40% to 50% is eliminated renally as unchanged drug and 40% as inactive metabolite in the urine.

Indications

1. Only in those individuals who respond inadequately to other AED treatments and whose epilepsy is so severe that a substantial risk of aplastic anemia and/or liver failure is deemed acceptable in light of the benefits conferred by its use

2. For either monotherapy or adjunctive therapy in the treatment of partial seizures with and without generalization, in adults with epilepsy, and as adjunctive therapy in the treatment of partial and generalized seizures associated with Lennox-Gastaut syndrome in children

Pediatric Use—The safety and effectiveness of FELBATOL in children other than those with Lennox-Gastaut syndrome has not been established.

Contraindications

1. Known hypersensitivity to the medication and its ingredients

2. Known sensitivity to other carbamates

3. History of any blood dyscrasia or hepatic dysfunction

Potential Side Effects

Body as a Whole—Weight increase, asthenia, malaise, influenza-like symptoms, fever, fatigue, weight decrease, pain, face edema neoplasm, sepsis, SIDS, sudden death, edema, hypothermia, rigors, hyperpyrexia.

Neurological System—Abnormal gait, ataxia, headache, dizziness, tremor, paraesthesia, migraine, stupor, paralysis, mononeuritis, cerebrovascular disorder, cerebral edema, coma, encephalopathy, nystagmus, choreoathetosis, extrapyramidal disorder, status epilepticus, dyskinesia, dysarthria, respiratory depression, apathy

Psychiatric Disorders—Anxiety, depression, agitation, psychological disturbance, aggressive reaction, somnolence, insomnia, nervousness, abnormal thinking, emotional lability, hallucination, euphoria, suicide attempt, delusion, impaired concentration, manic reaction, paranoid reaction, confusion, and psychosis

Cardiovascular System—Palpitation, tachycardia, atrial fibrillation, atrial arrhythmia, cardiac arrest, torsades de pointes, cardiac failure, hypotension, hypertension, flushing, thrombophlebitis, ischemic necrosis, gangrene, peripheral ischemia, bradycardia, Henoch-Schönlein purpura (vasculitis)

Respiratory System—Upper respiratory tract infection, pharyngitis, coughing, sinusitis, rhinitis, dyspnea, pneumonia, pneumonitis, hypoxia, epistaxis, pleural effusion, respiratory insufficiency, pulmonary hemorrhage, asthma

Gastrointestinal System—Dry mouth, anorexia, vomiting, constipation, hiccup, nausea, dyspepsia, constipation, diarrhea, abdominal pain, esophagitis, increased appetite

Hepatic System—Jaundice, hepatitis, increased SGOT and SGPT, hepatic failure

Hematological and Lymphatic Systems—Purpura, leukopenia, lymphadenopathy, leukocytosis, thrombocytopenia, granulocytopenia, increased and decreased prothrombin time, anemia, hypochromic anemia, aplastic anemia, pancytopenia, hemolytic uremic syndrome, increased mean corpuscular volume (MCV) with and without anemia, coagulation disorder, embolism-limb, disseminated intravascular coagulation, eosinophilia, hemolytic anemia

Metabolic System—Hypokalemia, hyponatremia, increased LDH and alkaline phosphatase, and hypophosphatemia

Muscular and Skeletal Systems—Myalgia, dystonia, arthralgia, muscle weakness, involuntary muscle contraction, rhabdomyolysis

Dermatologic System—Pruritus, rash, acne, urticaria, bullous eruption

Genitourinary System—Urinary incontinence, intermenstrual bleeding, urinary tract infection, menstrual disorder, acute renal failure, hepatorenal syndrome, hematuria, urinary retention, nephrosis, vaginal hemorrhage, abnormal renal function, dysuria, placental disorder

Special Senses—Otitis media, miosis, diplopia, taste perversion, abnormal vision, hemianopsia, decreased hearing, conjunctivitis

Potential Drug Interactions

1. FELBATOL causes an increase in steady state DILANTIN and DEPAKOTE plasma concentrations.

2. FELBATOL causes a decrease in the steady-state TEGRETOL plasma concentrations and an increase in the steady-state carbamazepine epoxide (a metabolite of TEGRETOL) plasma concentration. An increased level of this metabolite can result in clinical toxicity including diplopia, ataxia, and lethargy.

3. DILANTIN causes an approximate doubling of the clearance of FELBATOL at steady state. Therefore, the addition of DILANTIN causes an approximate 45% decrease in the steady-state trough concentrations of FELBATOL as compared to the same dose of FELBATOL given as monotherapy.

4. TEGRETOL causes an increase in the clearance of FELBATOL at steady state. Therefore, the addition of TEGRETOL results in an approximate 40% decrease in the steady-state trough concentrations of FELBATOL as compared to the same dose of FELBATOL given as monotherapy.

Potential Laboratory Tests Interactions

FELBATOL may cause slightly elevated serum cholesterol level in individuals receiving 2.6g/day.

Withdrawal Symptoms

FELBATOL should not be suddenly discontinued because of the possibility of increasing seizure frequency.

Laboratory Tests

The use of FELBATOL has been associated with a marked increase in the incidence of aplastic anemia. Among the cases who develop aplastic anemia, currently the estimate of overall fatality rates are in the range of 20% to 30%, but rates as high as 70% have been reported in the past. Hence, full hematologic evaluations should be performed before FELBATOL therapy, frequently during therapy, and for a significant period of time after discontinuation of FELBATOL therapy.

While it might appear prudent to perform frequent CBCs in individuals continuing on FELBATOL therapy, there is no evidence that such monitoring will allow early detection of marrow suppression before aplastic anemia occurs. But it will, in some cases, allow the detection of the hematologic changes before the aplastic anemia becomes clinically evident. Complete pretreatment blood counts including platelets and reticulocytes should be obtained as a baseline. If any hematologic abnormalities are detected during the course of treatment, immediate consultation with a hematologist is advised. FELBATOL should be discontinued if any evidence of bone marrow depression occurs.

Hepatic failure resulting in fatalities has been reported with a marked increase in frequency in individuals receiving FELBATOL. Hence, liver function tests (AST, ALT, bilirubin) should be done before FELBATOL is started and at one-to-two-week intervals while the patient is taking FELBATOL. If any liver abnormalities are detected during the course of treatment, FELBATOL should be discontinued immediately.

Serum therapeutic range for FELBATOL may be 40-100mg/mL. But it is not necessary to routinely monitor serum drug levels, since dose should be titrated to clinical response.

Dosage and Administration

FELBATOL has not been systematically evaluated as initial monotherapy in older adolescents and adults. Nevertheless, it is recommended to initiate FELBATOL at 1200mg/day in divided doses three or four times daily. The dosage can be increased in 600mg increments every two weeks to 2400mg/day based on clinical response and thereafter to 3600mg/day if clinically indicated.

When AEDs are converted to FELBATOL monotherapy in older adolescents and adults, initiate FELBATOL at 1200mg/day in divided doses three or four times daily while reducing the dosage of concomitant AEDs by 20% to 30%. At week 2, increase the FELBATOL dosage to 2400mg/day while reducing the dosage of other AEDs up to an additional 30% of their original dosage. At week 3, increase the FELBATOL dosage up to 3600mg/day and continue to reduce the dosage of other AEDs as clinically indicated.

As adjunctive therapy in older adolescents and adults, FELBATOL should be added at 1200mg/day in divided doses three or four times daily while reducing present AEDs by 20% in order to control plasma concentrations of concurrent DILANTIN, DEPAKOTE, TEGRETOL and its metabolites. Further reductions of the concomitant AEDs dosage may be necessary to minimize side effects due to drug interactions. Increase the dosage of FELBATOL by 1200mg/day increments at weekly intervals to 3600mg/day.

As an adjunctive therapy in children (2-14 years-of-age) with Lennox-Gastaut Syndrome, FELBATOL should be added at 15mg/kg/day in divided doses three or four times daily while reducing present AEDs by 20% in order to control plasma levels of concurrent DILANTIN, DEPAKOTE, and TEGRETOL and its metabolites. Further reductions of the concomitant AED dosage may be necessary to minimize side effects due to drug interactions. Increase the dosage of FELBATOL by 15mg/kg/day increments at weekly intervals to 45mg/kg/day divided three-to-four times/day.

Overdosage

The only adverse experiences reported were mild gastric distress and a resting heart rate of 100 bpm. No serious adverse reactions have been reported.

KEPPRA

(Levetiracetam)

Pharmacodynamics

The precise mechanism by which KEPPRA exerts its antiepileptic effect is unknown and does not appear to derive from any interaction with known mechanisms involved in inhibitory and excitatory neurotransmission. In vitro studies show that KEPPRA did not result in significant ligand displacement at known receptor binding sites. On the other hand, in vitro and in vivo recordings of epileptiform activity from the hippocampus seems to suggest that KEPPRA may selectively prevent hypersynchronization of epileptiform burst firing and propagation of seizure activity.

Pharmacokinetics

- KEPPRA is rapidly and almost completely absorbed after oral administration. The oral bioavailability of KEPPRA tablets is 100%.

- The peak plasma concentration occurs in about an hour following oral administration in fasted subjects.

- The extent of absorption and bioavailability of KEPPRA is not affected by food.

- KEPPRA is not protein bound (<10% bound) and its volume of distribution is close to the volume of intracellular and extracellular water.

- Steady state is achieved after two days of multiple twice-daily dosing.

- KEPPRA is not extensively metabolized in humans. The major metabolic pathway is the enzymatic hydrolysis of the acetamide group, and it is not dependent on any liver cytochrome P450 isoenzymes.

- Plasma half-life of KEPPRA is approximately six to eight hours. It is unaffected by either dose or repeated administration. KEPPRA is eliminated from the systemic circulation by renal excretion. Sixty-six percent of the dose is renally excreted unchanged. The mechanism of excretion is glomerular filtration with subsequent partial tubular reabsorption. KEPPRA elimination is correlated to creatinine clearance. The clearance of KEPPRA in children is approximately 40% higher than in adults. Because KEPPRA is primarily renally excreted and there are no important racial differences in creatinine clearance, pharmacokinetic differences due to race are not expected.

Indications

As adjunctive therapy in the treatment of partial complex seizures in adults

Pediatric Use—Safety and effectiveness in individuals below the age of 16 have not been established.

Contraindications

Hypersensitivity to KEPPRA or to any of the inactive ingredients in KEPPRA tablets

Potential Side Effects

Body as a Whole—Asthenia or fatigue, headache, infection, pain, abdominal pain, fever, flu syndrome, accidental injury

Neurological System—Amnesia, ataxia or coordination difficulties, dizziness, vertigo, tremor, paresthesia, convulsion, grand mal convulsion

Psychiatric Disorders—Anxiety, depression, emotional lability, hostility, nervousness, somnolence, insomnia, confusion, abnormal thinking

Respiratory System—Increased cough, pharyngitis, rhinitis, sinusitis, bronchitis, chest pain

Hematologic System—Ecchymosis, decreased WBC, decreased neutrophil count

Gastrointestinal System—Anorexia, nausea, dyspepsia, vomiting, gingivitis, diarrhea, gastroenteritis, constipation

Endocrine System—Weight gain

Genitourinary System—Urinary tract infection

Muscular and Skeletal Systems—Arthralgia, back pain

Dermatologic System—Rash, fungal infection

Special Senses—Diplopia, otitis media

Drug Interactions

KEPPRA is unlikely to produce, or be subject to, pharmacokinetic interactions with other drugs including other AEDs.

Interaction with Laboratory Tests

Although most laboratory tests are not systematically altered with KEPPRA treatment, there have been relatively infrequent abnormalities seen in hematologic parameters and liver function tests.

Withdrawal Symptoms

KEPPRA should be withdrawn gradually to minimize the potential of increased seizure frequency.

Laboratory Tests

The value of monitoring plasma concentrations of KEPPRA has not been established.

Dosage and Administration

KEPPRA is given orally with or without food. Treatment should be initiated with a daily dose of 1000mg/day, given as twice daily dosing. Additional dosing increments may be given (1000mg/day additional every two weeks) to a maximum recommended daily dose of 3000mg. There is no evidence that doses greater than 3000mg/day provide additional benefit.

Overdosage

Other than drowsiness, there were no adverse events in the few known cases of overdose.

KLONOPIN®

(Clonazepam)

Pharmacodynamics

KLONOPIN acts by depressing nerve transmission in the motor cortex and thus suppressing the spike-and-wave discharge in absence seizures.

Pharmacokinetics

- KLONOPIN is well absorbed following oral administration. About 85% is bound to protein.

- Onset of effect is about 20-60 minutes after oral administration.

- Time to peak serum concentration is about one-to-three hours.

- Duration of effect after each dose is up to 6-8 hours in infants and young children, and up to 12 hours in adults.

- Half-life in children is about 22-23 hours, and about 19-50 hours in adults.

- Steady state is reached within five to seven days.

- Less than 2% is excreted unchanged in urine.

Indications

1. For prophylaxis or treatment of petit mal, petit mal variant (Lennox-Gastaut), akinetic, and myoclonic seizures

2. Unlabeled use in the treatment of agitation with or without aggression, restless legs syndrome, neuralgia, multifocal tic disorders, parkinsonian dysarthria, acute manic episodes, and adjunct therapy for schizophrenia

Pediatric Use—Because of the possibility that adverse effects on physical or mental development could become apparent only after many years, a benefit-risk consideration of the long-term use of KLONOPIN in children is important.

Contraindications

1. History of sensitivity to benzodiazepines

2. Evidence of significant liver disease

3. Acute narrow angle glaucoma

Potential Side Effects

Neurological System—Abnormal eye movements, aphonia, choreiform movements, ataxia, coma, diplopia, dysarthria, dysdiadochokinesis, "glassy-eyed" appearance, headache, hemiparesis, hypotonia, nystagmus, respiratory depression, slurred speech, tremor, and vertigo

Psychiatric Disorders—Drowsiness, confusion, depression, amnesia, hallucinations, hysteria, increased libido, insomnia, and psychosis

Respiratory System—Chest congestion, rhinorrhea, shortness of breath, hypersecretion in upper respiratory passages

Cardiovascular System—Palpitations

Dermatologic System—Hair loss, hirsutism, skin rash, ankle and facial edema

Gastrointestinal System—Anorexia, coated tongue, constipation, diarrhea, dry mouth, hypersecretion of saliva, encopresis, gastritis, hepatomegaly, increased appetite, nausea, and sore gums

Genitourinary System—Dysuria, enuresis, nocturia, urinary retention

Muscular and Skeletal Systems—Muscle weakness, pains

Hematologic System—Anemia, leukopenia, thrombocytopenia, eosinophilia

Hepatic System—Transient elevations of serum transaminases and alkaline phosphatase

Miscellaneous—Dehydration, general deterioration, fever, lymphadenopathy, weight loss or gain

Potential Drug Interactions

1. Alcohol, narcotics, barbiturates, nonbarbiturate hypnotics, antianxiety agents, the phenothiazine, thioxanthene, and butyrophenone classes of antipsychotic agents, monoamine oxidase inhibitors, the tricyclic antidepressants, and other anticonvulsant drugs may potentiate the CNS-depressant action of KLONOPIN.

2. DILANTIN and barbiturates may increase KLONOPIN clearance and thus decrease its antiepileptic effect.

3. When used in individuals in whom several different types of seizure disorders coexist, KLONOPIN may increase the incidence or precipitate the onset of generalized tonic-clonic (grand mal) seizures.

4. The concomitant use of DEPAKOTE and KLONOPIN may produce absence status.

Withdrawal Symptoms

Following abrupt discontinuance of KLONOPIN taken continuously at therapeutic levels for several months, withdrawal symptoms such as dysphoria and insomnia may develop.

In individuals on long-term, high-dose therapy, the abrupt withdrawal of KLONOPIN may precipitate status epilepticus. Therefore, when discontinuing KLONOPIN, gradual withdrawal is essential.

Drug Abuse and Dependence

Addiction-prone individuals (such as drug addicts or alcoholics) should be under careful surveillance when receiving KLONOPIN because of the predisposition of such individuals to habituation and dependence.

Laboratory Tests

1. Periodic blood counts and liver function tests are advisable during long-term therapy with KLONOPIN.

2. At present, the relationship of blood levels to therapeutic effects of KLONOPIN is unclear, though it has been suggested as 5-70ng/mL. Serum levels higher than 80ng/mL tend to produce toxic effects.

Dosage and Administration

<u>Infants and Children</u>

In order to minimize drowsiness, the initial dose for infants and children (up to ten years-of-age or 30 kg of body weight) should be between 0.01 and 0.03mg/kg/day, but not to exceed 0.05mg/kg/day, given in two or three divided doses. Dosage should be increased by no more than 0.25 to 0.5mg every third day until a daily maintenance dose of 0.1-to-0.2mg/kg of body weight has been reached or until seizures are controlled or side effects preclude further increase. Whenever possible, the daily dose should be divided into three equal doses. If doses are not equally divided, the largest dose should be given at bedtime.

Adults: The initial dose for adults should not exceed 1.5mg/day divided into three doses. Dosage may be increased in increments of 0.5 to 1mg every three days until seizures are adequately controlled or until side effects preclude any further increase. Maintenance dosage must be individualized depending upon response. Maximum recommended daily dose is 20mg.

Overdosage

Symptoms and signs of overdose include somnolence, confusion, ataxia, diminished reflexes, or coma.

LAMICTAL®

(Lamotrigine)

Pharmacodynamics

The precise mechanism by which LAMICTAL exerts its anticonvulsant action is unknown. One proposed mechanism of action of LAMICTAL involves an effect on sodium channels: LAMICTAL inhibits voltage-sensitive sodium channels, thereby stabilizing neuronal membranes and consequently inhibiting presynaptic transmitter release of excitatory amino acids (e.g., glutamate and aspartate). It appears that LAMICTAL has a weak inhibitory effect on the serotonin 5-HT3 receptor.

Pharmacokinetics

- LAMICTAL is rapidly and completely absorbed after oral administration with negligible first-pass metabolism (absolute bioavailability is 98%).

- Bioavailability is not affected by food.

- LAMICTAL is approximately 55% bound to human plasma proteins.

- Because LAMICTAL is not highly bound to plasma proteins, clinically significant interactions with other drugs through competition for protein binding sites are unlikely. The binding of LAMICTAL to plasma proteins did not change in the presence of therapeutic concentrations of DILANTIN, LUMINAL, or DEPAKOTE. LAMICTAL does not displace other AEDs (TEGRETOL, DILANTIN, LUMINAL) from protein binding sites.

- LAMICTAL is metabolized predominantly by glucuronic acid conjugation; the major metabolite is an inactive 2-N-glucuronide conjugate.

- Peak serum level is reached one to four hours following drug administration.

- Half-life is about 24 hours when used alone; it decreases to 12-15 hours when used with other AEDs. When used with DEPAKOTE, the half-life is about 48 to 72 hours.

- LAMICTAL is eliminated in urine as the glucuronide conjugate.

Indications

1. Adjunctive therapy in adults and adolescents with partial and secondarily generalized epilepsy, as well as in a wide range of seizure types, including typical and atypical absence seizures, atonic seizures, myoclonic seizures, and in Lennox-Gastaut syndrome in children

2. Unlabeled treatment for bipolar disorder

Pediatric Use—Safety and effectiveness in pediatric patients below the age of 16 have not been established.

Contraindications

Hypersensitivity to the drug or its ingredients

Potential Side Effects

Body as a whole—Headache, faintness, accidental injury, flu syndrome, fever, abdominal pain, infection, neck pain, malaise, aggravated reaction, chills, allergic reaction, face edema, halitosis, enlarged abdomen, and abscess

Neurological System—Dizziness, somnolence, insomnia, ataxia, incoordination, tremor, convulsion, vertigo, nystagmus, dysarthria, speech disorder, abnormal gait, akathisia, apathy, aphasia, dyskinesia, hyperkinesia, hypesthesia, myoclonus, stupor

Psychiatric Disorders—Depression, dysphoria, euphoria, racing mind, anxiety, nervousness, irritability, agitation, hostility, emotional lability, decreased memory, amnesia, confusion, concentration disturbance, sleep disorder, abnormal dreams, abnormal thinking, depersonalization, hallucinations, panic attack, paranoid reaction, personality disorder, psychosis

Cardiovascular System—Hot flashings, palpitations, migraine, postural hypotension, syncope, tachycardia, and vasodilation

Gastrointestinal System—Tooth disorder, dry mouth, increased salivation, thirst, gingivitis, glossitis, gum hyperplasia, mouth ulceration, dysphagia, nausea, vomiting, dyspepsia, anorexia, increased appetite, constipation, diarrhea, abnormal liver function tests, stomatitis

Muscular and Skeletal System—Arthralgia, joint disorder, myasthenia, muscle spasm, twitching.

Respiratory System—Rhinitis, pharyngitis, cough, dyspnea, epistaxis, hyperventilation

Dermatologic System—Rashes including Steven-Johnson syndrome and toxic epidermal necrolysis (rare but potentially fatal), pruritus, alopecia, acne, dry skin, eczema, erythema, hirsutism, maculopapular rash, sweating, vesiculobullous rash, urticaria, photosensitivity

Hematologic and Lymphatic Systems—Anemia, ecchymosis, eosinophilia, leukocytosis, leukopenia, lymphadenopathy, petechia

Endocrine and Metabolic Systems—Weight gain, weight loss, alkaline phosphatase increase, peripheral edema, dysmenorrhea, amenorrhea, breast pain

Genitourinary System—Vaginitis, vaginal moniliasis, lactation, hematuria, polyuria, urinary frequency, urinary incontinence, urinary retention

Sexual Function—Impotence

Ocular System—Diplopia, blurred vision, vision abnormality, abnormality of accommodation, conjunctivitis, photophobia

Special Senses—Ear pain, tinnitus, taste perversion

Drug Interactions

1. LAMICTAL is eliminated more rapidly in individuals who have been taking AEDs including TEGRETOL, DILANTIN, LUMINAL, and MYSOLINE.

2. The addition of DILANTIN decreases LAMICTAL steady-state concentrations by approximately fifty percent.

3. TEGRETOL, LUMINAL, and MYSOLINE decrease LAMICTAL steady state concentrations by approximately forty percent.

4. DEPAKOTE increases LAMICTAL steady-state concentrations by slightly more than two-fold.

5. The addition of LAMICTAL to DILANTIN or TEGRETOL does not affect their steady-state plasma concentrations.

6. When LAMICTAL is administered to individuals already receiving DEPAKOTE, the steady state DEPAKOTE concentrations in plasma decreased by an average of 25% over a three-week period, and then stabilized. When it is to be administered to an individual receiving DEPAKOTE, LAMICTAL must be given at a reduced dosage, less than half the dose used in individuals not receiving DEPAKOTE.

Potential Laboratory Test Interactions

None known.

Drug Abuse and Dependence

The abuse and dependence potential of LAMICTAL have not been evaluated in human studies.

Withdrawal Symptoms

Unless safety concerns require a more rapid withdrawal, the dose of LAMICTAL should be tapered over a period of at least two weeks.

Laboratory Tests

1. The value of monitoring plasma concentrations of LAMICTAL has not been established, though the therapeutic range is considered to be 2-4 µg/mL.

2. Because of the possible pharmacokinetic interactions between LAMICTAL and other AEDs being taken concomitantly, monitoring of the plasma levels of LAMICTAL and concomitant AEDs may be indicated, particularly during dosage adjustments.

3. Because LAMICTAL binds to melanin, it could accumulate in melanin-rich tissues over time. This raises the possibility that LAMICTAL may cause toxicity in these tissues after extended use. Accordingly, although there are no specific recommendations for periodic ophthalmological

monitoring, an individual with ASD and his or her parents or guardians should be aware of the possibility of long-term ophthalmologic effects.

Dosage and Administration

The risk of nonserious rash increased when the recommended initial dose or the rate of dose escalation of LAMICTAL is exceeded. There are suggestions that the risk of severe, potentially life-threatening rash may be increased by

1. Co-administration of LAMICTAL with DEPAKOTE

2. Exceeding the recommended initial dose of LAMICTAL

3. Exceeding the recommended dose escalation for LAMICTAL

Cases have also been reported in the absence of these factors. Because of the increased risk of serious rash, the recommended initial dose and subsequent dose escalations of LAMICTAL should not be exceeded.

Individuals Receiving Other AEDs, but Not DEPAKOTE

In adults, the initial dose of LAMICTAL is 50mg once a day for two weeks, followed by 100mg/day given in two divided doses for two weeks. Thereafter, the usual maintenance dose is 300 to 500mg/day given in two divided doses. To achieve maintenance, doses may be increased by 100mg/day every one-to-two weeks. In children, the dose range is 2-15mg/kg/day in 2 divided doses.

Individuals with Concomitant DEPAKOTE Therapy

The initial dose of LAMICTAL is 25mg every other day for two weeks, followed by 25mg once a day for two weeks. Then titrate to maintenance dose of 50-200mg/day in one-to-two divided daily doses.

Discontinuation Strategy

For individuals receiving LAMICTAL in combination with other AEDs, a reevaluation of all AEDs in the regimen should be considered if a change in seizure control, or an appearance of worsening, or another adverse experience is observed. If a decision is made to discontinue therapy with LAMICTAL, a step-wise reduction of dose over at least two weeks (approximately 50% per week) is recommended unless safety concerns require a more rapid withdrawal.

Overdosage

Symptoms of overdosage include dizziness, headache, somnolence, and coma.

MEBARAL®

(Mephobarbital)

Pharmacodynamics

MEBARAL depresses monosynaptic and polysynaptic transmission in the CNS, depresses the sensory cortex, and increases seizure threshold.

Pharmacokinetics

- Approximately 50% of an oral dose of MEBARAL is absorbed from the gastrointestinal tract.

- MEBARAL is bound to plasma and tissue proteins to a varying degree with the degree of binding increasing directly as a function of lipid solubility.

- About 75% of a single oral dose of MEBARAL is converted to phenobarbital in 24 hours. Therefore, chronic administration of MEBARAL may lead to an accumulation of phenobarbital in plasma.

- Following oral administration, the onset of action of the drug is 30 to 60 minutes and the duration of action is 10 to 16 hours.

- Elimination half-life is about 36 hours.

- The primary route of MEBARAL metabolism is N-demethylation by the microsomal enzymes of the liver to form phenobarbital.

- Phenobarbital may be excreted in the urine unchanged or further metabolized to p-hydroxyphenobarbital and excreted in the urine as glucuronide or sulfate conjugates.

Indications

1. Anticonvulsant for the treatment of grand mal and petit mal seizures

2. Sedative for the relief of anxiety, tension, and apprehension

Contraindications

1. Hypersensitivity to MEBARAL, other barbiturates, or any component

2. Pre-existing CNS depression

3. Respiratory depression

4. History of porphyria

Potential Side Effects

Nervous System—Somnolence, agitation, headache, confusion, hyperkinesia, ataxia, CNS depression, nightmares, nervousness, psychiatric disturbance, hallucinations, insomnia, anxiety, dizziness, thinking abnormality

Respiratory System—Hypoventilation, apnea

Cardiovascular System—Bradycardia, hypotension, and syncope

Gastrointestinal System—Nausea, vomiting, constipation, liver damage

Hematologic System—Megaloblastic anemia

Dermatologic System—Hypersensitivity reactions (angioedema, skin rashes, exfoliative dermatitis)

Potential Drug Interactions

1. The effect of MEBARAL on the metabolism of DILANTIN appears to be variable. Because the effect of MEBARAL on the metabolism of DILANTIN is not predictable, DILANTIN and MEBARAL blood levels should be monitored more frequently if these medications are given concurrently.

2. DEPAKOTE and DEPAKENE appear to decrease MEBARAL metabolism; therefore, MEBARAL blood levels should be monitored and appropriate dosage adjustments made as indicated.

3. The concomitant use of other central nervous system depressants including other sedatives or hypnotics, antihistamines, tranquilizers, or alcohol may produce additive depressant effects.

4. Monoamine Oxidase Inhibitors (MAOI) prolong the effects of MEBARAL, probably because metabolism of MEBARAL is inhibited.

5. MEBARAL appears to enhance the metabolism of exogenous corticosteroids, probably through the induction of hepatic microsomal enzymes. Individuals stabilized on corticosteroid therapy may require dosage adjustments if MEBARAL is added to or withdrawn from their dosage regimen.

6. Pretreatment with or concurrent administration of MEBARAL may decrease the effect of estradiol by increasing its metabolism. There have been reports of individuals treated with antiepileptic drugs (e.g. phenobarbital) who become pregnant while taking oral contraceptives. MEBARAL may have similar effect.

7. MEBARAL may increase vitamin D requirements, possibly by increasing vitamin D metabolism via enzyme induction. Rarely, rickets and osteomalacia have been reported following prolonged use of barbiturates.

Drug Abuse and Dependence

MEBARAL is a controlled substance in Narcotic Schedule IV. It may be habit forming. Tolerance, psychological dependence, and physical dependence may occur especially following prolonged use of high doses of MEBARAL.

Treatment of MEBARAL dependence consists of cautious and gradual withdrawal of the drug. In all cases withdrawal takes an extended period of time. One method involves initiating treatment at the individual's regular dosage level and decreasing the daily dosage by 10% if tolerated by the individual.

Withdrawal Symptoms

The symptoms of MEBARAL withdrawal can be severe and may cause death. Minor withdrawal symptoms may appear 8 to 12 hours after the last dose of MEBARAL. These symptoms usually appear in the following order: anxiety, muscle twitching, tremor of hands and fingers, progressive weakness, dizziness, distortion in visual perception, nausea, vomiting, insomnia, and orthostatic hypotension. Major withdrawal symptoms (convulsions and delirium) may occur within 16 hours and last up to five days after abrupt cessation of these drugs. Intensity of withdrawal symptoms gradually declines over a period of approximately 15 days.

Status epilepticus may result from the abrupt discontinuation of MEBARAL, even when administered in small daily doses in the treatment of epilepsy.

Laboratory Tests

1. Prolonged therapy with MEBARAL should be accompanied by periodic laboratory evaluation of organ systems, including hematopoietic, renal, and hepatic systems.

2. Therapeutic plasma concentrations for MEBARAL have not been established.

Dosage and Administration

Treatment of Epilepsy

Average dose for adults is: 400mg to 600mg daily; for children over five years: 32mg to 64mg three or four times daily; for children under five years: 16mg to 32mg three or four times daily. MEBARAL is best taken at bedtime if seizures generally occur at night, and during the day if attacks are diurnal.

Treatment should be started with a small dose that is gradually increased over four or five days until the optimum dosage is determined. If the individual has been taking some other antiepileptic drug, it should be tapered off as the dose of MEBARAL is increased, to guard against the temporary marked attacks that may occur when any treatment for epilepsy is changed abruptly. Similarly, when the dose is to be lowered to a maintenance level or to be discontinued, the amount should be reduced gradually over four or five days.

Combination with Other Medications

MEBARAL may also be used with DILANTIN. In some cases, combined therapy appears to give better results than either agent used alone, since DILANTIN is particularly effective for the psychomotor types of seizure but relatively ineffective for petit mal seizure. When the medications are taken concurrently, the DILANTIN dose should be reduced, but the full dose of MEBARAL may be given. Satisfactory results have been obtained with an average daily dose of 230mg of DILANTIN plus about 600mg of MEBARAL.

Overdosage

The toxic dose of MEBARAL varies considerably. Acute overdosage with MEBARAL is manifested by CNS depression with unsteady gait, slurred speech, sustained nystagmus, respiratory depression with apnea, constriction of the pupils to a slight degree (though in severe poisoning they may show paralytic dilation), oliguria, tachycardia, hypotension, lowered body temperature, and coma.

In extreme overdose, all electrical activity in the brain may cease. This effect is fully reversible unless hypoxic damage occurs. Complications such as pneumonia, pulmonary edema, cardiac arrhythmias, congestive heart failure, and renal failure may occur.

MYSOLINE

(Primidone)

Pharmacodynamics

The mechanism of antiepileptic action is not known. MYSOLINE may decrease neuron excitability and raise seizure thresholds or alter seizure patterns.

Pharmacokinetics

- Protein binding is very high, about 99%.

- MYSOLINE is metabolized in the liver to two metabolites: Phenobarbital (active) and phenylethylmalonamide (PEMA).

- Bioavailability is 60% to 80%.

- Peak serum concentration after oral administration is reached within 4 hours.

- Elimination half-life is about 10-12 hours for MYSOLINE, 52-118 hours for phenobarbital, and 16 hours for PEMA.

- Urinary excretion of both active metabolites and unchanged MYSOLINE is about 15% to 25%.

Indications

1. MYSOLINE, used alone or concomitantly with other anticonvulsants, is indicated in the control of grand mal, psychomotor, and secondarily generalized seizures. It may control grand mal seizures refractory to other anticonvulsant therapy.

2. Unlabeled use for treatment of benign familiar tremor (essential tremor)

Contraindications

1. Individuals with porphyria

2. Individuals who are hypersensitive to phenobarbital

Potential Side Effects

Neurological System—Ataxia, vertigo, nystagmus, and drowsiness

Psychiatric Disorders—Fatigue, hyperirritability, and emotional disturbances

Gastrointestinal System—Nausea, anorexia, vomiting

Sexual Function—Impotency

Potential Drug Interactions

1. MYSOLINE may decrease serum concentrations of ZARONTIN and DEPAKOTE.

2. DILANTIN and RITALIN may decrease MYSOLINE serum concentration.

Withdrawal Symptoms

The abrupt withdrawal of MYSOLINE may precipitate status epilepticus.

Laboratory Tests

1. A complete blood count and a sequential multiple analysis-12 (SMA-12) test should be made every six months.

2. Serum therapeutic range of MYSOLINE is 10-30µg/mL.

Dosage and Administration

Dosage should be individualized to provide maximum benefit. In some cases, serum blood level determinations of MYSOLINE may be necessary for optimal dosage adjustment. The therapeutic efficacy of a dosage regimen takes several weeks before it can be assessed.

Individuals older than eight years-of-age who have received no previous treatment may be started on MYSOLINE according to the following regimen:

1. Days 1 to 3: 100 to 125mg at bedtime

2. Days 4 to 6: 100 to 125mg twice daily

3. Days 7 to 9: 100 to 125mg three times daily

4. Day 10 to maintenance: 250mg three times daily.

For most adults and children eight years-of-age and over, the usual maintenance dosage is 250mg three-to-four times daily. If necessary, an increase to 1500mg daily in divided doses may be made but doses should not exceed 2000mg/day.

In individuals already receiving other AEDs, MYSOLINE should be started at 100 to 125mg at bedtime and gradually increased to maintenance level as the other drug is gradually decreased. This regimen should be continued until satisfactory dosage level is achieved for the combination, or the other medication is completely withdrawn. When therapy with MYSOLINE alone is the objective, the transition from concomitant therapy should not be completed in less than two weeks.

In children under 8 years-of-age, the following regimen may be used:

1. Days 1 to 3: 50mg at bedtime

2. Days 4 to 6: 50mg twice daily

3. Days 7 to 9: 100mg twice daily

4. Day 10 to maintenance: 125mg to 250mg three times daily

Overdosage

Signs and symptoms of MYSOLINE overdose include: unsteady gait, slurred speech, confusion, jaundice, hypothermia, fever, hypotension, coma, respiratory arrest.

NEURONTIN®

(Gabapentin)

Pharmacodynamics

The mechanism by which NEURONTIN exerts its anticonvulsant action is unknown. NEURONTIN is structurally related to the neurotransmitter GABA, (gamma-aminobutyric acid) but it does not interact with GABA receptors. It is not converted metabolically into GABA or a GABA agonist, and it is not an inhibitor of GABA uptake or degradation.

Pharmacokinetics

- After oral administration, about 50% to 60% NEURONTIN is absorbed from the GI tract.

- Food has no effect on the rate and extent of absorption of NEURONTIN.

- NEURONTIN circulates largely unbound to plasma protein.

- The liver does not metabolize NEURONTIN.

- Elimination half-life is 5 to 7 hours and is unaltered by size of dose or by multiple dosing.

- NEURONTIN is eliminated from the systemic circulation by renal excretion as the unchanged drug.

Indications

1. Add-on therapy in individuals over 12 years-of-age for drug-refractory partial seizures with or without secondary generalized seizures

2. Unlabeled use in Bipolar Mood Disorder

Pediatric Use—Safety and effectiveness in children below the age of 12 years have not been established.

Contraindications

Hypersensitivity to the drug or its ingredients

Potential Side Effects

Body As A Whole—Fatigue, weight increase, back pain, peripheral edema

Neurological System—Dizziness, ataxia, abnormal coordination, hyperkinesia, paresthesia, decreased or absent reflexes, increased reflexes, nystagmus, tremor, dysarthria, amnesia, twitching, CNS tumors, syncope, aphasia, hypesthesia, intracranial hemorrhage, hypotonia, dysesthesia, paresis, dystonia, hemiplegia, facial paralysis, stupor, cerebellar dysfunction, positive Babinski sign, decreased position sense, subdural hematoma

Psychiatric Disorders—Anxiety, hostility, depression, somnolence, nervousness, abnormal thinking and dreaming, hallucination, agitation, paranoia, depersonalization, euphoria, feeling high, apathy, doped-up sensation, suicidal ideation, psychosis

Cardiovascular System—Hypertension, vasodilatation, hypotension, angina pectoris, peripheral vascular disorder, palpitation, tachycardia, migraine, murmur

Gastrointestinal System—Dry mouth or throat, dental abnormalities, gingivitis, gum hemorrhage, glossitis, thirst, stomatitis, increased salivation, dyspepsia, anorexia, flatulence, constipation, increased appetite, gastroenteritis, hemorrhoids, bloody stools, fecal incontinence, and hepatomegaly

Hematologic and Lymphatic System—Purpura, decreased WBC (leukopenia), anemia, thrombocytopenia, and lymphadenopathy

Muscular and Skeletal Systems—Arthralgia, myalgia, fracture, tendinitis, arthritis, joint stiffness, joint swelling

Respiratory System—Pneumonia, rhinitis, pharyngitis, coughing, epistaxis, dyspnea, apnea

Dermatologic System—Abrasion, pruritus, alopecia, eczema, dry skin, increased sweating, urticaria, hirsutism, seborrhea, cyst, herpes simplex

Genitourinary System—Hematuria, dysuria, urination frequency, cystitis urinary retention, urinary incontinence, vaginal hemorrhage, amenorrhea, dysmenorrhea, menorrhagia

Sexual Function—Impotence, decreased or lost libido, abnormal ejaculation, inability to climax

Special Senses—Abnormal vision, diplopia, amblyopia, cataract, conjunctivitis, dry eyes, eye pain, visual field defect, photophobia, bilateral or unilateral drooping of upper eyelid, eye hemorrhage, hordeolum, hearing loss, earache, tinnitus, inner ear infection, otitis, taste loss, unusual taste, eye twitching, ear fullness

Potential Drug Interactions

1. Antacids such as MAALOX reduce the bioavailability of NEURONTIN by about 20%. This decrease in bioavailability was about 5% when NEURONTIN was administered two hours after MAALOX. It is recommended that NEURONTIN be taken at least two hours following MAALOX administration.

2. TAGAMET may decrease clearance of NEURONTIN and cause toxicity.

Drug Abuse and Administration

The abuse and dependence potential of NEURONTIN has not been evaluated in human studies.

Laboratory Tests

The value of monitoring NEURONTIN blood concentrations has not been established, although the minimum effective serum concentration may be $2\mu g/mL$. Routine monitoring of clinical laboratory parameters is not necessary for the safe use of NEURONTIN.

Dosage and Administration

NEURONTIN is given orally with or without food. The effective dose of NEURONTIN in older adolescents and adults is 900 to 1800mg/day, and in children the dosage range is 10-30mg/kg/day. NEURONTIN should be given in divided doses (three times a day) using 300 or 400mg capsules.

Titration to an effective dose can take place rapidly, over a few days:

1. 300mg on day 1

2. 300mg twice on day 2

3. 300mg three times on day 3

To minimize potential side effects, especially somnolence, dizziness, fatigue, and ataxia, the first dose on day 1 may be administered at bedtime. If necessary, the dose may be increased using 300 or 400mg capsules three times a day up to 1800mg/day. Dosages up to 2400mg/day have been well tolerated in long-term clinical studies. Doses of 3600mg/day have also been administered to a small number of individuals for a relatively short duration, and have been well tolerated. The maximum time between doses in the T.I.D. schedule should not exceed 12 hours.

When NEURONTIN is discontinued or alternate anticonvulsant medication is added to the therapy, this should be done gradually over a minimum of one week.

Overdosage

Symptoms and signs of acute overdose of NEURONTIN include double vision, slurred speech, drowsiness, lethargy and diarrhea.

TEGRETOL®

(Carbamazepine)

TEGRETOL-XR

(Carbamazepine Extended-Release Tablets)

CARBATROL®

(Carbamazepine Extended-Release Capsules)

Pharmacodynamics

The mechanism of antiepileptic action remains unknown. But it appears that TEGRETOL acts by depressing activity in the nucleus ventralis of the thalamus, by decreasing synaptic transmission, or by decreasing summation of temporal stimulation leading to neural discharge by limiting influx of sodium ions across the cell membrane.

Pharmacokinetics

- TEGRETOL is slowly absorbed from the GI tract. TEGRETOL suspension, conventional tablets, and XR tablets delivered equivalent amounts of drug to the systemic circulation. However, the suspension was absorbed somewhat faster, and the XR tablet slightly slower, than the conventional tablet. The suspension provides higher peak levels and lower trough levels than those obtained from the conventional tablet.

- Following chronic oral administration of suspension, plasma levels peak at approximately one-and-a-half hours compared to four-to-five hours after administration of conventional TEGRETOL tablets and 3-12 hours after administration of TEGRETOL-XR tablets.

- TEGRETOL in blood is 75% to 90% bound to plasma proteins.

- TEGRETOL is metabolized in the liver. It induces a liver enzyme to increase metabolism and shorten half-life over time.

- Because TEGRETOL induces its own metabolism, the half-life is also variable. Initial half-life values range from 18-55 hours, decreasing to 12-17 hours (in adults) and 8-14 hours (in children) on repeated doses.

- Steady state blood level is established between five and ten days.

- About 1% to 3% TEGRETOL is excreted unchanged in urine.

Indications

1. For the prophylaxis or treatment of partial seizures with complex symptomatology (psycho-motor, temporal lobe), generalized tonic-clonic (grand mal) seizures, mixed seizure patterns, or other partial or generalized seizures

2. For the treatment of trigeminal neuralgia and in glossopharyngeal neuralgia

3. Unlabeled use in the treatment of bipolar disorder and other affective disorders

4. Unlabeled use in the treatment of rages with aggressions and destructive behaviors

5. Unlabeled use in restless leg syndrome

6. Unlabeled use in psychotic behavior with dementia

7. Unlabeled use in resistant schizophrenia

Contraindications

1. Individuals with a history of previous bone marrow depression

2. Individuals with hypersensitivity to TEGRETOL, or known sensitivity to any of the tricyclic compounds, such as amitriptyline, desipramine, imipramine, nortriptyline, etc.

3. Co-administration of TEGRETOL with an MAOI is not recommended. Before administration of TEGRETOL, MAOIs should be discontinued for a minimum of 14 days or longer if the clinical situation permits.

Potential Side Effects

Neurological System—Dizziness, drowsiness, disturbances of coordination, confusion, headache, fatigue, oculomotor disturbances, nystagmus, speech disturbances, abnormal involuntary movements, peripheral neuritis and paresthesias, isolated cases of neuroleptic malignant syndrome

Psychiatric Disorders—Visual hallucinations, depression with agitation, talkativeness

Hematologic and Lymphatic Systems—Aplastic anemia, agranulocytosis, pancytopenia, bone marrow depression, thrombocytopenia, leukopenia, leukocytosis, eosinophilia, acute intermittent porphyria, adenopathy or lymphadenopathy

Dermatologic System—Pruritic and erythematous rashes, urticaria, toxic epidermal necrolysis (Lyell's syndrome), Stevens-Johnson syndrome, photosensitivity reactions, alterations in skin pigmentation, exfoliative dermatitis, erythema multiforme and nodosum, purpura, aggravation of disseminated lupus erythematosus, alopecia, diaphoresis

Cardiovascular System—Congestive heart failure, edema, aggravation of hypertension, hypotension, syncope and collapse, aggravation of coronary artery disease, arrhythmias and AV block, thrombophlebitis, thromboembolism

Hepatic System—Abnormalities in liver function tests, elevated levels of cholesterol, HDL cholesterol, and triglycerides, cholestatic and hepatocellular jaundice, hepatitis

Respiratory System—Pulmonary hypersensitivity characterized by fever, dyspnea, pneumonitis, or pneumonia

Genitourinary System—Urinary frequency, acute urinary retention, oliguria with elevated blood pressure, azotemia, renal failure, impotence, albuminuria, glycosuria, elevated BUN, microscopic deposits in the urine

Gastrointestinal System—Nausea, vomiting, gastric distress and abdominal pain, diarrhea, constipation, anorexia, and dryness of the mouth and pharynx including glossitis, and stomatitis

Muscular and Skeletal Systems—Aching joints and muscles, leg cramps

Metabolic System—Fever, chills, inappropriate antidiuretic hormone (ADH) secretion syndrome, water intoxication, decreased serum plasma levels of sodium (hyponatremia) and calcium (hypocalcemia)

Special Senses—blurred vision, transient diplopia, scattered punctate cortical lens opacities, conjunctivitis, tinnitus, hyperacusis

Potential Drug Interactions

1. Medications that have been shown or that would be expected to increase plasma TEGRETOL levels include TAGAMET, ERYTHROMYCIN, CALAN, DEPAKOTE, and PROZAC.

2. Medications that have been shown or that would be expected to decrease plasma TEGRETOL levels include FELBATOL, MEBARAL, DILANTIN, MYSOLINE and medications containing theophylline salt.

3. TEGRETOL causes, or would be expected to cause, increased levels of ANAFRANIL, DILANTIN, and MYSOLINE.

4. TEGRETOL causes, or would be expected to cause, decreased levels of the following: XANAX, KLONOPIN, CLOZARIL, ZARONTIN, HALDOL, phensuximide, DILANTIN, DEPAKOTE, TYLENOL, oral contraceptives, theophylline, corticosteroids, and thyroid hormones.

5. Co-administration of TEGRETOL and lithium may increase the risk of neurotoxic side effects.

6. Breakthrough bleeding has been reported among individuals receiving concomitant oral contraceptives, and their reliability may be adversely affected.

Potential Test Interactions

TEGRETOL may increase BUN, AST, ALT, bilirubin, and alkaline phosphatase and may decrease calcium, T_3, T_4, and sodium.

Withdrawal Symptoms

Abrupt discontinuation of TEGRETOL in a responsive epileptic individual may lead to seizures or even status epilepticus with its life-threatening hazards.

Laboratory Tests

1. Complete blood counts, including platelets and possibly reticulocytes and serum iron, should be obtained before the start of treatment as well as periodically during the course of treatment.

2. Baseline and periodic evaluations of liver function, particularly in individuals with a history of liver disease, must be performed during treatment with TEGRETOL.

3. Baseline and periodic eye examinations including slit-lamp, funduscopy, and tonometry are recommended.

4. Baseline and periodic complete urinalysis and BUN determinations are recommended for individuals treated with TEGRETOL because of observed renal dysfunction caused by TEGRETOL.

5. Thyroid function should be monitored because thyroid function tests have been reported to show decreased values with TEGRETOL treatment.

6. Periodic monitoring of blood levels of TEGRETOL increases the efficacy and safety of its use. The established serum therapeutic range is 6-to-12 μg/mL.

Dosage and Administration

TEGRETOL should be taken with large amounts of water or food because it may cause GI upset. Dosage should be adjusted to the needs of each individual. A low initial daily dosage with a gradual increase is advised. As soon as adequate control is achieved, the dosage may be reduced very gradually to the minimum effective level.

Since a given dose of TEGRETOL suspension will produce higher peak levels than the same dose given as the tablet, it is recommended to start with low doses and to increase slowly to avoid unwanted side effects. Later, when converting from oral TEGRETOL suspension to TEGRETOL tablets, the same total daily mg dosage should be given in larger, less frequent doses (i.e., three times daily of suspension to twice daily of tablets).

TEGRETOL-XR is an extended-release formulation for twice-a-day administration. When converting from TEGRETOL conventional tablets to TEGRETOL-XR, the same total daily mg dose of TEGRETOL-XR should be administered. TEGRETOL-XR tablets must be swallowed whole and never crushed or chewed.

For the treatment of seizure disorders

Initial Dosage—The starting dosage in children younger than six years-of-age is 5mg/kg/day. Dosage may be increased every five to seven days to 10mg/kg/day, then up to 20mg/kg/day if necessary. The medication should be administered in two to four divided doses per day.

In children aged 6 to 12 years, the starting dosage is 100mg twice daily or 10mg/kg/day in two divided doses; increase by 100mg/day at weekly intervals depending upon response.

In children older than 12 years-of-age and adults, the initial dosage is 200mg twice daily; increase by 200mg/day at weekly intervals using a b.i.d. regimen of TEGRETOL-XR or a t.i.d. or q.i.d. regimen of the other formulations until the optimal response is obtained or therapeutic levels reached. Usual dosage is 800-1200mg/kg/day, but some individuals may require up to 1600-2400mg/day.

Dosage generally should not exceed 1000mg daily in children younger than 15 years-of-age and 1200mg daily in individuals older than 15 years-of-age.

Maintenance Dosage—Adjust dosage to the minimum effective level, usually 800-1200mg daily in adults, 400-800mg daily in children 6-12 years-of-age, below 20mg/kg/day in children under six years-of-age.

Treatment of Trigeminal Neuralgia

Initial Dosage—On the first day, a total dose of 200mg is administered. This daily dose may be increased by up to 200mg/day. Do not exceed 1200mg daily.

Maintenance Dosage—Control of pain can be maintained in older adolescents and adults with 400-800mg daily. However, some individuals may be maintained on as little as 200mg daily while others may require as much as 1200mg daily. At least once every three months throughout the treatment period, attempts should be made to reduce the dose to the minimum effective level or even to discontinue the drug.

Overdosage

The first symptoms appear after one-to-three hours of oral ingestion of TEGRETOL. Neuromuscular disturbances are the most prominent. Cardiovascular disorders are generally milder, and severe cardiac complications occur only when very high doses (>60g) have been ingested. There may be irregular breathing, respiratory depression, tachycardia, hypotension or hypertension, conduction disorders, motor restlessness, muscular twitching, tremor, athetoid movements, opisthotonos, ataxia, drowsiness, dizziness, mydriasis, nystagmus, psychomotor disturbances, hyper-reflexia followed by hyporeflexia, nausea, vomiting, anuria or oliguria, urinary retention, convulsions (especially in small children), shock, impairment of consciousness ranging in severity to deep coma.

Laboratory tests may show isolated instances of overdosage including leukocytosis, reduced leukocyte count, glycosuria, and acetonuria. EEG may show dysrhythmias.

TOPAMAX®

(Topiramate)

Pharmacodynamics

The precise mechanism by which TOPAMAX exerts its anti-seizure effect is unknown; however, electrophysiological and biochemical studies of the effects of TOPAMAX on cultured neurons have revealed three properties that may contribute to TOPAMAX's antiepileptic efficacy:

Action potentials elicited repetitively by a sustained depolarization of the neurons are blocked by TOPAMAX, suggesting a state-dependent sodium channel blocking action. TOPAMAX increases the frequency at which GABA activates $GABA_A$ receptors and enhances the ability of GABA to induce a flux of chloride ions into neurons, suggesting that TOPAMAX potentiates the activity of this inhibitory neurotransmitter. TOPAMAX also antagonizes the ability of kainate to activate a subtype of excitatory amino acid (glutamate) receptor.

Pharmacokinetics:

- Absorption of TOPAMAX is rapid, with peak plasma concentrations occurring at approximately two to four hours following an oral dose.

- The relative bioavailability of TOPAMAX from the tablet formulation is about 80% compared to a solution.

- The bioavailability of TOPAMAX is not affected by food.

- The mean plasma elimination half-life in adults is about 19-23 hours.

- Steady state is reached in about four days.

- TOPAMAX is not extensively metabolized and is primarily eliminated unchanged in the urine (approximately 70% of an administered dose). There is evidence of renal tubular reabsorption of TOPAMAX

Indications

1. Adjunctive therapy for the treatment of both partial and generalized seizures in adults

2. Orphan drug for the treatment of Lennox-Gastaut syndrome in children

3. Unlabelled use for the treatment of bipolar disorder

Pediatric Use—Safety and effectiveness in children have not been established.

Contraindications

History of hypersensitivity to the medication or component

Potential Side Effects

Body as a Whole—Fatigue, fever, influenza-like symptoms, hot flushes, body odor, edema, chest pain, enlarged abdomen, syncope

Neurological System—Dizziness, ataxia, abnormal coordination, headache, speech disorders, language problems, nystagmus, tremors, paresthesia, hypoesthesia, hyperesthesia, hypokinesia, vertigo, stupor, grand mal convulsions, hyperkinesia, hypertonia, leg cramps, hyporeflexia, hyperreflexia, neuropathy, migraine, apraxia, dyskinesia, dysphonia, ptosis, dystonia, delirium, coma, encephalopathy, upper motor neuron lesion

Psychiatric Disorders—Somnolence, insomnia, psychomotor slowing, nervousness, anxiety, difficulty with memory, confusion, depression, difficulty with concentration/attention, agitation, mood problems, aggressive reaction, apathy, depersonalization, emotional lability, personality disorder, hallucination, euphoria, psychosis, suicide attempt, paranoid reaction, paranoia, delusion, abnormal dreaming, neurosis

Gastrointestinal System—Dry mouth, increased saliva, gingivitis, gum hyperplasia, tooth caries, stomatitis, increased appetite, anorexia, nausea, vomiting, dyspepsia, dysphagia, gastroenteritis, abdominal pain, constipation, diarrhea, fecal incontinence, flatulence, hemorrhoids, melena, hiccups, gastroesophageal reflux, tongue edema, esophagitis

Liver and Biliary System—Increased SGPT and SGOT, gall bladder disorder

Muscular and Skeletal Systems—Myalgia, back pain, leg pain, involuntary muscle contractions, arthralgia, muscle weakness, arthrosis, osteoporosis

Endocrine and Metabolic Systems—Breast pain, breast discharge in males, dysmenorrhea, menstrual disorder, weight decrease, weight increase, goiter, thirst, hypokalemia, increase alkaline phosphatase, dehydration, hypocalcemia, hyperlipemia, acidosis, hyperglycemia, increased creatinine, hyperchloremia, menstrual bleeding, leukorrhea, menorrhagia, amenorrhea

Respiratory System—Upper respiratory infection, pharyngitis, sinusitis, rhinitis dyspnea, coughing, bronchitis, asthma, bronchospasm

Cardiovascular System—Hypertension, hypotension, postural hypotension, vasodilatation, palpitation, AV block bradycardia, bundle branch block

Hematologic and Lymphatic Systems—Leukopenia, anemia, epistaxis, gingival bleeding, purpura, thrombocytopenia, pulmonary embolism, lymphadenopathy, eosinophilia, lymphopenia, granulocytopenia, lymphocytosis

Dermatologic System—Rash, pruritus, increased sweating, decreased sweating, acne, alopecia, dermatitis, nail disorder, folliculitis, dry skin, urticaria, skin discoloration, eczema, photosensitivity reaction, erythematous rash, seborrhea, abnormal hair texture

Genitourinary System—Hematuria, urinary tract infection, vaginitis, micturition frequency, urinary incontinence, dysuria, renal calculus, urinary retention, face edema, renal pain, nocturia, albuminuria, polyuria, oliguria, kidney stones

Sexual Function—Impotence, decreased libido, ejaculation disorder

Ocular System—Diplopia, abnormal vision, scotoma, eye pain, visual field defect, conjunctivitis, abnormal accommodation, photophobia, abnormal lacrimation, strabismus, color blindness, myopia, mydriasis

Special Senses—Decreased hearing, tinnitus, taste perversion, taste loss, parosmia

Potential Drug Interactions

1. The addition of TOPAMAX to DILANTIN or DEPAKOTE may require an adjustment of the dose of DILANTIN or DEPAKOTE to achieve optimal clinical outcome because TOPAMAX may increase DILANTIN or decrease DEPAKOTE blood concentrations.

2. DILANTIN can decrease TOPAMAX serum level by as much as 48%; TEGRETOL reduces it by 40% and DEPAKOTE reduces TOPAMAX by 15%.

3. Because of the potential of TOPAMAX to cause CNS depression as well as other cognitive and neuropsychiatric adverse events, TOPAMAX should be used with extreme caution if used in combination with alcohol and other CNS depressants.

4. Efficacy of oral contraceptives may be compromised by topiramate.

5. Concomitant use of TOPAMAX with other carbonic anhydrase inhibitors, e.g., acetazolamide or DARANIDE (dichlorphenamide, for treatment of glaucoma), may create a physiological environment that increases the risk of *renal stone formation* and should therefore be avoided.

Withdrawal Symptoms

Adverse events associated with discontinuing therapy include somnolence, dizziness, anxiety, difficulty with concentration or attention, fatigue, and paresthesia and increased fatigue at dosages above 400mg/day. TOPAMAX should be withdrawn gradually to minimize the potential of increased seizure frequency.

Laboratory Tests

The value of monitoring plasma concentrations of TOPAMAX has not been established.

Dosage and Administration

TOPAMAX can be taken without regard to meals. Because of the bitter taste, tablets should not be broken. Addition or withdrawal of DILANTIN and/or TEGRETOL during adjunctive therapy with TOPAMAX may require adjustment of the dose of TOPAMAX.

In older adolescents and adults, the recommended total daily dose of TOPAMAX as adjunctive therapy is 400mg/day in two divided doses. In children, the recommended dosage range is 3-6mg/kg/day. It is recommended that therapy be initiated at 50mg/day followed by 50mg weekly titration (e.g., 50mg daily first week, 50mg twice a day second week, etc.) to an effective dose or target dose of 200mg twice daily. No evidence of tolerance has been demonstrated in humans. Doses above 400mg/day have not been shown to improve responses.

Overdosage

Symptoms of overdosage have not been reported by the manufacturer of TOPAMAX.

ZARONTIN®

(Ethosuximide)

Pharmacodynamics

ZARONTIN suppresses the motor cortex and elevates the threshold of the central nervous system to convulsive stimuli. Thus, the frequency of epileptiform attacks is reduced.

Pharmacokinetics

- Peak serum concentration of ZARONTIN is reached within two to four hours.

- Steady-state blood level is reached in five to eight days.

- About 80% of ZARONTIN is metabolized in the liver.

- Elimination half-life is 30 hours in children and 50-60 hours in adults.

- ZARONTIN is slowly excreted in urine as metabolites (50%) and as unchanged drug (10% to 20%); small amounts are excreted in feces.

Indications

ZARONTIN is indicated for the control of absence (petit mal), myoclonic, and atonic seizures.

Contraindications

History of hypersensitivity to ethosuximide

Potential Side Effects

Neurological System—Drowsiness, headache, dizziness, euphoria, hiccups, irritability, hyperactivity, lethargy, fatigue, ataxia, and increase in the frequency of grand mal seizures

Psychiatric Disorders—Disturbances of sleep, night terrors, inability to concentrate, aggressiveness, paranoid psychosis, an increased state of depression with overt suicidal intentions

Gastrointestinal System—Anorexia, vague gastric upset, nausea and vomiting, cramps, epigastric and abdominal pain, weight loss, diarrhea, hypertrophy and swelling of the tongue

Hematologic and Lymphatic Systems—Leukopenia, agranulocytosis, pancytopenia with or without bone marrow suppression, and eosinophilia

Hepatic System—Abnormal liver function

Dermatologic System—Urticaria, Stevens-Johnson syndrome, systemic lupus erythematosus, pruritic erythematous rashes, and hirsutism

Genitourinary System—Vaginal bleeding, microscopic hematuria, abnormal renal function

Sexual Function—Increased libido

Ocular System—Myopia

Potential Drug Interactions

1. DILANTIN, TEGRETOL, MYSOLINE, and LUMINAL may increase the hepatic metabolism of ZARONTIN and thus decreases the clinical effect of ZARONTIN.

2. Isoniazid may inhibit hepatic metabolism with a resulting increase in ZARONTIN serum concentration and thus increases risk of toxicity.

Potential Laboratory Tests Interactions

ZARONTIN may increase alkaline phosphatase value in a liver function test and it decreases serum calcium values.

Withdrawal Symptoms

It is important to proceed slowly when increasing or decreasing dosage of ZARONTIN as well as when adding or eliminating other medications. Abrupt withdrawal of anticonvulsant medication may precipitate absence (petit mal) status.

Laboratory Tests

1. Blood dyscrasias, including some with fatal outcomes, have been reported to be associated with the use of ZARONTIN; therefore, periodic blood counts should be performed. Should signs or symptoms of infection (e.g., sore throat, fever) develop, blood counts should be considered.

2. Abnormal liver and renal function studies have been reported in individuals who take ZARONTIN. Periodic urinalysis and liver function studies are advised for all individuals receiving the drug.

3. Since ZARONTIN may interact with concurrently administered AEDs, periodic serum level determinations of these drugs may be necessary. The serum therapeutic range of ZARONTIN is 40 to 100μg/mL.

Dosage and Administration

ZARONTIN is administered orally, and it should be taken with food. The initial dose for children three to six years-of-age is 250mg/day (or 15mg/kg/day) in two divided doses; for individuals six years-of-age and older, 250mg twice daily. Dosage should be increased by small increments. The daily dose is increased by 250mg every four to seven days until control is achieved with minimal side effects.

Maintenance dose for children is 15-40mg/kg/day for younger children and 20-40mg/kg/day for older children and adults in two divided doses. Dosages exceeding 1.5g daily in divided doses should be administered only under the strictest supervision of the physician.

The optimal dose for most children is 20mg/kg/day. This dose has given average plasma levels within the accepted therapeutic range of 40-100μg/mL. Subsequent dose schedules can be based on effectiveness and plasma level determinations.

Zarontin may be administered in combination with other anticonvulsants when other forms of epilepsy coexist with absence (petit mal) seizure.

Overdosage

A relationship between ZARONTIN toxicity and its plasma levels has not been established. Nevertheless, acute overdoses may produce nausea, vomiting, and CNS depression including ataxia, stupor, coma, hypotension, and respiratory depression.

Much of the above information was obtained from the *Physicians' Desk Reference* (PDR), published by the Medical Economics Company.

Glossary

Medicine uses technical terms that enable the clinician to identify the symptoms of disorders or side effects of medication and to communicate clearly with other colleagues. You may not be familiar with many of the technical terms in this book. I have attempted to keep such terms to a minimum, introducing medical and psychiatric terminology only for reasons of specificity or because you, as a caregiver, will encounter them in discussing your child's status with the prescribing physician. The definitions in the following pages are brief and intended to help your understanding of the technical terms. However, if this glossary does not provide adequate information for your needs, you should ask your child's doctor to explain the terms he is using.

Abscess. Collection of pus in the soft tissues of the body, forming a swelling that is warm, tender, and quite painful.

Absorption. Incorporation of substances into or across tissues of the body.

Accommodation. Spontaneously focusing the eyes.

Acidifier, urinary. Medicine that makes the urine more acidic.

Acidosis. Too much acidity or loss of alkalinity in the body fluids and tissues.

Acute. Rapid onset or of short duration.

Adenoids. Lymph tissue at the back of the throat (above the tonsils) that sometimes swells during childhood.

Adjunct treatment. An additional or secondary treatment that is helpful but is not necessary to treatment of a particular condition; not effective for that condition if used alone.

Adrenal cortex. Outer layer of tissue of the adrenal gland, which produces corticosteroid hormones.

Adrenal glands. Two organs located next to the kidneys. They produce the hormones epinephrine and norepinephrine and corticosteroid hormones such as cortisol.

Adrenaline. A hormone (also called epinephrine) secreted by the medulla of adrenal glands, that prepares the body to respond to stress. It raises blood pressure, increases heart rate, raises the output of the heart, and elevates the level of glucose (blood sugar) in the bloodstream. It has been synthesized for medical use and is commonly given as an emergency treatment for severe allergic reactions.

Adrenal medulla. Inner part of the adrenal gland, which produces epinephrine and norepinephrine.

Adrenocorticoids. Group of cortisone-like hormones, also called corticosteroids, that are secreted by the adrenal cortex and are critical to the body. The two major groups are glucocorticoids, which affect fat and body metabolism, and mineralocorticoids, which regulate salt/water balance.

Aerosol. Suspension of very small liquid or solid particles in compressed gas.

Agent. A substance capable of causing a change.

Agoraphobia. Fear of public places or open spaces.

Agranulocytosis. A severe decrease in the number of granulocytes, a type of white blood cell.

Alkaline. Having a pH of more than 7; the opposite of acidic.

Alkalizer, urinary. Medication that makes the urine more alkaline.

Alkalosis. Too much alkalinity or loss of acidity in the body fluids and tissues.

Alopecia. Loss or absence of hair from areas where it normally is present; baldness.

Amblyopia. Reduced vision from nonuse.

Amenorrhea. Absence of menstrual periods.

Analgesic. Medication that relieves pain without causing unconsciousness.

Anaphylaxis. The most severe form of an allergic reaction, characterized by severe difficulty in breathing, a drop in blood pressure, hives, and severe abdominal pain.

Androgen. Substance, such as testosterone, that stimulates development of male characteristics.

Anemia. An abnormally low concentration of red blood cells with a reduction of hemoglobin in the blood.

Anesthetic. Medication that causes a loss of feeling or sensation, especially of pain.

Angina. Pain, tightness, or feeling of heaviness in the chest, usually caused by lack of oxygen for the heart muscle.

Anorexia. Loss of appetite for food.

Anoxia. Absence of oxygen.

Antacid. Medication used to neutralize excess acid in the stomach.

Antagonist. Drug or other substance that blocks or works against the action of another.

Antianemic. Agent that prevents or corrects anemia.

Antianginal. Medication used to prevent or treat angina attacks.

Antianxiety agent. Medication used to treat anxiety.

Antiarrhythmic. Medication used to treat irregular heartbeats.

Antiasthmatic. Medication used to treat asthma.

Antibacterial. Medication that kills or stops the growth of bacteria.

Antibody. Special kind of blood protein that helps the body fight infection.

Antibulimic. Medication used to treat bulimia.

Anticoagulant. Medication used to prevent formation of blood clots in the blood vessels.

Anticonvulsant. Medication used to prevent or treat convulsions (seizure disorders).

Antidepressant. Medication used to treat depression.

Antidiabetic. Medication used to control blood sugar levels in patients with diabetes mellitus.

Antidiarrheal. Medication used to treat diarrhea.

Antidiuretic. Medication used to decrease urine formation.

Antidote. Medication used to prevent or treat harmful effects of another medication or a poison.

Antidyskinetic. Medication used to treat the loss of muscle control.

Antidysmenorrheal. Medication used to treat menstrual cramps.

Antiemetic. Medication that prevents or treat nausea and vomiting.

Antienuretic. Medication used to prevent bedwetting.

Antiflatulent. Medication used to help relieve excess gas in the stomach or intestines.

Antifungal. Medication used to treat infections caused by a fungus.

Antihemorrhagic. Medication used to prevent or help stop serious bleeding.

Antihistamine. Medications used to prevent or relieve the symptoms of allergies.

Antihypertensive. Medication used to treat high blood pressure.

Antihypocalcemic. Medication used to increase blood calcium levels.

Antihypoglycemic. Medication used to increase blood sugar levels.

Antihypokalemic. Medication used to increase potassium blood levels.

Anti-inflammatory. Medication used to relieve pain, swelling, and other symptoms of inflammation.

Anti-inflammatory, nonsteroidal. An anti-inflammatory medication that is not similar to a cortisone.

Anti-inflammatory, steroidal. A cortisone-like anti-inflammatory medication.

Antimuscarinic. Medication used to block the effects of a certain chemical in the body; often used to reduce smooth muscle spasms, especially abdominal or stomach cramps or spasms.

Antimyotonic. Medication used to prevent or relieve nighttime leg cramps or muscle spasms.

Antineuralgic. Medication used to treat neuralgia.

Antipsychotic. Medication used to treat certain nervous, mental, and emotional conditions.

Antipyretic. Medication used to reduce fever.

Antithyroid agent. Medication used to treat an overactive thyroid gland.

Antitremor agent. Medication used to treat tremors (trembling or shaking).

Anxiolytic. Medication used to treat excessive nervousness, tension, or anxiety.

Apnea. A temporary cessation (stopping) of breathing.

Appetite stimulant. Medication used to increase the desire for food.

Appetite suppressant. Medication used to decrease the desire for food.

Arrhythmia. Abnormal heart rhythm.

Arteritis. Inflammatory disease of the arteries.

Arthralgia. Pain in a joint.

Arthritis, rheumatoid. Chronic disease, especially of the joints, marked by pain and swelling.

Biliary. Relating to bile, the bile duct, or the gallbladder.

Bilirubin. A by-product of the breakdown of red blood cells. The liver processes and excretes bilirubin. An excess of bilirubin in the blood may cause jaundice.

Behavior modification. Method of treatment used to help children change behaviors by rewarding desired behaviors and establishing consequences for undesirable ones.

Bradycardia. Slow heart rate, usually less than 60 beats per minute.

Bronchodilator. Medication used to increase the flow of air by opening the bronchial tubes in the lungs.

Bruxism. Grinding or clenching of teeth during sleep.

Buccal. Relating to the cheek.

Bulimia. Disturbance in eating behavior marked by bouts of excessive eating followed by self-induced vomiting and diarrhea, hard exercise, or fasting.

Bursa. A fluid-filled sac found in various locations in the body where there is potential for friction to develop between two adjacent structures, such as a tendon and a bone.

Bursitis. Inflammation of a bursa, resulting in local pain, swelling, tenderness, and difficulty moving.

Candidiasis. An infection caused by the organism Candida albicans (a type of fungus) either on the skin surface or within the mouth or vagina.

Cardiac. Relating to the heart.

Cardiac arrhythmia. Irregularity or loss of the normal rhythm of the heartbeat.

Cataract. A clouding or loss of transparency of the lens of the eye.

Catatonia. Condition in which a person is unresponsive, immobile, unable to talk, and sometimes with rigid muscles

Central nervous system, CNS. The part of the nervous system that includes the brain and spinal cord.

Cholestasis. Retention of bile in the liver.

Choreiform movements. Jerking of multiple body parts.

Choreoathetoid movements. Jerking and writhing movements.

Chromosome. The structure in the cell nucleus that contains the DNA.

Chronic. Describes a condition of long duration, which may change slowly.

Cirrhosis. Chronic disease marked by destruction of liver cells and abnormal tissue growth.

Cognitive therapy. Method of psychotherapy used to decrease symptoms of depression and anxiety by examining negative thoughts and ideas associated with these feelings.

Cogwheeling movement. Slow, rigid movement of a body joint, like the jerky motion of a cogwheel.

Colic. Waves of sudden severe abdominal pain, which are usually separated by relatively pain-free intervals.

Congestive heart failure. Condition resulting from inability of the heart to pump strongly enough to maintain adequate blood flow; characterized by breathlessness and edema.

Convulsion. Sudden involuntary contraction or repeated jerking of muscles.

Corticosteroids. See adrenocorticoids.

Cortisol. Natural hormone produced by the adrenal cortex, important for carbohydrate, protein, and fat metabolism and for the normal response to stress; synthetic cortisol (hydrocortisone) is used to treat inflammations, allergies, collagen diseases, rheumatic disorders, and adrenal failure.

Croup. Inflammation and blockage of the larynx (voice box) in young children.

Crystalluria. Crystals in the urine.

Cushing's syndrome. Condition in which the adrenal gland produces too much cortisone-like hormone, leading to weight gain, round face, and high blood pressure.

Cyanosis. Bluish discoloration of skin caused by lack of oxygen in the blood.

Cyst. Abnormal sac or closed cavity filled with liquid or semisolid matter.

Cystitis. A bladder infection with stinging, burning, and frequent need to urinate.

Cytoplasm. The contents of a cell outside the nucleus.

Decongestant, nasal. Medication used to help relieve nasal congestion (stuffy nose).

Delusion. False and perhaps bizarre belief that cannot be changed by logical arguments or evidence.

Dermatitis herpetiformis. Skin disease marked by sores and itching.

Dermatitis, seborrheic. Type of eczema found on the scalp and face.

Dermatomyositis. Inflammatory disorder of the skin and underlying tissues, including breakdown of muscle fibers.

Diabetes insipidus. Disorder in which the patient produces large amounts of dilute urine and is constantly thirsty.

Diabetes mellitus. Disorder in which the body cannot process sugars to release energy; either because the body does not produce enough insulin or the body tissues are unable to use the insulin present. This leads to too much sugar in the blood (hyperglycemia).

Diplopia. Double vision.

Diuretic. Medication used to increase the amount of urine produced by helping the kidneys get rid of water and salt.

DNA. Deoxyribonucleic acid; the genetic material in the cell nucleus that controls heredity.

Dysfunction. Inadequate, impaired, or abnormal function.

Dyskinesia. Refers to abnormal, involuntary movement or a defect in voluntary movement.

Dysmenorrhea. Painful menstruation (menstrual cramps).

Dyspepsia. Indigestion.

Dysphagia. Difficulty in swallowing.

Dyspnea. Difficult or labored breathing.

Dystonia. Intermittent or sustained muscular contraction or spasm that may produce an abnormal posture or involuntary movements.

Dysuria. Painful urination.

Ecchymosis. Collection of blood in the tissues causing a black, blue, or yellow discoloration of the skin; a bruise.

Eczema. Inflammation of the skin, marked by a patchy rash that is dry, reddish, and very itchy.

Edema. A diffuse abnormal accumulation of fluid within a particular tissue or part of the body; usually the swelling is first noticed in the feet or lower legs.

Electrolyte. In medical use, chemicals (ions) in body fluids that are needed for normal functioning of the body. Body electrolytes include bicarbonate, chloride, sodium, potassium, etc.

Emesis. Vomiting.

Emphysema. Lung condition in which destructive changes occur in the air spaces, and air is not exchanged normally during the process of breathing in and out.

Encephalitis. Inflammation of brain tissue, usually caused by a virus.

Encephalopathy. Any degenerative disease of the brain.

Encopresis. Fecal soiling or leakage not due to illness or physical defect, which occurs past the age of normal toilet training.

Endocarditis. An inflammation of the internal lining of the heart, usually caused by an infection, leading to fever, heart murmurs, and heart failure.

Endocrine gland. A gland that has no duct and releases its secretion directly into the blood stream.

Enema. Method of bringing about a bowel movement by inserting fluid into the rectum.

Enteric coating. Coating on tablets which allows them to pass through the stomach unchanged before being broken up and absorbed in the intestine. Enteric coatings are used to protect the stomach from the medicine or the medicine from the stomach's acid.

Enteritis. Inflammation of the small intestine, usually causing diarrhea.

Enuresis. Involuntary passage of urine into the bed at night (bedwetting) or clothes during the day at least once or twice per month in a child who is at least five years -of-age.

Enzyme. Type of protein produced by cells that may bring about or speed up a normal chemical reaction in the body.

Eosinophil. One type of white blood cell, which is readily stained by the dye eosin and is important in allergic reactions and parasitic infections.

Eosinophilia. A condition (e.g., an allergic reaction or a parasitic infection) in which the number of eosinophils in the blood is abnormally high.

Epidural space. Area in the spinal column.

Epilepsy. A brain disorder featuring sudden attacks of seizures.

Epinephrine. See adrenaline.

Epistaxis. Nosebleed.

Erythema. Redness of the skin.

Esophagus. The hollow structure connecting the pharynx to the stomach that transports food from the throat to the stomach.

Estrogen. Principal female sex hormone necessary for the normal sexual development of the female.

Exanthem. A skin rash accompanied by an acute infection

Exophthalmos. Thrusting forward of the eyeballs in their sockets giving the appearance of the eyes sticking out too far; commonly associated with hyperthyroidism.

Expectorant. Medication used to promote removal of mucus or phlegm from the lungs by coughing or spitting.

Extrapyramidal symptoms (EPS). Movement disorders occurring with certain diseases or with use of certain drugs, including trembling and shaking of hands and fingers, twisting movements of the body, shuffling walk, and stiffness of arms or legs.

Fasciculation. Small, spontaneous contraction of a few muscle fibers, which is visible through the skin; muscular twitching.

Flatulence. Excessive production and passing of air or gas from the intestines.

Flushing. Temporary redness of the face and/or neck.

Galactorrhea. Excessive flow of milk from the breast.

Gastric. Relating to the stomach.

Gastritis. Inflammation of the stomach lining.

Gastroenteritis. Inflammation of the stomach and intestinal tract, usually resulting from an acute viral or bacterial infection, and sometimes called stomach flu.

Gastroesophageal reflux. Backward flow into the esophagus of the contents of the stomach and duodenum. The condition is often characterized by "heartburn."

Genital. Relating to the organs concerned with gender and reproduction.

Gilles de la Tourette syndrome. Disorder characterized by multiple motor tics along with vocal tics such as grunting, humming, tongue-clicking, and sniffing.

Gingiva. Gums.

Gingival hyperplasia. Overgrowth of the gums.

Gingivitis. Inflammation of the gums.

Glaucoma. A condition characterized by increased pressure within the eye. It can cause blindness if left untreated.

Glomeruli. Clusters of capillaries in the nephrons of the kidney that act as filters of the blood.

Glomerulonephritis. Inflammation of the glomeruli of the kidney not directly caused by infection.

Gluten. Type of protein found primarily in wheat and rye.

Goiter. Enlargement of the thyroid gland that is chronic, diffuse, and non-cancerous.

Gonadotropin. Any hormone that stimulates the activities of the ovaries or testes.

Granulation. Small, fleshy outgrowths on the healing surface of a wound or ulcer; a normal stage in healing.

Granulocyte. A class of white blood cell.

Granulocytopenia. Abnormal reduction of the number of granulocytes in the blood.

Gynecomastia. Excessive development of the breasts in the male.

Halitosis. Bad breath; usually indicates that an infection is present somewhere in the gums, throat, tonsils, adenoids, or sinuses.

Hallucination. A false perception involving any of the five senses without external stimulation, resulting from a disturbance in central nervous system function.

Hematemesis. Vomiting of blood.

Hematocrit. The percentage of whole blood that consists of red cells.

Hematuria. Presence of blood or red blood cells in the urine.

Hemiplegia. Paralysis of one side of the body.

Hemoglobin. Iron-containing substance found in red blood cells that transports oxygen from the lungs to the tissues of the body.

Hemolysis. The destruction or breakdown of red blood cells.

Hemolytic anemia. Type of anemia resulting from breakdown of red blood cells.

Hemostasis. Control of bleeding.

Hepatic. Relating to the liver.

Hepatitis. Inflammation of the liver.

Hirsutism. Excessive growth of body or facial hair, especially in women.

Hives. A generalized allergic response involving raised, reddened, irregular itchy patches of skin that may blanch (turn white) when pressure is applied. They may vary from dime-size to much larger areas of skin, and they change size and location.

Hodgkin's disease. Malignant condition marked by swelling of the lymph nodes with weight loss and fever.

Hormone. Substance produced in one part of the body (such as a gland), which then passes into the bloodstream and travels to other organs or tissues, where it carries out its effect.

Hydrocortisone. See cortisol.

Hydronephrosis. An enlargement of the kidneys caused by some degree of blockage to normal urine flow, sometimes called "water kidney."

Hypercalcemia. Too much calcium in the blood.

Hypercalciuria. Too much calcium in the urine.

Hypercholesterolemia. Excessive amount of cholesterol in the blood.

Hyperglycemia. Abnormally high blood sugar.

Hyperkalemia. Abnormally high amount of potassium in the blood.

Hyperkeratosis. Overgrowth or thickening of the outer horny layer of the skin.

Hyperlipidemia. An abnormally high level of any or all of the lipids in the blood.

Hyperopia (farsightedness). The ability of the eye to focus on distant objects more easily than on objects that are closer. See Myopia.

Hyperphosphatemia. Too much phosphate in the blood.

Hyperthermia. Abnormally high body temperature.

Hyperthyroidism. Excessive secretion of thyroid hormones by the thyroid gland.

Hyperventilation. Abnormally rapid and deep breathing that most commonly arises from emotional stress.

Hypnotic. Medication used to induce sleep.

Hypocalcemia. Too little calcium in the blood.

Hypoglycemia. Abnormally low blood sugar.

Hypokalemia. Abnormally low amount of potassium in the blood.

Hypotension, orthostatic. Excessive fall in blood pressure that occurs when standing or upon standing up.

Hypothalamus. Area of the brain that controls many body functions, including body temperature, certain metabolic and endocrine processes, and some activities of the nervous system.

Hypothermia. Abnormally low body temperature.

Hypothyroidism. Condition caused by thyroid hormone deficiency, which results in a decrease in the rate of metabolism.

Hypoxia. Condition in which an inadequate supply of oxygen is delivered to the tissues of the body.

Idiopathic. Arising from an unknown cause.

Immune system. Complex network of the body that defends against foreign substances or organisms that may harm the body.

Immunosuppressant. Medication that reduces the body's natural immunity; often used following organ transplantation.

Impetigo. A bacterial skin infection, usually caused by common strains of streptococcus or staphylococcus, in which an irregular honey-colored crusted eruption spreads over the face and/or upper body.

Impotence. Difficulty or inability of a male to have or maintain an erection of the penis.

Incontinence. Inability to control natural passage of urine or bowel movements.

Infertility. Medical condition which results in the difficulty or inability of a woman to become pregnant or of a man to cause pregnancy.

Inflammation. Pain, redness, swelling, and heat, usually in response to an injury or illness.

Inhalation. Medication that is used when inhaled into the lungs.

Inhibitor. Substance that prevents a process or reaction.

Insomnia. Inability to sleep or remain asleep.

Intra-arterial. Within an artery.

Intramuscular (IM). Injections given directly into muscle.

Intravenous (IV). Injections given directly into a vein.

Ion. Atom or group of atoms carrying an electric charge.

Ischemia. A condition caused by inadequate blood flow to a part of the body; usually caused by constriction or blocking of blood vessels that supply the part of the body affected.

Jaundice. Yellowing of the eyes and skin due to excess bilirubin in the blood.

Lacrimation. The secretion and discharge of tears.

Lactation. Secretion of breast milk.

Lactose. Type of sugar found in breast milk, cow's milk, and most non-soy infant formulas.

Larynx. Organ containing the vocal cords that serves as an air passage from the pharynx to the lungs.

Lavage. The washing out of an organ such as the stomach or bowel.

Laxative. Medication used to increase bowel movements.

Lennox-Gastaut syndrome. Type of childhood epilepsy.

Lethargy. Lack of energy; feeling of tiredness or listlessness.

Leukocyte. White blood cell.

Leukoderma. A condition identified by patches of skin that do not contain pigment, thus appearing white; also called vitiligo.

Leukopenia. An abnormal reduction in the number of leukocytes (white blood cells) in the blood.

Lipid. Term applied generally to dietary fat or fatlike substances not soluble in water.

Lupus erythematosus, systemic. Chronic inflammatory disease most often affecting the skin, joints, and various internal organs; also called lupus or SLE (systemic lupus erythematosus).

Lymph. Fluid that bathes the tissues. It is formed in tissue spaces in all parts of the body and is circulated by the lymphatic system.

Lymphadenopathy. Swollen lymph nodes.

Lymphatic system. Network of vessels that conveys lymph from the spaces between the cells of the body back to the bloodstream.

Lymph nodes. Small collections of cells that assist in the body's immune response. The nodes act as filters for the lymph by keeping bacteria and other foreign particles from entering the bloodstream. They also produce lymphocytes.

Lymphocyte. White blood cells found in the blood, lymph, and lymphatic tissues. They are involved in immunity.

Macula (of the eye). Central part of the retina responsible for detailed vision.

Magnetic resonance imaging (MRI). A type of imaging study that utilizes a strong magnetic field to create detailed cross-sectional views of an area of the body.

Mast cells. Cells in the connective tissue that store histamine; they release substances that bring about inflammation and produce signs of allergic reactions.

Megavitamin therapy. Taking very large doses of vitamins to prevent or treat medical problems.

Meninges. The membrane that covers and protects the brain and spinal cord.

Meningitis. Inflammation of the tissues that surround the brain and spinal cord.

Menorrhagia. Heavy bleeding during menstruation.

Miotic. Medication used in the eye that causes the pupil to become smaller.

Mononucleosis. Infectious viral disease occurring mostly in adolescents and young adults, marked by fever, sore throat, swelling of the lymph nodes in the neck and armpits, and severe fatigue.

Mucous membrane. Moist layer of tissue surrounding or lining many body structures and cavities, including the mouth, lips, inside of nose, anus, and vagina.

Mucus. Thick fluid produced by the mucous membranes and glands.

Myalgia. Muscle pain.

Mydriasis. Prolonged dilation of a pupil of the eye.

Mydriatic. Medication used to dilate (enlarge) the pupil of the eye.

Myocardial infarction. Interruption of blood supply to the heart, leading to sudden, severe chest pain and damage to the heart muscle; a heart attack.

Myopia. Nearsightedness; the inability to see distant objects clearly.

Myositis. Inflammation of one or more muscle groups, resulting in pain, tenderness, and/or weakness.

Nasal. Relating to the nose.

Necrosis. Death of tissue, cells, or a part of a structure or organ, surrounded by healthy parts.

Neoplasm. New, abnormal, uncontrolled, and progressive growth of tissue; a tumor.

Nephron. Unit of the kidney that acts as a filter of the blood in forming urine.

Neuralgia. Severe stabbing or throbbing pain along the course of one or more nerves.

Neuralgia, trigeminal. Severe burning or stabbing pain along nerves in the face; tic douloureux.

Neuritis. Swelling or inflammation of a nerve.

Neuritis, optic. Disease of the nerves in the eye.

Neuritis, peripheral. Inflammation of terminal nerves or the nerve endings, usually associated with pain, muscle wasting, and loss of reflexes.

Neurobiological. Regarding the biology of the nervous system.

Neurology. Medical specialty concerned with the function and malfunction of the nervous system.

Neurotransmitter. Chemical messenger that transmits information across the junction (synapse) that separates one nerve cell (neuron) from another nerve cell or a muscle.

Neutropenia. Abnormally small number of neutrophils in the blood.

Neutrophil. The most common type of white blood cell that is specifically associated with the body's immune response and is important in the body's protection against infection.

Nightmare. A "bad dream," the contents of which arouse fear or anxiety.

Night terrors. Harmless sleep disorder that causes the child to scream out and behave uncontrollably; usually of short duration with no memory of the event the next day.

Nocturia. Urination at night.

Nodule. Small, rounded mass, lump, or swelling.

NSAID. Nonsteroidal anti-inflammatory drug. See anti-inflammatory, nonsteroidal.

Nucleus. The part of the cell that contains the chromosomes.

Nystagmus. Rapid, rhythmic, involuntary movements of the eyeball; may be from side to side, up and down, or around.

Occiput. The lower portion of the back of the head where it merges with the neck.

Ocular. Having to do with the eyes.

Oligomenorrhea. Abnormally infrequent and/or scanty menstruation.

Ophthalmic. Relating to the eye.

Oral. Relating to the mouth.

Osteomalacia. Softening of the bone due to a calcium or vitamin D deficiency or kidney disease.

Osteomyelitis. A serious bacterial infection of bone.

Osteoporosis. Loss of calcium from bone tissue, which leaves bones brittle and easily fractured.

Otic. Relating to the ear.

Ototoxicity. Harmful to the organs or nerves of the ear that enable hearing and balance.

Pallor. Pale appearance of the skin.

Palpebra. The eyelid.

Palpitation. The sensation that the heart is beating too rapidly, irregularly, or strongly.

Pancreatitis. Inflammation of the pancreas.

Pancytopenia. Reduction in the number of red blood cells, white blood cells, and platelets.

Papule. A small, solid, raised skin lesion.

Paralytic ileus. Failure or loss of contraction in the intestine

Parenteral. A term applied to medications or fluids that are given by injection into a vein, muscle, or fatty layer below the skin using a needle and syringe.

Paresis. Partial paralysis or weakness of a specific muscle.

Paresthesia. Abnormal burning, prickling, or tingling ("pins and needles") sensation on the skin.

Parkinsonism. See Parkinson's disease.

Parkinson's disease. Brain disease marked by tremor (shaking), stiffness, and difficulty in moving.

Paroxysm. A sudden attack (such as coughing).

Pemphigus. Skin disease marked by successive outbreaks of blisters.

Peptic ulcer. Open sore in esophagus, stomach, or duodenum.

Pericarditis. Inflammation of the sac that surrounds the heart.

Peritoneum. Membrane sac lining the abdominal wall and covering the liver, stomach, spleen, gallbladder, and intestines.

Petechiae. Flat, purple to red, pinhead-sized spots that appear in the skin or mucous membranes as a result of leakage of blood from tiny blood vessels.

Pharynx. Space just behind the mouth that serves as a passageway for food from the mouth to the esophagus and for air from the nose and mouth to the larynx.

Phlebitis. Inflammation of a vein.

Phlegm. Thick mucus produced in the respiratory passages.

Phobia. Persistent and irrational fear of particular objects, people, animals, or situations.

Photophobia. An abnormal intolerance of light.

Pituitary gland. Pea-sized body located at the base of the skull. It produces a number of hormones that are essential to normal body growth and functioning.

Platelets. The tiny, disk-shaped structures in the blood that play an important role in the blood clotting process.

Pleura. Membrane covering the lungs and lining the chest cavity.

Polydipsia. Excessive thirst.

Polyuria. Excessive urination.

Porphyria. A group of uncommon, usually inherited diseases of defective porphyrin metabolism.

Porphyrin. One of a number of pigments occurring in living organisms throughout nature. Porphyries are constituents of bile pigment, hemoglobin, and certain enzymes.

Postictal. A prolonged state after a seizure attack during which the child sleeps, is very sluggish, or has transient weakness of an arm or leg.

Precocious puberty. Signs of sexual maturation prior to age eight years.

Priapism. Prolonged abnormal, painful erection of the penis.

Progesterone. Natural steroid hormone responsible for preparing the uterus for pregnancy. If fertilization occurs, progesterone's actions maintain the pregnancy.

Prolactin. Hormone secreted by the pituitary gland that stimulates and maintains milk flow in women following childbirth.

Prophylactic. Medications used to prevent the occurrence of a specific condition.

Proteinuria. Protein in the urine.

Psychopharmacology. Medical specialty concerned with the use of psychoactive medications to alleviate symptoms of emotional, behavioral, or mental disorders.

Ptosis. Drooping of the upper eyelid.

Purpura. Condition marked by bleeding into the skin; skin rash or spots are first red, darken to purple, then fade to brownish-yellow.

Purulent. Containing, or consisting of, pus.

Pustule. A small nodule, cyst, or blister that contains pus.

Pyelonephritis. A kidney infection

Rapid eye movement (REM). Description of activity of closed eyes during a particular stage of sleep during which dreams occur. This stage of sleep is also called REM sleep.

Raynaud's syndrome. Condition marked by paleness, numbness, and discomfort in the fingers when they are exposed to cold.

Rectal. Relating to the rectum.

Reflux. A backflow of liquid caused by a valve or sphincter failing to close.

Renal. Relating to the kidneys.

Retina. The cellular membrane covering the back inner surface of the eyeball. The retina contains the light-sensing cones and rods that are necessary for vision and connects directly to the brain via the optic nerve.

Retinopathy. Disorder of the retina.

Rheumatic heart disease. Heart disease marked by scarring and chronic inflammation of the heart and its valves, occurring after rheumatic fever.

Rhinitis. Inflammation of the mucous membrane inside the nose.

Scleroderma. Chronic disease first characterized by hardening, thickening, and shrinking of the skin. Certain organs are affected later.

Scotoma. Area of decreased vision or total loss of vision in a part of the visual field; blind spot.

Sebaceous gland. Skin gland that secretes sebum.

Seborrhea. Skin condition caused by the excess release of sebum from the sebaceous glands, accompanied by dandruff and oily skin.

Sebum. Fatty secretion produced by sebaceous (oil) glands of the skin.

Sedative-hypnotic. Medication used to treat excessive nervousness, restlessness, or insomnia.

Sedation. A profoundly relaxed or calmed state.

Sepsis. Bacteria induced toxic condition.

Seizure. A sudden attack or convulsion, as in epilepsy or other disorders.

Serotonin. Neurotransmitter (chemical messenger) involved in regulation of sleep, mood, appetite, and sexual function.

Serum. The liquid portion of blood that does not contain blood cells or the protein fibrinogen, which is involved in clotting.

SIADH. Secretion of inappropriate antidiuretic hormone syndrome; disease in which the body retains more fluid than normal.

Skeletal muscle relaxant. Medication used to relax certain muscles and help relieve the pain and discomfort caused by strains, sprains, or other injury to the muscles.

Soluble. Able to be dissolved in a fluid.

Spasticity. Increase in normal muscular tone, causing stiff, awkward movements.

Stomatitis. Inflammation of the inner surface of the mouth.

Stridor. Harsh, raspy breathing usually caused by the narrowing of the larynx or trachea.

Subcutaneous. Under the skin.

Sublingual. Under the tongue. A sublingual medicine is taken by placing it under the tongue and letting it slowly dissolve.

Suppressant. Medication that stops an action or condition.

Suspension. A form of medication in which the drug is mixed with a liquid but is not dissolved in it.

Syncope. Passing out; loss of consciousness due to inadequate blood flow to the brain; fainting.

Systematic desensitization. Behavioral therapy technique in which the patient is presented with a graduated hierarchy of anxiety provoking stimuli; a treatment for phobias.

Tachycardia. A rapid heart rate, usually at a rate over 100 beats per minute in adults.

Tachypnea. A rapid rate of breathing.

Teratogenic. Causing abnormal development in an embryo or fetus resulting in birth defects.

Testosterone. Principal male sex hormone.

Tetany. Condition marked by spasm and twitching of the muscles, particularly those of the hands, feet, and face.

Thought disorders. Disorders characterized by an impairment of thinking including disorganized, incoherent, or vague speech, delusions, hallucinations, or paranoia.

Thrombolytic agent. Substance that dissolves blood clots.

Thrombophlebitis. Inflammation of a vein accompanied by the formation of a blood clot.

Thrush. See Candidiasis of the mouth. Appears as a white film or patches on the tongue, inner surfaces of the cheeks, or roof of the mouth. It may be confused with milk coating the mouth, but leftover milk can be scraped off easily with a cotton swab.

Thyroid gland. Gland in the lower front of the neck. It releases thyroid hormones, which control body metabolism.

Thyrotoxicosis. Condition resulting from excessive amounts of thyroid hormones in the blood, causing increased metabolism, fast heartbeat, tremors, nervousness, and increased sweating.

Tics. Involuntary, repetitive muscle contractions, involving any muscle group but most commonly the face, eyes, or neck.

Tic douloureux. See neuralgia, trigeminal.

Tinea. Fungus infection of the surface of the skin, particularly the scalp, feet, and nails; ringworm.

Tinnitus. A noise heard in the ear described as a ringing, buzzing, or clicking sound.

Tone. The slight, continuous tension present in resting muscles.

Topical. For local effects when applied directly to the skin.

Tourette syndrome. See Gilles de la Tourette syndrome.

Tranquilizer. Medication that reduces anxiety, agitation, or emotional tension.

Transdermal. A means of administering medication into the body by use of skin patches or ointment; medication contained in the patch or the ointment is absorbed through the skin.

Triglyceride. A molecular form in which fats are present in food and the body; triglycerides are stored in the body as fat.

Tyramine. Chemical present in many foods and beverages. Its structure and action in the body are similar to epinephrine.

Urticaria. Hives; an eruption of itching wheals on the skin.

Urinary urgency. The sensation of needing to urinate immediately.

Vascular. Relating to the blood vessels.

Vasculitis. Inflammation of blood vessels.

Vasodilator. Medication that dilates the blood vessels, permitting increased blood flow.

Ventricular fibrillation. Fine, quivering, and irregular movements of many individual muscle fibers of the ventricular muscle of the heart that replace the normal heart beat and interrupt pumping function; potentially life-threatening.

Ventricle. A small cavity, such as one of the two lower chambers of the heart or one of the several cavities of the brain.

Vertigo. A spinning sensation, either of oneself or of one's surroundings, that often results in nausea.

Vitiligo. See leukoderma.

Wheal. Temporary, small, raised area of the skin, usually accompanied by itching or burning; welt.

Wheezing. A whistling sound made when there is difficulty in breathing.